D0897861

Studying
Lives
Through
Time
Personality and
Development

Studying Lives Through Time
Personality and Development

Edited by David C. Funder, Ross D. Parke,
Carol Tomlinson-Keasey, and Keith Widaman

American Psychological Association • Washington, DC

Published by the
American Psychological Association
750 First Street, NE
Washington, DC 20002

Copies may be ordered from
APA Order Department
P.O. Box 2710
Hyattsville, MD 20784

Typeset in Century Book by Techna Type, Inc., York, PA

Printer: Edwards Brothers, Inc., Ann Arbor, MI
Cover Designer: Janice Wheeler
Cover Illustrator: Margaret Scott
Technical/Production Editor: Paula R. Bronstein
Copy Editor: Christine P. Landry

Library of Congress Cataloging-in-Publication Data

Studying lives through time : personality and development / edited
    by David C. Funder ... [et al.].
        p.   cm.
    Based on papers presented at a conference sponsored by the
    Science Directorate of the American Psychological Association, the
    Murray Research Center of Radcliffe College, and the Dept. of
    Psychology and the Center for Family Studies of the University of
    California, Riverside, held in the fall of 1991 in Palm Springs, Calif.
    in honor of Jack Block.
    Includes bibliographical references and index.
    ISBN 1-55798-193-0 (acid-free paper)
    1. Personality development—Longitudinal studies—Congresses.
2. Personality development—Research—Methodology—
Congresses.   3. Personality assessment—Methodology—
Congresses.   I. Funder, David Charles.
BF637.P4S88   1993
155.2′5—dc20   93-2980
                                                                CIP

Printed in the United States of America
First Edition

APA Science Volumes

A PA expects to publish volumes on the following science topics:

The Contributions of Psychology to Mathematics and Science
    Education
Emotion and Culture
Maintaining and Promoting Integrity in Behavioral Science Research
Sleep Onset: Normal and Abnormal Processes
Stereotypes: Brain–Behavior Relationships
Temperament: Individual Differences in Biology and Behavior
Women's Psychological and Physical Health

As part of its continuing and expanding commitment to enhance the dissemination of scientific psychological knowledge, the Science Directorate of the APA established a Scientific Conferences Program. A series of volumes resulting from these conferences is jointly produced by the Science Directorate and the Office of Communications. A call for proposals is issued several times annually by the Science Directorate, which, collaboratively with the APA Board of Scientific Affairs, evaluates the proposals and selects several conferences for funding. This important effort has resulted in an exceptional series of meetings and scholarly volumes, each of which individually has contributed to the dissemination of research and dialogue in these topical areas.

The APA Science Directorate's conferences funding program has supported 24 conferences since its inception in 1988. To date, 17 volumes resulting from conferences have been published.

William C. Howell, PhD   Virginia E. Holt
Executive Director   Scientific Conferences Manager

Contents

Part Two: Weighing the Evidence

Contributors

Tommy Andersson, Stockholm University

Jack Block, University of California, Berkeley

Elizabeth Carlson, Institute of Child Development, University of Minnesota, Minneapolis

Avshalom Caspi, University of Wisconsin, Madison

Seymour Epstein, University of Massachusetts, Amherst

David C. Funder, University of California, Riverside

Norman Garmezy, University of Minnesota, Minneapolis

Per F. Gjerde, University of California, Santa Cruz

Lewis R. Goldberg, University of Oregon, Eugene and Oregon Research Institute

David M. Harrington, University of California, Santa Cruz

Ravenna Helson, Institute of Personality and Social Research, University of California, Berkeley

Jacquelyn B. James, Henry A. Murray Research Center, Radcliffe College

Eva Klohnen, University of California, Berkeley

Jane Loevinger, Washington University (St. Louis)

David Magnusson, Stockholm University

Daniel J. Ozer, University of California, Riverside

Ross D. Parke, University of California, Riverside

Elizabeth L. Paul, Trenton State College

Shmuel Shulman, Tel Aviv University

L. Alan Sroufe, Institute of Child Development, University of Minnesota, Minneapolis

Avril Thorne, University of California, Santa Cruz

Bertil Törestad, Stockholm University

Carol Tomlinson-Keasey, University of California, Davis

Keith Widaman, University of California, Riverside

Preface

Personality psychology and developmental psychology should be natural partners. The first is concerned with how to characterize and understand an individual's personality, and the second is concerned with the factors that created the personality and continue to shape it over a lifetime. Although historically the two fields sometimes have proceeded along rather separate tracks, in recent years their common interests have begun to yield richly integrated studies of personality and its evolution over the life course. As in all successful partnerships, both personality and developmental psychology bring special strengths to their union. This book is intended to highlight what we see as the most essential of those strengths: the theory and methodology of personality assessment and the longitudinal approach to the study of psychological development.

The potential of the longitudinal approach for illuminating processes of personality development is increasingly being realized. It is the method of choice for answering many critical questions. How can personality change for the better? How can individuals avoid negative outcomes? When faced with adversity, which qualities or childhood influences cause some individuals to adapt and some to crumble?

The following chapters document several themes. One central message is that the essence of personality development from early childhood through adulthood is not consistency but rather coherence. This coherence is the result of a process by which early experience forms a template for the interpretation of later experiences in life, and by which aspects of personality that develop early can affect how people select and change their social environments. The essential basis of developmental coherence, therefore, lies in the interaction between the individual personality and the wider social world.

A second theme is that personality is a multifaceted construct that must be examined through numerous and diverse methods. The contributors to this book describe studies that employ self-reports, observer judgments, direct behavioral observations, and life outcomes as sources of data. In addition, the book includes state-of-the-art surveys of the methodology of longitudinal research in personality development. The focus is on conceptual methodology and techniques for data gathering rather than exclusively on statistical issues, and our hope is to provide some nuts-and-bolts direction for the researcher who wishes to select the best possible methods for exploring the kinds of continuity and change that characterize individuals across the life span.

Jack Block, a champion of methodological, scholarly, and statistical rigor, has long demonstrated how important insights can emerge when the concerns and methods of personality and developmental psychology are joined. With his late wife, Jeanne, he initiated a longitudinal study of personality development with a diverse sample of individuals that has continued for more than two decades and remains a rich source of scientific data. Their research has impressively documented the coherence of personality over the course of development, along with the central and wide-ranging role of the personality dimensions of ego-control and ego-resiliency. Perhaps an even more important influence of the Blocks and their work has been on the lives, careers, and scientific outlooks of several generations of psychologists.

The foundation of this book was a research conference on personality and development held in honor of Jack Block in the fall of 1991 in Palm Springs, California. The conference was cosponsored by the Science Directorate of the American Psychological Association, the Murray Research Center of Radcliffe College, and the Department of Psychology and the Center for Family Studies of the University of California, Riverside.

It is our intention that this book further the understanding of research methodology, personality assessment, and the unique virtues of the longitudinal method for the study of personality development. Through this contribution we hope to honor Jack Block, Jeanne Block, and their seminal work in the study of lives through time.

The editors are grateful to the individuals who provided reviews of the chapters in this volume: Lisa Bridges, University of California, Riverside; P. Lindsay Chase-Lansdale, University of Chicago; C. Randall Colvin, University of California, Berkeley; Carol E. Franz, Boston University; Stuart Hauser, Harvard Medical School; Ravenna Helson, University of California, Berkeley; Rick Ingram, San Diego State University; Dan McAdams, Northwestern University; Robert R. McCrae, National Institute on Aging; Steven Reise, University of California, Riverside; William Revelle, Northwestern University; Ronald Siefer, Brown University; Everett Waters, State University of New York, Stony Brook; and Stephen West, Arizona State University. The editors also acknowledge the assistance of numerous graduate students from the University of California, Riverside, in staging the conference that was the foundation of this volume. Outstanding staff support for budgeting and organizing was provided by Dianne Fewkes of the Department of Psychology, University of California, Riverside. Finally, the editors thank Mary Lynn Skutley and Paula R. Bronstein of APA Books for their thoughtful and efficient contributions to the production of this volume.

David C. Funder
Ross D. Parke
Carol Tomlinson-Keasey
Keith Widaman

Introduction

CHAPTER 1

Studying Lives Through Time: About This Book

David C. Funder, Ross D. Parke, Carol Tomlinson-Keasey, and Keith Widaman

Is the set of character fixed early or late or never? Is the parenting a child receives influential in shaping how, as an adult, life is lived? Can especially fortunate or tragic or otherwise interesting life outcomes be anticipated early on? What are the conditions and consequences of personality change? Do we all proceed through the life course in more or less the same way or are alternative, psychologically tenable routes taken? If so, why? What are the pushes and pulls, the surges and the abatements characterizing the inexorably encountered stages of a human life? What are the adaptive functions, common and different, by which individuals respond to and on their changing world and self-recognitions? In short and simply put, Why do people turn out the way they do? (Block, this volume, p. 10)

A s this quotation from Jack Block implies, the study of personality and the study of development are natural partners. Implicit in every question about an individual's personality is another question: How did the person get this way? And, implicit in every question about child development is another question, What kind of adult will be the eventual result?

These reasons for the mutual relevance of personality and developmental psychology are timeless. Other, more timely considerations also are promoting an integration of these two fields of research. Personality psychology, historically one of the oldest and most central parts of the discipline, is at last coming out of the shadow of two decades of debate. In its new emergence, it is beginning to address new and important substantive and methodological issues. Among the most important are those concerned with the development of personality (e.g., the contribution of genetic factors, cognitive processing, methods for personality assessment at different ages, and the study of individual life trajectories as a unit of analysis). At the same time, significant advances in the understanding of personality development across the life course are being attained through a growing emphasis within developmental psychology on longitudinal research.

We believe that research in both of these traditions could profit from closer interaction. Developmental psychology's increasing emphasis on longitudinal study could enhance the ability of personality psychology to contribute to the understanding of the ways in which central aspects of personality develop over time. By the same token, personality psychology's strong tradition in psychometrics and measurement could enhance longitudinal research by improving the level of sophistication of measurement of central constructs of interest.

The purpose of this book is to promote just such an integration. The book contains state-of-the-art contributions from personality and developmental psychologists and those who are trying to integrate the two fields. And, the book's two major sections represent work concerned with methodological and statistical issues that go to the heart of the integrative enterprise, as well as work that contributes to the resolution of some of the pressing substantive issues in the emerging field of developmental–personality psychology.

Following this brief introduction, the book begins with a chapter by Jack Block that provides an incisive overview of personality development from the unique perspective garnered from his program of longitudinal research. The chapter strikes many themes that are echoed later in the book, including the indispensability of longitudinal data and, more subtly but just as strongly, the importance of methodological, statistical, and conceptual rigor when tackling the complex issues entailed by the study of personality development. The first group of chapters that follows emphasizes methodological issues. The second group of chapters addresses a variety of specific topics concerning the development and manifestation of personality.

Examining the Methods

The methodological section begins with a chapter by Jacquelyn James and Elizabeth Paul, who discuss the valuable data resources available in research archives across the United States and around the world. James and Paul point out that it is not necessary to wait many years for the insights that only longitudinal research can offer because there are numerous data sets already available that contain a wealth of underused information. In the following chapter, Carol Tomlinson-Keasey describes more specifically the nuts and bolts of working with archival data sets, including problems of subject attrition, cohort effects, and ethical concerns that are unique to this still-unusual style of research.

The next chapter, by Ravenna Helson, tackles the thorny issues involved in comparing results from different longitudinal data sets. Sometimes seemingly different findings—such as the finding of personality stability in one study and personality change in another—can be reconciled by close attention to differences in samples and data-gathering methods. Helson also describes methods such as the Q-sort that can be used to transcend the differences in specific data gathered by different longitudinal studies and enhance direct comparison between them.

David Funder, in the next chapter, discusses observer judgments of personality, which are a widely used form of data in both personality and developmental psychology research. He defends such data from critics who see judgments as being so prone to error as to be useless and outlines a program of research that is delineating the circumstances under which observer data are more and less likely to be accurate. Next, Daniel Ozer considers more specifically the Q-sort, a widely used technique for operationalizing human judgments in research contexts. He provides a much needed, up-to-date primer on the technique, discussing different styles of data analysis with the Q-sort, the assessment of reliability, and some specific advantages of this increasingly widely used technique.

Lew Goldberg's contribution contrasts hierarchical and vertical representations of the language of traits that is at the heart of much of the study of personality development. He concludes that although both structural representations have their merits, a horizontal approach—which considers the relative similarities of traits at the same level of generality—is superior for providing a theoretical explanation of the meaning of traits.

Jane Loevinger, in the following chapter, raises an important issue concerning the putative similarity and overlap of two particular personality constructs: conformity and conscientiousness. She outlines how the two are often lumped together in conventional factor analyses but how a long cultural and religious tradition insists on their separation. She describes how a culturally informed psychological analysis can supplement what might otherwise be a "purely technological fix" on semantic similarity.

In the final piece in the methodological section of this book, David Magnusson considers how the contribution of specific factors to development can be overestimated when they are measured separately from the more general factors they instantiate. As he points out, "one aspect of dynamic processes is their holistic character" and to study one influence in isolation can lead to seriously misleading results. Magnusson challenges researchers to capture larger pieces of the holistic, dynamic factors that influence personality development.

Weighing the Evidence

To begin the substantive, empirical section of this book, Avril Thorne presents the first of three chapters based on data from the landmark longitudinal study of personality development initiated by Jack Block and Jeanne Block. Thorne elicited important personal memories from the subjects in this study at ages 18 and 23, and traced backward the antecedents of the themes that emerged. Thorne presents a compelling case for the analysis of personal memories as a key to understanding the course and themes of personality development. The second "Block project" chapter, by Per Gjerde, is a prospective examination of the roots of depression. He finds an importantly different pattern among boys and girls, and attributes this difference to sex-typed patterns of child rearing and socialization. The third chapter from the Block project, by David Harrington, operationalizes Alice Miller's popularly influential construct of "poisonous pedagogy." In a compelling and sobering analysis, Harrington describes how harmful patterns of child rearing can have consequences that persist across generations.

Alan Sroufe's emphasis in the next chapter is on the development of attachment relationships, another early influence on later personality. He traces the beneficial effects of an early secure attachment up to middle childhood and finds the harm caused by an insecure attachment relationship to be mediated, in part, by the social worlds that insecurely attached children construct for themselves. Avshalom Caspi, in the next chapter, describes a similar process by which maladaptive behavioral patterns can persist throughout much of life. People with explosive or aggressive personalities, for example, create for themselves social worlds that help to perpetuate their problems. Caspi presents a modern and insightful integration of the genetic-, cognitive-, reinforcement-, and environment-based explanations for the continuity of personality. He concludes his chapter with a list of factors, based on this analysis, that can be expected to promote positive personality change. Norman Garmezy, in the next chapter, builds on this list with his own discussion of the factors that can promote the development of healthy personality and psychological "resilience" even in the presence of obvious environmental difficulties.

The final chapter in this section, by Seymour Epstein, presents his "cognitive–experiential self-theory" of personality. In this theory three separate, basic psychological systems—rational, experiential, and primary process—work to satisfy and balance four basic needs. Epstein particularly focuses on the experiential system and describes an innovative use of fantasy to access and possibly change for the better the contents of this system.

The prospect for a more complete integration of personality and developmental psychology has created excitement among researchers and clinicians in both fields. We hope that some of that excitement is conveyed by this book.

CHAPTER 2

Studying Personality the Long Way

Jack Block

Ways of Construing the Science of Psychology

There are many ways to be a psychologist and, indeed, in the last decade or two, the range of inquiry and the kinds of approaches used in the psychological sciences have broadened astonishingly. Thus, in my own department at the University of California, Berkeley, there are colleagues superbly studying the spatial frequency selectivity of cells in the macaque visual cortex, the neurogenesis of motoneurons in the sexually dimorphic spinal nucleus of the bulbocavernosus in rats, factors

This chapter is based partly on the G. Stanley Hall Award presentation given at the 99th Annual Convention of the American Psychological Association held in San Francisco in August 1991. The title paraphrases a line from Robert W. White (1981), a personality psychologist I greatly respect.

The study described herein was supported by National Institute of Mental Health Grant MH 16080 to Jack Block and Jeanne H. Block.

influencing the detection of interaural differences of time in high-frequency trains of clicks, the temperature dependence of in vitro androgen production in the testes of hibernating ground squirrels, the relation of enkephalin hydrolysis in plasma to escape performance in rats, and so on.

The layperson is often surprised by what it is many scientific psychologists do because their work seems frequently to be far removed from the root meaning of the word *psychology*. Lay interest in psychology focuses on very different matters, on homely human concerns, hopes, fears, pleasures, sadnesses, and the ways and experiences of living. Nonpsychologists, in their naïveté, seem to view psychology as the field that might explain why people, in their everyday existences, do what they do and feel what they feel.

In particular, when laypeople reflect historically on their own lives or the lives of other people, they expect the science of psychology to have the promise of responding to such poignant questions as: Is the set of character fixed early or late or never? Is the parenting a child receives influential in shaping how, as an adult, life is lived? Can especially fortunate or tragic or otherwise interesting life outcomes be anticipated early on? What are the conditions and consequences of personality change? Do we all proceed through the life course in more or less the same way or are alternative, psychologically tenable routes taken? If so, why? What are the pushes and pulls, the surges and the abatements characterizing the inexorably encountered stages of a human life? What are the adaptive functions, common and different, by which individuals respond to and on their changing world and changing self-recognitions? In short, and simply put, the layperson wishes to know, Why do people turn out the way they do?

Questions such as these—responding to persistent human wonderings—lie behind the wide and demanding lay interest in psychology. Academic and research psychologists sometimes forget, or do not recognize, that these lay questions are fair questions ultimately, even if sometimes ingenuously framed. They deserve far more serious scientific attention than has yet been granted them by the busily preoccupied field of scientific psychology.

As psychology has enormously expanded its scientific reach, it has seemed to me that, concomitantly, psychologists have tended to become ever more specialized and to turn often from psychological matters having relevance for lives as they are led and experienced. I do not mean to suggest that basic psychological research must be "relevant" in order to be justified. I recognize the importance of research not directed by immediate concerns for usefulness but instead motivated by theoretical questions and even the aesthetics of curiosity. Such basic research often enough has proved to be the quickest way to achievements relevant by anyone's definition. It is worthwhile to remember, however, that research that lacks relevance is not thereby necessarily basic.

In academic and research circles, the currently celebrated vision of psychological science has been oriented toward four separable but often intertwined approaches for advancing the field: (a) It has turned its focus onto neural, hormonal, and physiological matters; (b) it has stressed the importance of nomothetic functioning and influences on the average individual, with little concern manifested for the meaning and implication of interindividual differences; (c) it has placed its faith on controlled experimentation per se as the method for achieving understanding, with little interest in studying variation and covariation occurring in the natural, uncontrolled world; and (d) it has emphasized the microanalysis of psychological phenomena of relatively brief duration with little attention being addressed to the macroanalysis of psychological relations discernible only over long periods of time.

I value and do not question the importance, frequent necessity, and, often, the elegance of the neurohormonal, nomothetic, experimental, microanalytic approaches to psychology as a science (I myself have done research of all four kinds). The accomplishments of this kind of psychology have been many (although sometimes, I must say, these pursuits have captured only small game and have seemed to me more scientistic than scientific).

However, there are many central concerns of the broader field of psychology—psychology conceived of as the science of human mental states and behaviors, their underlying processes, and their development— that simply do not admit of access in these ways, modeled as they are after a special and idealized view of the physical sciences. The neuro-hormonal approach may identify the physiological mechanisms influencing or being influenced by experience and behavior. However, there is a logical chasm involving context and meaning between these two levels of observation that simply cannot be bridged, even in principle; the mind is a function of the brain, but the two cannot be made coordinate (see Hyland, 1985). Nomothetic findings, so often based on group averages that presume individual differences are only "nuisance variance," may or may not misrepresent the behavior of the normative individual (Tucker, 1966). Indeed, as Underwood (1975) has observed, nomothetic findings may well require resorting to the "crucible" of evaluation via individual differences in order to achieve a proper understanding of the underlying processes involved. The orthogonalizing requirements of research designs may impose a procedural artificiality and ecosystem unrepresentativeness on experimental manipulations. As a consequence, we may be led to misunderstand the conditions actually influencing behavior and experience in the natural world. And, just as the study of particle physics has little to say about plate tectonics because of their profound differences in focus and time scales, a microanalytic approach to psychology has little to contribute to a developmental understanding of the perceptions, experience, and behaviors that constitute a personality: One cannot see a mountain with a supercollider.

The limitations of the neurohormonal, nomothetic, experimental, and microanalytic approaches in coping with the matters of psychological meaning and context on which behavior is predicated and for understanding the diverse patterns and trajectories of personality and cognitive development need not require giving up scientific efforts to study what cannot be isolated and closely manipulated in the laboratory. The idea of scientific method is not tied to a particular content area or a particular research strategic presumption or a particular analytical method or a particular scale of measurement (Fiske & Shweder, 1986). The scientific method continues to apply in more naturalistic, less controllable, extended time-scale domains, although its form and rules of inference may change. Astronomy, geology, and meteorology are all serious and important but not neat sciences; systematic observation and theory building characterize these sciences, although they are not particularly experimental in nature. Recognition of the diverse ways one can be scientific compels a choice, wittingly or not, for would-be psychologists as to what kind of psychologist one wishes to be and what aspects of psychology one wishes to study.

For various reasons, some of them overdetermined, it has seemed to me necessary to study people in the large, as they exist in their natural and real world, and the way and the why of their differences. And, to satisfyingly pursue this goal, the longitudinal study of personality development has seemed to me the compelled approach. By *longitudinal study*, I mean the close, comprehensive, systematic, objective, sustained study of individuals over significant portions of the life span. Such study permits unique and crucial scientific recognitions regarding human development and the factors influencing human development.

Longitudinal studies, once embarked on, perhaps inevitably become career investments of great personal significance and meaning to the investors. The commitment of self to so protracted a research enterprise runs the risk of distorting and subverting the subsequent scientific possibilities of the inquiry. It is also the case that such cathexis is required if the venture is to be carried through with care to a time of fruition and of harvest of what can be known in psychology no other way. No one longitudinal study will answer all the questions of developmental psychology, but also there is no alternative scientific approach that can begin to discern and disentangle the specific influential factors conjoining, interweaving, and reciprocating with each other as the individual reaches out to life, is enveloped by circumstance, and forges character. When we, as developmental or personality psychologists deign to observe a few conveniently accessible behaviors, here and there, now and then, for a moment or two, we are likely to be touching on or sampling rather little of the basis for comprehending a human life. It is the special merit of the longitudinal approach that by its scope, by its persistence, and by its analytical orientation toward the study of lives through time, it can perhaps permit a greater understanding of why it is people turn out as they do.

Aspirations for a Longitudinal Study of Personality Development

In 1968, my late wife, Jeanne, and I decided to initiate a longitudinal study of personality development. For a variety of reasons, each itself insufficient but in their sum compelling, it seemed like the thing to do and the time to do it. After an academic hiatus consequent upon child having and child rearing, Jeanne had reestablished herself as a psychologist with her studies on the psychosomatics of asthma (see, e.g., J. H. Block, 1968; J. H. Block, Jennings, Harvey, & Simpson, 1964), for which she won the Hofheimer Prize of the American Psychiatric Association, and her series of papers on the nature of student activism (see, e.g., J. H. Block, 1972; J. H. Block, Haan, & Smith, 1969).

I was completing the decade-long data analyses and the solitary writing that culminated in my book, *Lives Through Time* (J. Block, 1971). We had both become powerfully impressed by the logic and possibilities of the longitudinal approach. We were interested in studying developmentally for the first time two personality constructs—ego-control and ego-resiliency—that, from our graduate student days, we believed to be of central theoretical and behavioral importance. We felt we were old enough and young enough, old enough to have developed the necessary cautionary perspectives on so risky and so difficult a research enterprise and young enough to be able to look forward optimistically to an abundant scientific harvest. We were smart and energetic and aspiring. We were beyond the tenure trap because I already had tenure while Jeanne, limited by nepotism fears at Berkeley, had sought and received a Career Development Research Award from the National Institute of Mental Health. Perhaps most important, we danced very well together.

It will provide context for our study to recall just what the issues and orientations of psychology were like in 1968, the watershed year when we happened to begin our venture. Mischel's astonishingly influential book had just appeared, wherein he argued that there was little point in maintaining interest in the concept of personality. His "clear conclusion," presented as empirically driven, was that "behavioral consistencies have not been demonstrated, and the concept of personality traits as broad response predispositions is thus untenable" (Mischel, 1968, p. 146). Moreover, and of special interest, Mischel's gloomy view regarding the possibility of discerning behavioral consistencies even extended to his own preferred cognitive social learning approach: "the discriminativeness and idiosyncratic organization of behavior are facts of nature, not limitations unique to trait theories" (Mischel, 1973, p. 265). Because the behaviors of an individual are exquisitely and uniquely dependent on or controlled by discriminated features of the environments encountered, Mischel argued, no broad ways of dimensionalizing or classifying individuals can prove useful. This line of argument and conclusion proved especially attractive to the then-burgeoning field of experimental social psychology, which vigorously opposed the study of individual differences.

In developmental psychology, Kagan (1976) extended the Mischelian argument of behavioral inconsistency by adding the dimension of time: Discontinuity rather than continuity was said by him to characterize development; there were no or few long-term implications of the early years for the later years. He, too, pointed to weak evidence from studies of developmental continuities. From the claim that the concept of personality was not especially useful, there was now the claim that the idea of coherent paths of personality development was irrelevant. Again, knowledge of current stimulus conditions, of the surrounding environment, of normative maturation at different rates, and of the immediate pushes and pulls on the individual were said to be all one could, and should, invoke to explain the behavior being observed.

In the midst of this discouraging *zeitgeist,* my wife and I committed ourselves to a longitudinal venture. We were moved to this commitment because we believed there was indeed an essential *coherence,* a deep structure to personality functioning and in personality development. Sure, it was crucial to recognize the ways in which the immediate environmental context influenced behavior, as personality psychologists Henry Murray (1938), Kurt Lewin (1946), Robert White (1959), and others earlier had observed. However, stimulus situations alone could not provide, we believed, a sufficient basis for understanding behavior. Human beings are not simply linear response systems effectively at the mercy of the situations they encounter. Besides making exquisite and unique discriminations, humans develop broad and adaptively functional, consistently applied generalizations. These constructed generalizations are shaped by a common evolutionary heritage, by modal perceptual and action patterns, and by commonly encountered environmental contingencies. Because of these constructed generalizations, individuals vary reliably and meaningfully and can be usefully dimensionalized or classified regarding the ways they perceive and react upon their world. We believed, 20 years ago, that the generally dismal state of empirical evidence for this proposition existed because, too often, the underlying coherence had not been sought well. In particular, we believed that consistency or continuity in behavior will not be found if one looks for expressions of personality consistency and continuity in ways that are conceptually obtuse or methodologically insufficient or empirically constrained. We thought we could do better and wanted to give it a try. We were by no means certain that, in our optimism, our faith would be fulfilled. We were certain, however, that those who would not try for coherence would not lead the way to understanding.

We sat down one evening to begin to list the desiderata for a longitudinal study of personality development. Gradually, as we thought about what had been done in the past and what we believed should be done in the future, we evolved a set of criterion dimensions in terms of which we planned our own effort.

Desiderata for a Longitudinal Study of Personality Development

1. *A longitudinal study should be an intentional rather than an accidental study, not a study begun for other reasons and only subsequently (and belatedly) declared to be a longitudinal study.* Some well-known longitudinal studies initially had not been conceived to be or to become long-term inquiries. Because of this lack of anticipation, various simple, obvious, crucial kinds of research planning and data gathering had not been done at the outset, the one and only time when planning could have been effective or certain kinds of data could have been gathered. I am

not referring to deficiencies of research design or research implementation easily and unfairly identified by cheap and virtuous retrospective wisdom. Instead, I have in mind omissions of data collection and failures of research design that could have been known at the time to be attenuating or vitiating of later analyses and hoped-for understandings. Our study, therefore, was to be deliberately longitudinal. Of course, intentionality did not prevent us from making our own mistakes, but it did permit us to avoid some important errors of the past.

2. *A longitudinal study should make public and communicable just what was done during the course of the study, how observations were made, how categories or numbers were generated, and how conclusions and interpretations were formulated.* We had observed that longitudinal investigators sometimes were carried away and infatuated by the aura of potential understanding that surrounds this well-regarded, if rarely used, approach. Too often, declamations and interpretations from longitudinal inquiries have been offered into the scientific literature on impressionistic and unspecifiable bases and, because of the positive aura surrounding longitudinal inquiry, have had unwarranted influence (see J. Block, 1981, for an account of one such unfortunate incident). Our longitudinal study, therefore, was to be one in which later psychologists could know what we had done, our rationales, the nature of our data and analyses, and the bases of our conclusions.

3. *A longitudinal study should be sufficiently extended in time so that developmental processes, continuities, and changes can be discerned.* Protracted, laborious, controlling of the researchers though a proper longitudinal study may be, there is not much point to a study so brief it cannot track development. Because of the cachet that now surrounds the term *longitudinal,* one sometimes encounters the oxymoron of "short-term longitudinal" studies. Our own plan and aspiration, therefore, was to conduct a long-term longitudinal study from early childhood (age 3 years) through the completion of high school (ages 17–18) and perhaps beyond. Although we viewed the then-incoming and increasingly popular emphasis on development throughout the life span to be salutary for those who had not earlier attained that important recognition, our

own theoretical concerns were centered on the childhood and adolescent years, a time when personality development is relatively rapid and, as we believed, consequential.

4. *A longitudinal study should involve a sample of reasonable initial and continuing size, of reasonable relevance, and of both sexes seen a number of aptly selected times.* Given the diversity of personality development and the omnipresent noise in assessment measures, a sample size sufficient to permit discernment of relationships is crucial if this difficult game is to be worth the candle. Yet, one cited longitudinal study involved a sample of 3 subjects that, when reassessed a final time 1 year later, showed a 33% attrition rate. Regarding sample relevance, in another longitudinal study the investigators apparently enlisted mothers from among their friends and friends of friends with the consequence that 78% of their subjects came from Jewish, professional, urban, economically comfortable families. Certainly, one cannot aspire to a random or representative sample of subjects (representative of what, pray tell?) when close and continued study of development is being pursued, but certainly also, unusual, severely disproportionate subject selection that could well be relationship distorting is to be avoided. Other longitudinal researchers have considered subjects of only one sex, usually males; surely, this kind of exclusion is limiting of psychological understanding.

5. *A longitudinal study should have a conceptual or theoretically integrating rubric directing its doings and progression rather than be blandly or blindly eclectic.* In ranging widely in its coverage, a longitudinal study need not forsake theoretical pursuits. Indeed, the incisiveness and implicativeness of theoretical constructs are better seen when a wide array of behaviors can be evaluated. Jeanne and I had developed some large, organizing personality constructs, ego-control and ego-resiliency, during our thesis days at Stanford University and demonstrated their behavioral implications in a variety of concurrent circumstances. Our constructs seemed to relate in intrinsic ways to other constructs formulated and studied by other investigators, encouraging us to think we were onto something of appreciable theoretical and behavioral importance. However, our constructs (and related ones) had never been studied developmentally. Obviously, to deepen understanding it was crucial to do

so. We wished, therefore, to see how boys and girls over time evolved their personal systems for the modulation of motivations and the achievement of adaptive resourcefulness and perhaps to identify the environmental factors that differentially influenced these parameters of living. So, we oriented our longitudinal study to examine developmentally our particular theoretical constructs.

6. *A longitudinal study should be comprehensive, intensive, systematic, and scientifically contemporary in coverage of its chosen conceptual domains.* Instead of being narrow and shallow, longitudinal inquiries should be broad and deep. They should involve *close psychological inquiry*, not just epidemiologically oriented surveys. Longitudinal studies are so rare that, although an already difficult research burden becomes even more difficult, a scientific responsibility is placed on the investigators to be catholic rather than parochial in designing and implementing their study. With broad and continuing assessments on the same set of subjects, there devolves the opportunity—which should not be missed—of relating within one sample research approaches customarily kept separate. Thereby, linkages among bodies of psychological research usually kept compartmentalized may possibly be established. The relationships, longitudinal or perhaps only concurrent, that subsequently may be discerned if there has been breadth of the research scan should have wide and cumulative import and speak to many psychological questions. Therefore, our longitudinal venture was to range widely in the constructs to be covered and was to be alert to current thinking and procedures in the ongoing field of personality development. We expected to spend appreciable time with each of our subjects during each assessment for, as Robert White once informally remarked, one must look at personality in order to study it.

7. *A longitudinal study should be methodologically competent and display craftsmanship in its implementation.* Methodological competence should not be taken to mean simply and only knowledge of statistics; psychologists often incorrectly make this equivalence. Rather, methodological competence should mean competence of several kinds, invoked sequentially, with the recognition that later analytical possibilities depend crucially on earlier sensible decisions appropriately implemented. Com-

petence with sophisticated or at least pertinent statistical methods is certainly required in the ultimate effort to discern relationships. However, prior to the invocation of such methods, a proper longitudinal research design must have been employed so that, from one time to another or from one context to another, data can be known to be absolutely independent and the subsequently obtained relationships indisputably can be recognized as inferentially clean. Prior to these considerations of research design, the measures being used must achieve sufficient psychometric status in terms of reliability and consequent discriminating power. Elaborate statistical analysis of logically independent measures will fail or will issue dismayingly null findings unless the measures employed are dependable. Finally, prior to concerns regarding measure dependability, it is essential to worry about the construct validity of the measures being used: Do they have the sweet reasonability and the supporting nomological network they must have if they are to represent the constructs the psychologist has in mind? Historically, longitudinal studies have been methodologically innocent and therefore interpreted sinfully. Measures have been awarded auspicious but unearned labels, with the consequence that subsequently observed relationships have been portrayed in misleading ways. Aware of these different aspects of methodology and their logical sequence, we aspired, in our longitudinal effort, to a higher standard in this realm than previously had been achieved.

8. *A longitudinal study should seek to be innovative.* I mention this virtuous and grandiose aspiration, which modesty should perhaps cause me to conceal, to register my view that longitudinal studies often had been carried through in plodding, unthinking ways. Because head circumference was easy to measure, it was measured. In the home economics version of child psychology that prevailed prior to the 1950s, such parentally frowned-on behaviors as nail biting, eating problems, and enuresis were important topics and were longitudinally studied. Because the Rorschach Inkblot Test and the Thematic Apperception Test had become popular, they were administered. In short, a characteristic of previous longitudinal studies was that they brought together an agglomeration of readily available and unthought-about measures without much consideration being given to the concepts and issues to be studied and the

necessary formulation of relevant assessment procedures bearing on these matters. A corollary of this passive, uncritical, atheoretical approach to longitudinal research is that when longitudinally studied subjects were followed-up, it was too often the case that measures were reflexively, unthinkingly repeated *because they had been administered before* no matter how useless they had proved themselves to be or how age inappropriate they had become. We were determined to avoid such prosaicness in our longitudinal study. We therefore tried to seek out or create assessment procedures and concept-representing measures that were new, age appropriate, theoretically interesting, technically sound, and perhaps even elegant.

9. *A longitudinal study should be able to sustain the quality of the enterprise over the long period of time required.* An endemic disease of longitudinal studies seems to be that, after a time, they reach a point where they begin to falter, lose their vitality, and perhaps even their *raison d'être.* Staff demoralization occurs, and there is busyness without purpose. In part, this anomie may develop because the longitudinal idea takes so long before payoff. Also, some personnel replacements may be seeking a job rather than a purpose and so do not contribute to the necessary sense of meaning that must undergird the longitudinal enterprise. An especially troubling problem arises because longitudinal studies typically exist outside of academic departments and are supported by "soft" funds. In this insecure context, longitudinal researchers are hampered in their efforts to attract high-caliber research individuals for more than a few productive years. Understandably, such people must seize on ultimately more satisfying academic opportunities as they arise. Our longitudinal venture sought to forfend these problems by selecting and maintaining an intelligent, resourceful, dedicated cadre of professional staff, by encouraging an elan and group sense of meaning, by renewing and reinvigorating this small group over the years via carefully chosen replacements, and—perhaps primarily—by our very awareness that these problems could be expected to arise.

Taken altogether, these criteria for a longitudinal study represented a grandiose, quite adolescent ambition. I will not say that we achieved all of these worthy goals (indeed, I wish to be the first to criticize our enterprise), but these were the standards we set out for ourselves. I will leave to others and for another time the evaluation of how well we achieved our aspirations.

What, Indeed, Did We Do?

We began with 128 children from two nursery schools in Berkeley, a heterogeneous sample with regard to socioeconomic status, parental education, and ethnic background. Extensive individual assessments of these children were conducted at ages 3, 4, 5, 7, 11, 14, 18, and, most recently, at age 23. These time periods were selected for assessment because of our sense of when, developmentally, it would be most incisive to study our subjects. At age 23, we assessed 104 subjects. This small amount of subject attrition is due to the great attention we gave to motivating subjects and their parents, to repeated friendly contacts we initiated between assessment periods, to maintaining up-to-date records on subject locations, to paying the subjects a nominal sum for their participation once they entered adolescence, and to having the prescience to carry out such a study in the San Francisco Bay Area, from which there is a decided tendency not to move. Having interviewed just about all of our subjects during our most recent assessment, I have alerted them to our plans to see them again in their late 20s, after another eventful 5 years of life. By then, I no longer will be the prime mover of this enterprise; I hope to be involved, but the study will have been transferred to several younger and more energetic colleagues.

During each of the eight assessment periods, every child (or adolescent or young adult) individually experienced an extensive battery of widely ranging procedures involving 10- or 11-hour-long sessions at ages 3 and 4, 4 or 5 longer sessions at ages 5 and 7, and 6 two-hour (or longer) sessions at ages 11, 14, 18, and 23.

Various methodological or design principles guided our effort. We were oriented toward employing various kinds of data, not just life history, school, or demographic information (L-data); not just ratings of our subjects by teachers or parents or knowledgeable observers (O-data); not just formal experimental procedures or standardized tests (T-data); and not just questionnaires or other self-report techniques (S-data). Rather, we sought to include all (L-, O-, T-, and S-data) of these various approaches to generating useful data. Early on, we emphasized T-data in assessments because young children in their experimental and test behaviors rather directly express their motivations and characteristics. As our subjects moved into preadolescence and became "interiorized," we shifted to a greater use of S-data. Throughout our assessments, we collected various kinds of L-data information from the parents, school records, and the subjects themselves. And throughout the study we relied heavily on O-data, context-recognizing evaluations of our subjects at various ages, evaluations contributed by observers who had observed the subjects in diverse, often intimate situations, and often for appreciable periods of time.

We were also oriented toward the use of multiple measurements within each kind of data so as to achieve dependability and generalizability of our measures. Instead of measuring the fidgetiness of a child by a single behavioral time sample, we measured fidgetiness on a number of occasions and developed an averaged index, which, of course, displayed much better reliability and subsequent relations with other variables. When measures were not sensibly repeatable, such as when we sought to study a broad construct such as style of categorizing, we sampled the conceptual domain using diverse measures of categorizing, which we then composited so as to rise above the problem of method variance. When we relied on observer evaluations of personality or interactions, we relied on a composite judgment of several independent observers—never just one—encoded by the Q-sort method so as to ensure observer comparability in the way they used numbers and to lessen the influence of response sets.

In successive assessments we used entirely different crews of assessors so that absolute independence was maintained between the data gathered at these different times. The T-procedures that were specifically repeated, such as the Witkin Rod-and-Frame Test, were not influenceable by prior testing or were separated by enough time so that memory could not play a vitiating role.

We used various data-reduction procedures with the thousands of variables that accumulated (e.g., factor analysis, hierarchical regression analysis, the compositing of standard scores derived from variables all conceptually or empirically linked, the generation of prototype scores to reflect how well a constellation of obtained scores fits a conceptual standard). In our analyses, we were sensitive to the problem of chance significance and applied an early version of the bootstrap method (J. Block, 1960) to our results and also catalyzed a method developed by truly mathematical statisticians (Alemayehu & Doksum, 1990) to further deal with the data analysis problems besetting us. Our most persuasive way of analyzing data, however, was to seek for and to find convergence of relationships from different kinds of data sets and from different times of assessment.

Routinely, we analyzed our data for the two sexes separately. It is crucial to do so. When the same pattern of findings characterizes both boys and girls, both young men and young women, one has a cross-validated result. However, when, as happens surprisingly often, reliably different correlational patterns characterize the two sexes, a sex difference has been found that requires attention and thought. Over the years, I have been profoundly impressed by the differences between the sexes not so much in their respective mean levels on whatever is being measured as in the differences in the correlational *patterns* that characterize males as compared with females.

I now present an inundating listing (a sampling, really) of the measures and procedures and situations we imposed on our subjects over the years. The reader should not try to truly incorporate the meaning of the many measures so tersely mentioned; a sense of the scope and ambition of our effort is all that is needed.

Thus, we used measures of activity level; delay of gratification; distractability; vigilance; exploratory behavior; motor inhibition (Simon Says!); susceptibility to priming; satiation and cosatiation; planfulness; curiosity; instrumental behavior when confronted by barriers or frustrations; dual focus (the ability to split attention); susceptibility to perceptual illusions; risk taking; level of aspiration; utilization of feedback; the Wechsler Intelligence Scale at ages 4, 11, and 18; the Raven Progressive Matrices; Piagetian measures of conservation; semantic retrieval; the Lowenfeld Mosaic Test; divergent thinking and other indexes of creativity; chained word association to index associative drift; various cognitive styles such as field dependence–independence, reflection–impulsivity, category breadth, and perceptual standards; sex role typing; egocentrism; physiognomic perception; incidental learning; the Stroop Color and Word Test; the Kogan Metaphor Test for metaphor comprehension; metaphor generation; short-term memory via digit span; memory for sentences; and memory for narrative stories; moral development; Loevinger's Washington University Sentence Completion Test to measure ego development; Kelly's Role Construct Repertory Test; skin conductance while lying, when startled, and recovery rate from startle; the phenomenology of emotions; Spivack and Shure's interpersonal problem-solving measure; free play at age 3 and free play again at age 11 (patterned after Erik Erikson's approach); self-concept descriptions; descriptions of ideal self, of mother, of father, and of sought-for love object; decision time and decision confidence in situations varying in the intrinsic difficulty of decision; enacting a standard set of expressive situations (videotaped); experience sampling for a week via a beeper; blood pressure and heart rate in response to a set of stressors; depressive realism; false consensus; health indexes; activity and interest indexes; long and intensive clinical interviews (videotaped) relating to, among other topics, adult attachment, ways of knowing and ego development, and core conflict relationship themes; Diagnostic Interview Schedule screening so as to connect with the revised third edition of the *Diagnostic and Statistical Manual of Mental Disorders (DSM–III–R)* classification system; and hundreds of questionnaire and inventory items relating to dozens of personality scales.

Both the mothers and fathers of our subjects also participated in the study in various ways, contributing several kinds of data over the years. We have information at various times of their child-rearing orientations, their self-descriptions, their characterizations of the child, their responses to a personality inventory, home interviews and characterizations of the home environment, and videotapes of their interactions with their child during the preschool years and also during early adolescence.

In assembling and administering this array of procedures, there was continual concern for the age appropriateness of the procedures used. Some measures of conceptual interest sensibly could be repeated in later years, such as the Rod-and-Frame Test, which we administered in six different assessments; others could not be, such as our procedure to measure delay of gratification by having nursery school children work for M&Ms. We were also attentive, as we went along, to the ongoing psychological literature, introducing into our assessments new topics and new measures that attracted our interest and to ensure continued contemporaneity of our broad-gauge inquiry. I offer as an observation and not as a boast that there is not another sample in psychology so extensively and intensively assessed for so long a period.

What Have We Found Out?

A little. As yet, we have barely begun to explore the analytical possibilities residing in our data bank. Partly, this is because of the press of longitudinal work. Because one cannot stop time, the pressures are incessant and in ways beyond usual mention in formal publications (e.g., making curtains for a mobile home or talking to school counselors or putting down carpet or locating a lost subject through the Department of Motor Vehicles). When problems emerge and impinge, and the study depends on responding to them, there is not much choice: One must do then and there what needs to be done. Before one is through evaluating the implications of an assessment, it is necessary to plan for and ready another assessment. If one is to maintain funding, papers and chapters need to be written and need to be properly impressive.

Also, there were unpredictable but inevitable human problems, fluctuations in our efficiency at various times and intrusions of health problems, in particular the tragic illness that swept away my partner, Jeanne. Technocratically evaluated, it is clear we could have done better.

These excuses having been offered, let me also say that I think we have found out enough to have justified our effort. Let me select for brief presentation a half dozen diverse and, I suggest, nonobvious findings, all of which depended crucially on the *longitudinality* of our data, findings not establishable without introducing the dimension of time, of extended time. Within this particular chapter, I of necessity make declarations about our results rather than seriously justify my remarks. Substantiation will be found in a number of referenced articles and in forthcoming papers.

Of course, the work I cite is not mine alone; I have benefited immensely from long collaborations with a large number of fine research colleagues.

1. *Self-concept and self-esteem over time* (J. Block & Robins, in press). Psychologists have long studied the self because one's self-perceptions are both a reflection of the life that has been led and an influence on the life that will be lived. In our longitudinal inquiry, as our subjects moved into adolescence and began to develop an articulated self-reflectiveness, we sought "snapshots" of their evolving self-concepts. Subjects provided self-descriptions at ages 11, 14, 18, and 23 and descriptions of their ideal self at ages 14, 18, and 23. The same Q-sort method was used throughout. Self-esteem at a given age was indexed by the degree of congruence between the way a subject described the personally perceived self and the way that, a week later, the ideal self was described. To the extent one sees oneself as being close to one's ego ideal, one can be said to have self-esteem. This congruence index is a long-used and well-accepted measure.

Interestingly and implicatively, the sexes diverged in self-esteem over time, primarily in the period from ages 14 to 18. They were just about equal in mean self-esteem at age 14, differed significantly at age 18 ($p < .03$), and differed even more significantly at age 23 ($p < .006$). The mean self-esteem scores of the boys for ages 14, 18, and 23 were .53, .62, and .61, respectively, rising during adolescence; the mean self-esteem scores of the girls for the three ages were .53, .53, and .48, decreasing somewhat during the course of adolescence. The self-esteem of girls showed good continuity from ages 14 through 18 to 23 (correlations of about .5). The self-esteem of boys showed marked restructuring from age 14 to age 18 ($r = .08$) and reasonable continuity from ages 18 to 23 ($r = .38$). For both sexes, self-esteem correlated about zero with Wechsler Adult Intelligence Scale IQ and also did not relate to social class.

Personality evaluations of the subjects were available, made by independent observers. For each sex separately, these were correlated with self-esteem. Vis-à-vis self-esteem, there were many correlational similarities for the two sexes. Thus, young women and young men scoring high on self esteem both were independently characterized by observers as resilient, having rapid tempos, assertive rather than submissive, undiscouraged by adversity, without fluctuating moods, decisive, having a sense of personal meaning, initiating of and responsive to humor, and unpreoccupied by ruminative fantasy. This is an interesting and coherent set of characteristics, and there is no conceptual problem in seeing how these personality qualities are conducive to or expressive of self-esteem in either sex.

However, there were many instances in which the correlation of self-esteem with an independently evaluated personality characteristic in one sex was significantly different from the corresponding correlation for the other sex, suggesting that self-esteem is imbedded in highly different characterological contexts for the two sexes. Thus, attending to these sex differences in correlations, young women scoring high on self-esteem also tended to be evaluated as relatively warm, giving, protective, sympathetic, gregarious, talkative, conventional, moral, straightforward, cheerful, poised, and interested in the opposite sex. Young men scoring high on self-esteem also tended to be viewed as relatively critical, self-defensive, hostile, keeping people at a distance, sensitive to demands, concerned about their personal adequacy, likely to have unconventional thought processes, and likely to be aesthetically sensitive. These young men with self-esteem impressed observers as being relatively intelligent although, as already noted, self-esteem did not correlate with an index of IQ.

Although there was a personality core to self-esteem common in the two sexes, young women with high self-esteem scores seemed happy, warmly extraverted, and deeply concerned about interpersonal relationships. Young men with high self-esteem seemed self-focused and defensively critical, uneasy, and unready for a connection with others.

2. *The personality of children prior to divorce* (J. H. Block, Block, & Gjerde, 1986). Over the past decade, a number of studies of the effects of divorce have appeared and have had wide influence. Typically in such studies, children (usually young adolescents) who have experienced divorce have been contrasted with children who have not experienced divorce. The findings have suggested that boys experiencing divorce were relatively unsocialized, troublesome, undercontrolled, aggressive, and characterized by excessive energy. The findings relating to girls have been

unclear or weak, perhaps (in my conjecture) because possible effects of divorce in girls are more likely to be observed later when they have become young women and focus on establishing intimate, long-term relationships of their own.

In our longitudinal study, about half of the children experienced divorce. When we compared boys who had experienced divorce with boys who had not experienced divorce, we identified distinguishing personality characteristics similar to those reported by previous investigators and, again, uncertain results for the girls. However, because our study was longitudinal and previous studies had not been longitudinal, we were able to analyze our data in an unprecedented way: We could compare boys who were going to experience divorce but had not yet with boys who were not going to experience divorce. Tellingly, this comparison revealed that boys who were going to experience divorce sometime in their future, when contrasted with boys who were not going to experience divorce in their future, were characterized by undercontrol of impulse, aggressiveness, and excessive energy, and were generally more troublesome. That is, a finding previously said to be a *consequence* of divorce was found to exist *prior* to the fact of divorce. Children's behavioral problems may be present years before the formal divorce actually occurs. Indeed, the family discord often characterizing the period before parental separation may well have serious consequences for the children involved. This is not to say that the subsequent experiences of divorce, with all the life changes that are entailed, have no additional or special influence on the lives and character of the children of divorce. It is to say that the examination of families only after divorce has occurred is a demonstrably insufficient means of comprehending the complex interpersonal processes influencing character development. To approach a more complete understanding of divorce and its subsequent import, it is necessary to study families years before there is a divorce, while the family is still intact.

3. *Longitudinally foretelling drug usage in adolescence: Early childhood personality and environmental precursors* (J. Block, Block, & Keyes, 1988; see also Shedler & Block, 1990). One of the great concerns of our cultural epoch is the problem of understanding the factors under-

lying substance abuse. During these times, it was inevitable that, within the course of our prolonged longitudinal study, a number of our subjects would become involved with some of the drugs widely available in American society. We were able to develop well-based information regarding the drug usage of our subjects and could relate the degree and kind of drug usage in early adolescence to concurrent and preschool personality characteristics. The personality concomitants and antecedents of drug use differed somewhat as a function of gender and the drug used. For both sexes at age 14, the use of marijuana was related to ego-undercontrol, whereas the use of harder drugs reflected an absence of ego-resiliency with undercontrol also a contributing factor. Of special interest, at ages 3–4, subsequent adolescent drug usage in girls was related to both undercontrol and lower ego-resiliency; in boys it was related to undercontrol, with resiliency having no long-term implications. Overall, preschool children subsequently using drugs at age 14 were characterized as restless and fidgety, emotional labile, disobedient, lacking in calmness, domineering, behaving immaturely when under stress, reluctant to yield and give in, aggressive, overreactive to frustration, teasing, and unable to recoup after stress. Early family environment related to adolescent drug usage in girls but not boys. These early antecedents of drug usage are important for contemporary views regarding adolescent drug usage and, consequently, social policy. It would appear that the roots of adolescent substance abuse are discernible, and perhaps modifiable, in early childhood.

4. *Personality antecedents of depressive tendencies in 18-year-olds* (J. Block, Gjerde, & Block, 1991). Depression is a major human problem. Understanding why certain individuals are especially susceptible to depressive moods while others cheerily go through life is an important scientific task. In our longitudinal study, we had the opportunity, which is continuing, to study individual differences in depressive tendencies, seeking to identify some of the antecedent factors contributing to this mood disorder. Depressive tendencies, from which the correlated contribution of anxiety was partialed, were evaluated and related to prior longitudinal data. Many significant correlations, coherent within each sex but differing crucially as a function of gender, were found, going back to

middle and even early childhood. Subsequently depressed girls at age 7 tended to be shy and reserved, oversocialized, intropunitive, and over-controlled. Subsequently depressed boys at age 7 and even as early as age 3 tended to be unsocialized, aggressive, and undercontrolled in a self-aggrandizing way. IQ related positively to subsequent depression in girls and negatively in boys. Currently, with our age 23 data, we are following-up on these findings to evaluate whether these sex differences persist and, furthermore, seeking to distinguish between two kinds of depression: depression precipitated by anguish regarding a no-longer-available love object and depression precipitated by the individual's sense of agentic failure.

5. *Personality antecedents of political orientation* (J. Block, 1992). Psychologists and political scientists have long been interested in the relations between personality and politics (see, e.g., Christie & Jahoda, 1964; Greenstein, 1975; McClosky, 1958). However, studies of the person-ality correlates of political orientations have made little headway because of methodological problems and perhaps because political scientists, given the premises of their field, have been disinclined to give credence to the empirical psychological connections that have been brought for-ward. Although conservatism–liberalism have been measured and related to concurrent or subsequent behavior, there has been little interest in studying the antecedents of political orientation, except for identifying various epidemiological factors. Our longitudinal study has permitted an unprecedented analysis in this area. At age 23, our subjects were admin-istered measures of conservatism–liberalism via direct query and a scale of various items dealing with issues such as abortion, expenditures for welfare, national health insurance, the rights of suspected criminals, pro-gressive income tax increases, meeting energy needs by risking offshore oil spills, and so on. The measures used were reliable. Relating these measures to our data collected when the subjects were aged 3–4 revealed many antecedent correlations. Preschool children (both boys and girls) subsequently relatively conservative at age 23 were described as being significantly more likely to be easily victimized; easily offended; indecisive and vacillating; fearful, anxious, and rigid, especially in unpredictable, stressful environments; inhibited; and constricted. Preschool children

who, 20 years later, were relatively liberal were more likely to develop close relationships, be self-reliant, be energetic, and be somewhat dominating. IQ did not relate to conservatism–liberalism. Although much more needs to be done to refine these analyses, these connections between personality at an early age and subsequent political orientation obviously provide much food for thought regarding the psychodynamic underpinnings of political values.

6. *Ego-resiliency and ego-control over time.* As a last, more detailed example of a significant developmental finding discernible only by longitudinal inquiry, consider the questions driven by the conceptual framework from which our study began: What is the consistency of ego-resiliency and ego-control over time? Are children who are relatively ego-resilient or relatively ego-controlled at an early age relatively ego-resilient or relatively ego-controlled at later ages (i.e., in middle childhood, in preadolescence, adolescence, and young adulthood)? This is *not* a question about what is so often unfortunately called *stability.* The individuals may change and indeed do change. Twenty-three-year-olds were more resilient and more controlled than 3-year-olds, so they were not "stable." Our question really is, Do these individuals tend to maintain their *relative* position with respect to ego-resiliency and ego-control? To what extent, despite all the life experiences accruing over time, do children tend to preserve through adolescence and into young adulthood their relative order with respect to the widely relevant behavioral dimensions of ego-resiliency and ego-control? There has not previously been reasonable developmental information regarding such questions. Indeed, at the time we started our study, in the late 1960s and as already noted, the accepted view of psychologists was that little or no continuity of personality functioning existed from early childhood into the later years.

For our longitudinally followed subjects, we had reliable and independent indexes of ego-resiliency and ego-control at ages 3, 4, 7, 11, 14, 18, and 23, based on prototype scoring of the Q composites available for them at each age. Table 1 shows the ego-resiliency intercorrelations, uncorrected for the lowering effect of attenuation for the two sexes separately, as well as the ego-control intercorrelations.

Regarding ego-resiliency, the correlations were consistently positive for the boys or young men throughout the years. Many of the correlations

TABLE 1

The Longitudinal Consistency of Ego-Undercontrol and Ego-Resiliency

Age	3	4	7	11	14	18	23
				Age at personality assessment			
				ego-undercontrol			
3	—	.70***	.47**	.22	.40**	.22	.31
4	.82***	—	.56***	.35*	.56***	.42**	.40*
7	.58***	.48**	—	.46**	.66***	.37**	.35*
11	.34*	.53***	.58***	—	.58***	.51***	.47**
14	.49**	.47***	.50***	.74***	—	.72***	.67**
18	.42**	.26	.44**	.43**	.51***	—	.76**
23	.54**	.42*	.31	.46**	.62***	.49**	—
				ego-resiliency			
3	—	.68***	.19	.19	.00	−.06	.08
4	.65***	—	.38**	−.02	−.28	−.23	−.16
7	.34*	.47**	—	.37**	.28	.21	.07
11	.35*	.46**	.41**	—	.58***	.40**	.21
14	.23	.37*	.42**	.65***	—	.58***	.53**
18	.31*	.47**	.58***	.58***	.60***	—	.56**
23	.22	.42*	.23	.39*	.38*	.54**	—

Note. Results for girls are above the diagonal; results for boys are below the diagonal. Sample sizes for girls ranged from 39 to 52; sample sizes for boys ranged from 37 to 50.
*p < .05.   **p < .01.   ***p < .001.

are at a level psychologists would consider quite high. For males, this evidence clearly indicates that individual differences in ego-resiliency are identifiable from an early age and largely continue over the next 20 years.

The ego-resiliency correlations for the girls presented a much different picture, however. These correlations between adjacent time periods were reasonably positive and even high. In the early childhood years, there was reasonable ordering consistency. From adolescence on, there was reasonable, even impressive ordering consistency. However, between these two periods, there was really no relation: For girls, being resilient (or brittle) during the childhood years carried no implication for being ego-resilient (or brittle) in adolescence and beyond. There appears to be a sliding transformation over time, especially marked as girls enter puberty, that obliterates the connection between level of ego-resiliency in the childhood years and level of ego-resiliency during adolescence and young adulthood.

What does this difference between the sexes mean? Is it yet another instance of how psychological findings bounce around and are difficult to replicate? Or is this difference between the sexes in the longitudinal pattern of ego-resiliency believable and therefore seriously implicative and warranting of interpretation? For added perspective, consider the findings surrounding ego-control.

Regarding ego-control, the correlations were consistently positive for both sexes. The size of these correlations was perhaps impressively high considering attenuating factors, the great length of time involved, and life circumstances fostering personality change. This is strong evidence, replicated across the sexes, that from an early age individual differences in the level of ego-control are identifiable and continue to distinguish people for at least the next 20 years and, from the evidence of other studies (see J. Block, 1971), even beyond.

Considering the correlational results for ego-resiliency and ego-control for both sexes, in three of the four comparisons longitudinal continuity of individual differences was to be observed. In all four of the analyses, the same methodology was used. I suggest, therefore, that it becomes difficult to attribute the discrepant ego-resilience results for girls to methodological or sampling fluctuations. The failure of ordering continuity of ego-resilience for the girls (in the larger context of ordering continuity for the boys and the ordering continuity of ego-control for both sexes) would appear to represent a real finding and not a vagary of our data. Some other findings from our longitudinal study further reinforce my view that this difference between the sexes in regard to their longitudinal patterns of resiliency continuity is truly based and not easily explained away (e.g., see the depression findings, mentioned earlier).

What happened to the girls as they left childhood and moved into puberty? One clue may perhaps be provided by the relations between ego-resiliency and ego-control over time. For the boys, over more than 20 years from ages 3 through 23, ego-resiliency and ego-control were essentially unrelated, with the correlations averaging not quite zero (.02), with little variation. For girls, the relationship between ego-resiliency and ego-control was essentially zero at ages 3, 4, and 7. However, at age 11, there suddenly appeared a substantial negative correlation between ego-resiliency and overcontrol. This relationship diminished somewhat during the subsequent adolescent years and by the early 20s, it became low again. However, during the preadolescent and adolescent years, ego-resiliency in girls appeared to be appreciably related, reciprocally, to overcontrol. During this re-formative period, ego-resiliency in girls went along with a lessening of overcontrol.

How is this connection between ego-resiliency and ego-control to be developmentally explained? Speculation is required here; my own interpretation goes along the following lines. The literature on the differential socialization of the sexes indicates that girls grow up in a more structured and directive world than boys (J. H. Block, 1983). Girls experience more parental supervision, more restrictions on exploration, more emphases on maintaining proximity, and more frequent (often unnecessary) help in problem-solving situations. These various sex-differentiating influences combine to create a more canalized and predictable environment for girls than for boys, whose encounters with the world outside of the home are both more extensive and less managed. These formal differences in the learning environments provided to girls as compared with boys can be expected to have cumulative, powerful, and generalizing effects on the adaptive strategies invoked when the world in which one has been living changes in fundamental ways.

The onset of puberty, of internal transformations that also transform how the world reacts to one's strangely different yet much the same self is such a fundamental change. Because of the differential socialization of the sexes (and likely, too, because of the earlier age at which girls physically mature), the changes catalyzed by puberty may well present a larger and more abrupt adaptational problem for girls than for boys. For girls in particular, the necessary changes require restructuring of previously sufficient modes of adaptation, an emergence from the cocoons of security and restriction in which they have grown up.

The ability to achieve this restructuring is, of course, encompassed by the construct of ego-resiliency. Also, however, the leaving of previous constrictive adaptations and the absence of behavioral perseveration are indicators that the individual is not, or no longer, overcontrolled. Thus, girls confronting adolescence who display resiliency in their adaptive modes necessarily have moved away from overcontrol, thus accounting for the empirical relationships we have observed.

Coda

For quite a few years now, the longitudinal method, charting the lives of people over time and across circumstances, has been recognized as being essential for the investigation of crucial questions regarding psychological development. However, such studies have been criticized as being, by their very nature, relatively sprawling, untidy, costly, difficult to integrate both with respect to data processing problems and conceptual matters, and sometimes excessively prolonged. (In one famous criticism, longitudinal studies were characterized as "issuing promissory notes that were never redeemed.")

Such criticisms are true, more or less. How compelling these criticisms are should depend on the personal orientation of the investigator. Sprawl also offers reach, untidiness tends to accompany large intentions, considerations of cost must also be accompanied by considerations of benefit, data are bothersome, concepts are difficult to think about, and who is to say while lives go on how long a longitudinal study should continue?

Although there certainly are daunting difficulties and uncertainties along the way, it seems to me that the strategy of longitudinal inquiry can now be seen in a new, more assertively *positive* light, one that illuminates a better way developmental psychologists might proceed. If a longitudinal study has been carried along far enough and at a decent level of competence, I wish to argue that the longitudinal strategy will, surprisingly often, be more science-effective, more cost-effective, and more time-effective than the approach presently characterizing so much of developmental psychology: numerous, small, compartmentalized, incomplete, hit-and-run studies that often do not seem to build toward a cumulative science.

The longitudinal strategy is more science-effective, I suggest, because it provides a richer road to developmental understandings. The number of conceptually important analytical possibilities becomes extraordinary; concepts usually carefully kept separate can now be related or indeed established to be unconnected; serendipitous recognitions often follow from the many unprecedented data explorations that become feasible. For example, the Stroop Color and Word Test, a measure of the ability to resist interference usually studied only in information-processing contexts, proved in our longitudinal study to have extensive personality correlates in both male and female adolescents.

The longitudinal strategy is more cost-effective, I suggest, because it is a cheaper, more energy-efficient road to developmental understandings. In an extensive and prolonged longitudinal inquiry, there is exponential growth in the number of analytical possibilities. As a consequence, the cost in money and in energy for each different yet often important analysis can become impressively small. For example, it cost us almost nothing to develop information from our subjects regarding their patterns of drug usage (J. Block et al., 1988; Shedler & Block, 1990) and their political orientations, whereupon the consequent, immediately feasible, computationally trivial analyses revealed incontestable connections with early childhood personality characteristics that are of great implication.

The longitudinal strategy is more time-effective, I suggest, because, paradoxically, it is a quicker way to developmental understandings. Motley, unrelated, limited studies that are not followed through cannot resolve conceptual issues or methodological concerns, and so these questions may linger indefinitely in the field. A well-planned and well-monitored longitudinal study—by the range of its assessments, by its opportunity for repeated testing to establish the dependability of a finding, and by its planning in subsequent assessments to clarify interpretative ambiguities left over from an earlier assessment—can close in on and resolve debates in the field that otherwise would go on forever. For example, our longitudinal approach to the Matching Familiar Figures Test, which had been presented as a sufficient index of the influential construct of reflection–impulsivity, showed that this previously popular measure did not have construct validity at any of the various ages when it was used (J. Block, Block, & Harrington, 1974; J. Block, Gjerde, & Block, 1986; Gjerde, Block, & Block, 1985). On the other hand, the Rod-and-Frame Test, when longitudinally evaluated, proved to have many of the correlates, albeit with some important exceptions, that its creator proposed (J. Block, 1983; Kogan & Block, 1991).

If it is taken as a given that longitudinal inquiry is necessary to study certain developmental questions, then it follows that the vicissitudes encountered by longitudinal studies in practice should be acknowledged, understood, fended off by anticipation, and worked on; they should not be viewed as vitiating.

Historically, longitudinal studies, so often called for, have been infrequently undertaken and carried through. Why has this been so?

One reason, I suggest, is the dilemma faced by the would-be longitudinal investigator, tentatively considering a heavy and long-term personal career commitment. Longitudinal research goes on principally in academic institutions where the generally prevailing basis for career advancement is evidence of research productivity. The psychologist at the beginning or even the middle of a career understandably fears a judgment of unproductivity will be rendered on him or her. A ten-year project is not a tenure project. The young psychologist interested in longitudinal research readily can be discouraged by the academic risks that will have to be run before a long research investment issues palpable products demonstrating there has been important, albeit quiet, research productivity all along. Academic evaluative criteria, as often applied, thus can cripple longitudinal research. I hope, but I am not optimistic, that universities will come to recognize alternative, equally valid ways of being "productive" and therefore help foster commitment to longitudinal research.

Another contributing factor to the sparseness of longitudinal studies, especially in these straitened times, is the problem of funding. Universities, the natural home of long-term investigations, do not enjoy the economic resources to maintain such studies. Recourse for support therefore must be made to various federal granting agencies concerned with human development. In many ways, for much time, somehow, in one way or another, federal support for longitudinal studies often has been forthcoming. However, the seeking of funding has been a disruptive and draining task for longitudinal investigators. Of course, longitudinal studies should not be granted perpetuity as a natural right; support must be earned. However, the vagaries of the federal budget and federal policies, together with an absence of recognition by some research review committees of the special support requirements of the longitudinal approach, can be disheartening. I can offer no solution for this problem except, perhaps, to suggest that certain private foundations take on the programmatic responsibility of supporting well-guided longitudinal research programs.

A third reason why longitudinal research is relatively infrequent stems from a controlling feature of so much contemporary psychological research. We are all naturally attracted to the study and analysis of psychological phenomena that are conveniently and quickly accessible. Why not? Life is short and, in principle, there is no necessary connection between the importance of a psychological question and how easy it is to study that question. Nevertheless, the preoccupation of psychologists with short-term, conveniently addressable questions may mean neglect of important psychological understandings discernible only inconveniently and only after long periods of time. Indeed, the implicit research requirement that a problem be conveniently and quickly studied may in effect introduce an unfortunate inverse relation between research convenience and the conceptual importance of the consequent research. Rather soon, most of the research possibilities conjointly convenient and important are likely to have been explored. If convenience and quickness continue to be insisted on, only relatively unimportant possibilities will then exist. Fishing may provide psychologists an apt analogy: If a line is cast only into the shallow waters of a nearby pond, only little fish will be caught. For the big fish, it is necessary to venture out into deep water. I urge psychologists to go for the big fish.

References

Alemayehu, D., & Doksum, K. (1990). Using the bootstrap in correlation analysis, with applications to a longitudinal data set. *Journal of Applied Statistics, 17*, 357–368.

Block, J. (1960). On the number of significant findings to be expected by chance. *Psychometrika, 25*, 369–380.

Block, J. (1971). *Lives through time.* Berkeley, CA: Bancroft Books.

Block, J. (1981). From infancy to adulthood: A clarification. *Child Development, 51*, 622–623.

Block, J. (1983, April). *The longitudinal study of cognitive styles.* Paper presented at the meeting of the Society for Research in Child Development, Detroit, MI.

Block, J. (1992, July). *Early childhood personality antecedents of liberalism-conservatism in young adulthood.* Paper presented at the meeting of the International Society of Political Psychology, San Francisco.

Block, J., Block, J. H., & Harrington, D. M. (1974). Some misgivings about the Matching Familiar Figures Test as a measure of reflection–impulsivity. *Developmental Psychology, 10,* 611–632.

Block, J., Block, J. H., & Keyes, S. (1988). Longitudinally foretelling drug usage in adolescence: Early childhood personality and environmental precursors. *Child Development, 59,* 336–355.

Block, J., Gjerde, P. F., & Block, J. H. (1986). More misgivings about the Matching Familiar Figures Test as a measure of reflection–impulsivity. *Developmental Psychology, 22,* 820–831.

Block, J., Gjerde, P. F., & Block, J. H. (1991). Personality antecedents of depressive tendencies in 18-year-olds: A prospective study. *Journal of Personality and Social Psychology, 60,* 726–738.

Block, J., & Robins, R. W. (in press). A longitudinal study of consistency and change in self-esteem from early adolescence to early adulthood. *Child Development.*

Block, J. H. (1968). Further considerations of psychosomatic predisposing factors in allergy. *Psychosomatic Medicine, 30,* 202–208.

Block, J. H. (1972). Generational continuity and discontinuity in the understanding of societal rejection. *Journal of Personality and Social Psychology, 22,* 333–345.

Block, J. H. (1983). Differential premises arising from differential socialization of the sexes. *Child Development, 54,* 1335–1354.

Block, J. H., Haan, N., & Smith, M. B. (1969). Socialization correlates of student activism. *Journal of Social Issues, 25,* 143–177.

Block, J. H., Jennings, P. H., Harvey, E., & Simpson, E. (1964). The interaction between allergic predisposition and psychopathology in childhood asthma. *Psychosomatic Medicine, 26,* 307–320.

Block, J. H., Block, J., & Gjerde, P. F. (1986). The personality of children prior to divorce: A prospective study. *Child Development, 57,* 827–840.

Christie, R., & Jahoda, M. (Eds.). (1964). *Studies in the scope and method of "The Authoritarian Personality."* New York: Free Press.

Fiske, D. W., & Shweder, R. A. (Eds.). (1986). *Metatheory in social science.* Chicago: University of Chicago Press.

Gjerde, P. F., Block, J., & Block, J. H. (1985). The longitudinal consistency of Matching Familiar Figures Test performance from early childhood to preadolescence. *Developmental Psychology, 21,* 262–271.

Greenstein, F. (1975). *Personality and politics.* New York: Norton.

Hyland, M. (1985). Do person variables exist in different ways? *American Psychologist,* *40,* 1003–1010.

Kagan, J. (1976). Emergent themes in human development. *American Scientist, 64,* 186–196.

Kogan, N., & Block, J. (1991). Field dependence-independence from early childhood through adolescence: Personality and socialization aspects. In S. Wapner & J. Demick (Eds.), *Field dependence-independence: Cognitive style across the life span* (pp. 177–207). Hillsdale, NJ: Erlbaum.

Lewin, K. (1946). Behavior and development as a function of the total situation. In L. Carmichael (Ed.), *Manual of child psychology* (pp. 918–970). New York: Wiley.

McClosky, H. (1958). Conservatism and personality. *American Political Science Review, 52,* 27–45.

Mischel, W. (1968). *Personality and assessment.* New York: Wiley.

Mischel, W. (1973). Toward a cognitive social learning reconceptualization of personality. *Psychological Review, 80,* 252–283.

Murray, H. A. (1938). *Explorations in personality.* New York: Oxford University Press.

Shedler, J., & Block, J. (1990). Adolescent drug use and psychological health: A longitudinal inquiry. *American Psychologist, 45,* 612–630.

Tucker, L. R. (1966). Learning theory and multivariate experiment: Illustration by determination of generalized learning curves. In R. B. Cattell (Ed.), *Handbook of multivariate experimental psychology* (pp. 476–501). Chicago: Rand McNally.

Underwood, B. J. (1975). Individual differences as a crucible in theory construction. *American Psychologist, 30,* 128–134.

White, R. W. (1959). Motivation reconsidered: The concept of competence. *Psychological Review, 66,* 297–333.

White, R. W. (1981). Exploring personality the long way: The study of lives. In A. I. Rabin, J. Aronoff, A. M. Barclay, & R. A. Zucker (Eds.), *Further explorations in personality* (pp. 3–19). New York: Wiley.

PART ONE

Examining the Methods

CHAPTER 3

The Value of Archival Data for New Perspectives on Personality

Jacquelyn B. James and Elizabeth L. Paul

The past 20 years in the field of personality research has been characterized by concern over whether the field is foundering or flourishing (Pervin, 1985; Rorer & Widiger, 1983), whether it is attending to the complexities of the "person" (Carlson, 1971; Levenson, Gray, & Ingram, 1976), and whether there is any unity beneath the diverse elements of the field (Buss, 1991). At the same time, there has been enormous change in the social forces at work in the lives of men and women, and calls for attention to the context in which personality is embedded. These events have combined to suggest a need for new and creative approaches for examining personality in general and "lives through time" in particular. We believe that one such creative approach is secondary analysis of existing data to address new research questions. Especially valuable for secondary analysis is the availability of original records that can be re-

Our thanks go to Anne Colby, Erin Phelps, and Avshalom Caspi for helpful comments on earlier drafts of this chapter. We also appreciate the assistance of Sarah Igo in preparing the chapter.

coded in countless ways. In this chapter we demonstrate that some of the areas of concern just mentioned can be studied most advantageously by the reuse of original records.

Our purpose is to (a) describe the advantages and challenges of secondary analysis, including the use of qualitative data; (b) present examples from three areas within personality that have been illuminated by the use of secondary qualitative data; and (c) suggest some useful methods for "recycling" existing qualitative data. Because Jack Block and Jeanne Block and their colleagues have been pioneers in many of these areas and have a continuing influence in the field, we draw heavily from the Blocks' work in our examples.

Advantages of Secondary Analysis

The use of existing data sources for new research questions has gained prominence in several fields in recent years (Brooks-Gunn, Phelps, & Elder, 1991; Colby, 1982; McCall & Appelbaum, 1991; Sieber, 1991; Stewart & Platt, 1982). Colby and Phelps (1990) have pointed out a number of advantages to this procedure, the most obvious of which is the ability to address original research questions without collecting new data. They also pointed out the value of secondary analysis for open scientific inquiry in that original findings can be verified, refuted, or refined (see J. Block & Lanning, 1984, for an excellent example). Other advantages include the possibility of extending research questions to larger or differently constituted samples, the possibility of conducting follow-ups of existing cross-sectional or longitudinal studies, pilot testing and question–hypothesis generation before collecting new data (Paul, 1990), and so on. Also important in times when research funds are scarce is the way that secondary analysis makes it possible to conduct ambitious studies with limited funds.

We argue in this chapter that many important questions in the field of personality are difficult to answer adequately without using existing data. This is true, at least in part, because so many of the questions require long-term longitudinal data. Researchers, for example, who seek to examine how person, situation, and time interact to affect behavior almost require longitudinal data. Longitudinal data are also needed for research that seeks to understand problems of immediate practical significance such as the links over time between personality and health, the development of detrimental effects of divorce on children's personality development, or the personal and situational antecedents of catastrophic outcomes such as suicide. Indeed, longitudinal data have long been recognized as being essential for the study of sequences of events and patterns of change over time. Especially beneficial for all of these questions is longitudinal data that include open-ended responses or interview material.

These qualitative data are crucial for secondary analyses because of their versatility for recasting and recoding to assess constructs of relevance to the research question. Even if a specific measure that would be useful to the researcher is not available within a given data set, many times it can be gleaned from open-ended materials (see, e.g., Peterson, Bettes, & Seligman, 1985; Winter, 1982). An added value of qualitative data for longitudinal analyses is the ability to extract comparable data from sometimes-inconsistent records. It is often the case with longitudinal studies that paper-and-pencil measures become outdated and are changed, rendering cross-time analyses of the construct of interest untenable. With methods for recoding qualitative records, such as the Q-sort (pioneered by Jack Block), these cross-time comparisons are made possible. Indeed, qualitative data can be recoded or content analyzed in numerous ways, creating a "new" set of quantitative data to analyze (see Stewart & Healy, 1989).

Yet, long-term longitudinal studies with qualitative materials are hard for investigators to conduct in their own lifetimes. As a result, these studies are relatively rare. In addition, the primary investigators of these studies cannot possibly address all of the questions afforded by these extensive data. Even if they could do so at any given time, new questions are continually being generated as the field progresses. These factors combine to suggest the importance of preserving these studies and making them accessible to other researchers for new questions. This, in turn, provides the basis for longitudinal approaches to more and more issues, leading to a more rapidly advancing field than would be possible if each investigator had to wait to collect his or her own longitudinal data. Thus, the demand for longitudinal approaches to a host of questions in personality psychology goes hand in hand with the increase in the practice of data sharing and secondary analysis.

Some examples of research that have made use of original records from existing longitudinal studies to shed light on some of the issues outlined earlier may be helpful in illustrating our points. We have chosen three highly different areas of inquiry to exemplify the versatility of secondary analysis for examining a range of issues. We have also included some secondary analyses conducted by the original investigators along with those conducted by new investigators. We considered any recoding of old data for new questions to be useful in exemplifying the general approach. In so doing, we hope to show the ways in which personality research is advancing more quickly, and perhaps coalescing, through the reuse of existing data.

The Nature of Personality: Person–Situation Interactionism and Coherence Over Time

The person–situation debate in personality psychology is age old yet still compelling. Although most contemporary personality psychologists would agree that aspects of both the person and the situation influence behavior (Pervin, 1985), the particular ways in which characteristics of persons and situations interact are still poorly understood. Some see the chief difficulty as being conceptual; there is a lack of thoughtful conceptual models of person–situation interactionism (Rorer & Widiger, 1983). Others say that the lack of methodological sophistication necessary for testing complex interactional models (Jenkins, 1982) is the biggest road block. Pervin (1985) viewed the problem as being embedded in the debate itself in that "it does not begin to provide us with answers concerning what and how—what in the person, interacts how, with what in the environment?" (p. 104). The complexity of person–situation interactionism has been augmented by those who have argued for consideration of a third important dimension thought to influence behavior: time. Indeed, Jack Block and Jeanne Block have been catalytic in the surge of interest in personality development and coherence over time.

In addressing some of the aforementioned issues involved in the study of person–situation interactionism, important conceptual and empirical contributions in this debate have been made recently (e.g., Caspi, 1987; Ozer & Gjerde, 1989). Moreover, because of the availability of rich, qualitative, multimethod longitudinal data sets, such progress has often relied on secondary analysis of existing data, enabling empirical progress to keep pace with conceptual advancements. In the following section, we provide a few examples of the ways in which existing data have been recast to make possible tests of new models that refine the understanding of person–situation interactionism.

Life-Course Model of Personality Development

Caspi (1987) contributed to the person–situation debate in his efforts to build a "framework for the study of personality that addresses the whole person living in a historically changing social world" (p. 1211). He explained that:

> anyone who has followed the trials and tribulations of personality psychology knows that the only survivors are interactionists, firm in the belief that both personality and context matter for social behavior (Bem, 1983). Beyond this, however, there is little agreement about the appropriate framework for the exploration of personality across time and circumstance. (Caspi, 1987, p. 1210)

Thus, Caspi (1987) asserted the need for attention to simultaneous temporal and situational parameters of personality development: the need to study "what specific people do in specific situations at specific times in the developmental process" (p. 1207). This life-course framework encompasses three primary elements: (a) the consideration of individuals in a historical context as indicated by their age cohorts; (b) the delineation of different life patterns, differentiated by age and cohort; and (c) the continual role of personality in negotiating life choices and transitions. To operationalize the temporal and situational dimensions of personality, Caspi advocated the use of life record data to construct life-course trajectories. Life-course trajectories reflect "a sequence of interactions of personality with age-graded roles and social transitions in historically changing environments" (p. 1210). He claimed (following J. Block, 1981) that

> If personality does have lawful implications for behavior in the age-graded life course, it should be evident in how experience is registered, how environments are selected, and how the stages of life are negotiated. In short, it should be reflected in how the individual confronts the agenda provided by his or her cultural and historical unit. (p. 1210)

As an application of this life-course framework, Caspi, Elder, and Bem (1987, 1988) drew on data from the Guidance Study (GS) of the Institute of Human Development, University of California, Berkeley, to explore the temporal and situational factors involved in maintaining the long-term coherence of the personalities of explosive, undercontrolled children (1987) and shy, withdrawn children (1988) in different social roles. Caspi and his colleagues relied on qualitative life records from the GS, which covers 40 years and canvasses multiple situations to construct life-course trajectories of involvement in various social roles. These consisted of education, military experience, work, marriage, and parenting. For each role, behavioral outcomes were selected from the GS data that were thought to reflect the adult manifestation of an explosive personality in childhood (e.g., unemployment or chaotic career trajectories, marital instability or divorce, inadequate parenting) or a shy childhood personality.

Even as different life situations were encountered, coherence of personality across 40 years was evident for both ill-temperedness and shyness. This coherence was evident for both men and women, although it was expressed in different domains. Many of the ill-tempered boys experienced life disorganization in adulthood, including deteriorating socioeconomic status and an erratic work history, whereas ill-tempered women were more likely to experience marital relationship deterioration in adulthood, as well as parenting difficulties. Similarly, childhood shyness persisted into adulthood and had predictable consequences, although different ones for men and women. Caspi et al. (1987, 1988) speculated that these findings reflected the more sex-segregated circumstances characteristic of the post-World War II era, the historical context in which these subjects grew up.

These secondary analyses of ill-temperedness and shyness are excellent examples of the usefulness of existing data for demonstrating the strength of a new conceptual framework. Without the availability of rich life record data across a 40-year time span in the GS, these authors would have had either to forego the study, collect cross-sectional or short-term longitudinal data (and thereby revise and limit their questions), or postpone their analyses for 40 years while collecting the necessary longitudinal data. By using longitudinal archival data, they successfully demonstrated the confluence of person, situation, and time as important dimensions in long-term personality development and coherence. Moreover, their use of life record data, unusual in personality consistency research, afforded the capturing of complexities of the "person" not possible with paper-and-pencil assessments of personality characteristics. Indeed, it is in this new direction of the study of personality development in context that the benefits of secondary analysis of existing data can be realized most fruitfully.

A Pattern Approach to Studying Personality Consistency and Change

Whereas Caspi et al. (1987, 1988) focused on continuity of individual differences over time, Ozer and Gjerde (1989) conducted a secondary analytic study to assess within-person trajectories of consistency *and* change over time.

At the outset, Ozer and Gjerde (1989) drew a distinction between variable-centered and person-centered approaches to studying personality development. The variable-centered approach involves an assessment of the same personality variables at different points in time for a sample of individuals. This aggregate-level approach yields an index of the degree of consistent ordering of individuals on these personality characteristics over time. By contrast, the person-centered approach, as developed by J. Block (1971), assesses the degree of consistent patterning of a set of characteristics within individuals over time.

Ozer and Gjerde (1989) cautioned that person- and variable-centered approaches do not yield the same results: "The relation between consistency and change at the aggregate level does not represent the relation between consistency and change which exists at the individual level" (p. 485). Furthermore, each approach has advantages and disadvantages, which suggests the importance of some combination of the variable- and person-centered approaches for clearer understanding.

Ozer and Gjerde (1989) drew on the J. Block and Block (1969/1980) data to (a) demonstrate one use of the person-centered approach; (b) explore associations between person- and variable-centered approaches; and (c) identify possibilities for combining the two. The Blocks' data lent themselves to these aims given the availability of ipsative Q-sort data at five time points over a 15-year time frame.

For their analyses, Ozer and Gjerde (1989) computed Q correlations between consecutive Q-sorts from the five waves of data collection (resulting in four Q correlations) and then cluster analyzed the vectors of Q correlations to identify "trajectories of consistency and change" over time (p. 506). They concluded that "persons differ markedly from one another in their degree of personality consistency and change over time. This effect, in some ways so obvious, is too often ignored in studies of personality development" (p. 506). Ozer and Gjerde added that one way in which person- and variable-centered approaches can be combined is by using person-centered measures of consistency as individual-difference variables in aggregate-level analyses.

Ozer and Gjerde (1989) brought considerable creativity to their secondary analytic study and as a result made a substantial contribution to the thinking about personality characteristics over time. Again, the availability of an abundance of qualitative materials within the data from the subjects themselves, their parents, teachers, and other observers made possible vivid portraits of the study participants. Moreover, their use of the Q-sort to bring across-wave consistency to otherwise noncomparable data is in itself a valuable contribution. Finally, these researchers' ingenuity in devising a new data-analytic strategy is evidence of the potential for creativity inherent in high-quality secondary analyses.

All of these studies (Caspi et al., 1987, 1988; Ozer & Gjerde, 1989) have contributed to clarification of some of the issues involved in the study of person–situation interactions. Taken separately, each addressed a neglected area of study. If each of these models were applied to the other data sets (or considered together), one might begin to draw cross-study comparisons that would allow more far-reaching conclusions and greater unity within the field. There are other much different areas of debate that have also profited from the use of secondary analysis. Some of these have important implications for interventions and treatment as well as theoretical significance.

Linking Personality and Health

Ever since the connection was made, however controversial, between the Type A behavior pattern and coronary heart disease (Rosenman & Friedman, 1974), an issue of major concern has been the link between various aspects of personality and health outcomes, both physical and emotional. A "disease-prone" personality type has even been identified (Friedman & Booth-Kewley, 1987). In general, the personality that is "hardy" (Kobasa, 1982), efficacious (Bandura, 1982), and optimistic (Peterson & Seligman, 1987) has been related to positive health outcomes, but these are mostly relationships examined at one point in time. It is hard to tell whether the personality contributed to the health or whether health status contributed to the personality; the need for clarifying the long-term effects of personality types on physical well-being has been great.

To address this issue, Peterson, Seligman, and Vaillant (1988) conducted a secondary analysis of data from a group of physically and mentally healthy men from the Study of Adult Development (Vaillant, 1977) to examine the relationship over time between "explanatory style" and physical health. Although explanatory style, the way that a person makes sense of bad events, is usually derived from a questionnaire, Peterson et al. developed a system referred to as *content analysis of verbatim explanations* (CAVE) for content analyzing the interview data for this personality characteristic (see Peterson et al., 1985; Peterson, Luborsky, & Seligman, 1983).

Again, the availability of life record data amenable to recoding potentiated new research in much the same way as described for the person–situation debate. The men of the Adult Development Study, recruited when they were university undergraduates in the early 1940s, have been followed ever since, contributing extensive interview data and submitting to health assessments by physicians. Thus, the interview data contained questions that made it possible to determine the extent to which one's explanatory style was optimistic, pessimistic, internal, or global. Health status was easily obtained from the physicians' records.

Results indicated that there was a relation between a pessimistic explanatory style at age 25 and physical health 35 years later. Thus, Peterson et al. (1988) were able to demonstrate that "the person who habitually explains bad events by stable, global, and internal causes in early adulthood is at risk for poor health in middle age" (p. 27).

Similarly, in a reanalysis of a follow-up of the Sears, Maccoby, and Levin (1957) data,[1] Franz, McClelland, Koestner, and Weinberger (1992) studied the relation of health to "agency motivation"—a personality characterized by proactivity, self-direction, and confidence—over a 10-year period for a group of 31-year-olds. Within these data were projective tests for assessing agency indirectly and self-ratings of health over time. They found that agency motivation (coupled with low stress) was related to health 10 years later.[2]

Interestingly, neither of the two studies described here showed a relation between the personality characteristic and *concurrent* health status. The authors of both studies concluded that personality did in fact influence health, but only over a time during which the personality exerted its influence on health-promoting habits, either in a positive (agentic) or negative (pessimistic) way.

Taken together, these two studies go a long way toward clearing up some of the controversy in the link between personality and health by considering time as a factor. Both studies used innovative coding schemes (for explanatory style, agency motivation), which depend on qualitative data. The studies would not have been possible without the longitudinal data and the secondary analysts' creative, conceptually clear, and methodical approaches to the data.

---

[1]Permission to conduct a follow-up of this study was granted to David McClelland and his colleagues in 1988 by the Henry A. Murray Research Center, the only archive that permitted recontacting study participants.
[2]Neither agency motivation nor low stress alone predicted health.

Personality Development and Life Events

Another matter of concern within personality research involves identifying antecedents and consequences of different life outcomes for personality development, both positive and negative (e.g., parental divorce during childhood, drug usage, unusual accomplishments, etc.). Much of this research is biased by the use of retrospective accounts of these experiences, oversampling of clinical cases, or the failure to include comparison groups. For valid results these studies require prospective studies that provide "baseline data essential for evaluating initial status, change and later outcome" (J. H. Block, Block, & Gjerde, 1986, p. 828), yet these types of problems rarely lend themselves to designing new prospective studies. Consider, for example, researchers who seek to understand the impact of divorce on children's personality development. One cannot randomly assign children to families that will divorce sometime in the future in order to study its impact on their development. One can, however, search for existing studies that may have sufficient incidence of divorce and relevant data about the children involved.

J. H. Block et al. (1986), for example, made use of their ongoing longitudinal study begun in 1968 containing extensive assessments of children and the status of their parents' marriage during six different times between the ages of 3 and 14. In this way they had data about children before divorce; they had a matched comparison group of children whose parents were not divorced; and they had multiple assessments of the children several years after the parents' separation. They found that children who experienced parental divorce exhibited distressed personalities *prior to* the divorce that seemed similar to the distress often associated with the aftermath of divorce. They concluded that some of the detrimental effects often associated with divorce for children have to do with their "conflicting and inaccessible parents" during the time preceding the divorce.

Using a similar design, J. Block, Block, and Keyes (1988) discovered antecedents and consequences of drug usage (see also Shedler & Block, 1990) and depressive tendencies (J. H. Block, Gjerde, & Block, 1991) in adolescents. Shneidman (1971) and Tomlinson-Keasey, Warren, and Elliott

(1986) identified several "signatures" of suicide using this design and a case method approach to a reanalysis of the Terman Genetic ᴗɑudies of Genius (Terman, 1925). Vaillant (1983) used the Study of Adult Development to examine the antecedents of alcoholism. This kind of design can also be used to predict more positive outcomes such as unusual accomplishments in the areas of education, work, intellect, and personal adjustment (Tomlinson-Keasey & Little, 1990). They would not be possible without the existence of well-designed, well-maintained, and available longitudinal studies. More important, they would not be possible without qualitative data that are amenable to the kinds of recoding involved in these highly creative efforts.

Some Challenges of Secondary Analysis

Having provided examples of what can be accomplished with secondary analysis, we now offer a few precautionary comments about some of its limitations and the barriers to its use. One such barrier is the perception that relevant data for reuse are not easily accessible. Colby and Phelps (1990) pointed out that "data archives are more numerous than most researchers realize, and individual data sharing is becoming more common" (p. 252). There are different types of archives, some of which contain data from a few related studies, such as the Institute of Human Development at the University of California, Berkeley, which oversees data collection, organization, and analysis of information from the Berkeley and Oakland longitudinal studies. Other archives house data from a large number of individual investigators in order to make them available to other researchers. Representative of this group are the Interuniversity Consortium for Political and Social Research at the University of Michigan, which provides computer data from hundreds of studies to consortium members, and the Henry A. Murray Research Center of Radcliffe College, which focuses on longitudinal studies and archives original records as well as computer data. (See also Young, Savola, & Phelps, 1991, for a complete listing of longitudinal studies, brief descriptions of the studies and the measures used, and where they are available for reanalysis if they are available.)

Probably the most obvious barrier and the one that comes to mind first is the problem of not locating available data pertinent to one's question of interest. If this is really the case, it is indeed an insurmountable problem and the investigator must proceed to collect new data. Sometimes, however, this is more of a mindset (or lack of know-how) than a reality. More often than one realizes, some time spent digging through data archives and creative thinking about how to recast the data can yield rich rewards. For example, the Terman study (1925) (mentioned earlier) was not designed to study suicide, the Study of Adult Development was not designed as a study of alcoholism, but, as we have shown, all of these data were used to examine the development of these outcomes over the life span. The data were there, but not in an obvious way; they had to be "excavated."

It is important to note that the studies we have highlighted here are not simple recombinations of variables. All required the researcher to radically restructure or "recast" (Elder, Pavalko, & Clipp, 1992) the data in such a way as to make them amenable to addressing new questions. The most important aspect of approaching the data for a reanalysis involves having a clear research question. This needs to be followed by patience, perseverance, and a willingness to "sit with the data" (Elder, et al., 1992). The kinds of reanalyses that will advance the field require versatility, creativity, and conceptual clarity.

Methods for Secondary Analysis

A lack of knowledge of methods in these areas can be perceived as yet another obstacle. There have been, however, in recent years considerable advances in methods available to secondary analysts, both "how-to" publications (Elder et al., 1992; Sieber, 1991) and published studies exemplifying these methods (see Brooks-Gunn & Chase-Lansdale, 1991). The researchers whose work has been described in this chapter have developed and used numerous techniques for recasting and recoding existing qualitative data so that data collected for entirely different purposes could be used to address their questions, which would otherwise require far greater expenditures of time, money, and effort.

One such method, although not new, is the Q-sort technique, which has been used successfully by several personality researchers (e.g., J. Block, 1971; Ozer & Gjerde, 1989) and represents an excellent approach to recoding case records that contain nonequivalent materials from one case to another. The Q-sort is particularly valuable for use with longitudinal data in which inconsistencies in measurement occur across waves. Furthermore, Q-sorts are useful within a multiple-method approach in which observer evaluations and subjective and objective assessments are wanted.

J. Block's (1971) approach to recasting the Oakland and Berkeley archival data created "new" data sets consisting of uniform and comparable data across waves to which various coding approaches could be applied. There are examples of similar approaches to other longitudinal data (Helson, Elliott, & Leigh, 1989; Helson, Mitchell, & Moane, 1984; James, 1990; Stewart & Salt, 1983). Such innovative approaches highlight the special value of qualitative archival data—which includes open-ended responses, interviews, and observations—for creating meaningful trajectories.

An increasing variety of content-analytic schemes are also available for application to existing data. The CAVE technique for assessing explanatory style, mentioned earlier, can be applied to interview data that contain information about an individual's experience of a bad event. For the Study of Adult Development data, the question about the men's wartime experiences was used for the assessment (see also Nelson, 1990, for another example of an application of CAVE).

Similarly, Winter (1982) developed a method for coding motives (achievement, power, affiliation) from interview data, speeches, literary works, and any other kind of imaginative material. This method has been used to assess the motives of presidents (Winter, 1987), presidential candidates (Winter, 1988) and Supreme Court justices (Aliotta, 1988). It can also be used to assess the motives of less famous subjects for whom relevant materials have been collected.

These and other content-analytic schemes can be used with qualitative data for assessing personality "at a distance" (Winter, 1982). They also can be extremely valuable in overcoming some of the barriers, both real and imagined, to successful secondary analysis.

Conclusion

It is impressive to note all of the design issues relevant to Carlson's (1971) famous question—"Where is the person in personality?"—that are redressed in the studies we have described. All were multiple observations of study participants over a substantial period of time; all involved data collected in participants' natural context; none were samples of college sophomores; most analyzed gender differences in theoretically relevant ways; all contained participants' own thoughts and open responses to questions; and all used coding strategies to render these "soft" methods more rigorous and useful. Clearly, these are some of the ways to incorporate the complexities of human functioning in the study of personality.

Moreover, the availability of these and other studies for reuse has much potential for assessing convergence in the field on a number of issues. This is true of the relation between personality and health, as we have shown. It is also true of theoretical models in need of empirical validation (see Harrington, chapter 13 in this book; Harrington, Block, & Block, 1987; Helson, Mitchell, & Hart, 1985). It is especially advantageous when the use of multiple data sets can be used to conduct cross-study comparisons that disentangle agè and cohort effects (Elder, 1974; Stewart & Healy, 1989; Stewart, Lykes, & LaFrance, 1982).

With the development of these integrative efforts, it seems that personality researchers are beginning to address some of the concerns raised by Carlson (1971) and many before her (Allport, 1937; Murray, 1938; Rogers & Skinner, 1956; Sanford, 1965). There are, of course, other areas of debate within the field of personality than we have mentioned and many other fine examples of secondary analytic studies than we have provided. Our aim was to suggest that secondary analysis should be higher in the "habit hierarchy" of methods available to personality researchers for addressing many of the controversies before them. If this becomes more the case, researchers of personality should have few worries about "foundering."

References

Aliotta, J. (1988). Social backgrounds, social motives and participation on the U.S. Supreme Court. *Political Behavior, 10*, 267–284.

Allport, G. W. (1937). *Personality: A psychological interpretation.* New York: Holt.

Bandura, A. (1982). Self-efficacy mechanisms in human agency. *American Psychologist, 37*, 122–147.

Bem, D. J. (1983). Constructing a theory of the triple typology: Some (second) thoughts on nomothetic and idiographic approaches to personality. *Journal of Personality, 51*, 566–577.

Block, J. (1971). *Lives through time*. Berkeley, CA: Bancroft Books.

Block, J. (1981). Some enduring and consequential structures of personality. In A. I. Rabin, J. Aronoff, A. M. Barclay, and R. A. Zucker (Eds.), *Further explorations in personality* (pp. 27–43). New York: Wiley.

Block, J., & Block, J. H. (1980). *The California Q-Set*. Palo Alto, CA: Consulting Psychologists Press. (Original work published 1969)

Block, J., Block, J. H., & Keyes, S. (1988). Longitudinally foretelling drug usage in adolescence: Early childhood personality and environmental precursors. *Child Development, 59*, 336–355.

Block, J., & Lanning, K. (1984). Attribution therapy requestioned: A secondary analysis of the Wilson-Linville study. *Journal of Personality and Social Psychology, 46*, 705–708.

Block, J. H., Block, J., & Gjerde, P. F. (1986). The personality of children prior to divorce: A prospective study. *Child Development, 57*, 827–840.

Block, J. H., Gjerde, P. F., & Block, J. H. (1991). Personality antecedents of depressive tendencies in 18-year-olds: A prospective study. *Journal of Personality and Social Psychology, 60*, 726–738.

Brooks-Gunn, J., & Chase-Lansdale, P. L. (Eds.). (1991). Secondary data analysis in developmental psychology [Special section]. *Developmental Psychology, 27*, 899–951.

Brooks-Gunn, J., Phelps, E., & Elder, G. H., Jr. (1991). Studying lives through time: Secondary data analyses in developmental psychology. *Developmental Psychology, 27*, 899–910.

Buss, D. M. (1991). Evolutionary personality psychology. *Annual Review of Psychology, 42*, 459–491.

Carlson, R. (1971). Where is the person in personality research? *Psychological Bulletin, 75*, 203–219.

Caspi, A. (1987). Personality in the life course. *Journal of Personality and Social Psychology, 53*, 1203–1213.

Caspi, A., Elder, G. H., Jr., & Bem, D. J. (1987). Moving against the world: Life-course patterns of explosive children. *Developmental Psychology, 23*, 308–313.

Caspi, A., Elder, G. H., Jr., & Bem, D. J. (1988). Moving away from the world: Life-course patterns of shy children. *Developmental Psychology, 24*, 824–831.

Colby, A. (1982). The use of secondary analysis in the study of women and social change. *Journal of Social Issues, 38*, 119–123.

Colby, A., & Phelps, E. (1990). Archiving longitudinal data. In D. Magnusson & L. R. Bergman (Eds.), *Data quality in longitudinal research* (pp. 249–262). Cambridge, England: Cambridge University Press.

Elder, G. H., Jr. (1974). *Children of the Great Depression*. Chicago: University of Chicago Press.

Elder, G. H., Jr., Pavalko, E. K., & Clipp, E. C. (1992). *Studying lives: Working with archival data*. Newbury Park, CA: Sage.

Franz, C., McClelland, D. C., Koestner, R., & Weinberger, J. (1992). *The role of agency motivation in maintaining health over time: A longitudinal study*. Unpublished manuscript.

Friedman, H. S., & Booth-Kewley, S. (1987). The "disease-prone personality": A meta-analytic view of the construct. *American Psychologist, 42*, 539–555.

Harrington, D. M., Block, J. H., & Block, J. (1987). Testing aspects of Carl Rogers's theory of creative environments: Child-rearing antecedents of creative potential in young adolescents. *Journal of Personality and Social Psychology, 52*, 851–856.

Helson, R., Elliott, T., & Leigh, J. (1989). Adolescent personality and women's work patterns. In D. Stern & D. Eichorn (Eds.), *Adolescence and work: Influences of social structure, labor markets, and culture* (pp. 259–289). Hillsdale, NJ: Erlbaum.

Helson, R., Mitchell, V., & Hart, B. (1985). Lives of women who became autonomous. In A. J. Stewart & M. B. Lykes (Eds.), *Gender and personality* (pp. 169–197). Chapel Hill, NC: Duke University Press.

Helson, R., Mitchell, V., & Moane, G. (1984). Personality and patterns of adherence and nonadherence to the social clock. *Journal of Personality and Social Psychology, 46*, 1079–1096.

James, J. B. (1990). Women's employment patterns and midlife well-being. In N. L. Chester & H. Y. Grossman (Eds.), *The meaning and experience of work in women's lives* (pp. 103–120). Hillsdale, NJ: Erlbaum.

Jenkins, S. R. (1982). *Personal-situation interaction and women's achievement-related motives*. Unpublished doctoral dissertation, Boston University, Boston.

Kobasa, S. C. (1982). The hardy personality: Toward a social psychology of stress and illness. In G. S. Sanders & J. Suls (Eds.), *Social psychology of health and illness* (pp. 3–32). Hillsdale, NJ: Erlbaum.

Levenson, H., Gray, M. J., & Ingram, A. (1976). Research methods in personality five years after Carlson's survey. *Personality and Social Psychology Bulletin, 2*, 158–161.

McCall, R. B., & Appelbaum, M. I. (1991). Some issues of conducting secondary analyses. *Developmental Psychology, 27*, 911–917.

Murray, H. A. (1938). *Explorations in personality*. New York: Oxford University Press.

Nelson, D. C. (1990). *Control, instrumentality, explanatory style for negative events, and optimism in relation to wellness in low and middle income women*. Unpublished doctoral dissertation, Boston University, Boston.

Ozer, D. J., & Gjerde, P. F. (1989). Patterns of personality consistency and change from childhood through adolescence. *Journal of Personality, 57*, 483–507.

Paul, E. L. (1990, July). *Secondary analysis of existing data: A promising approach for personal relationships research*. Paper presented at the Fifth International Conference on Personal Relationships, Oxford, England.

Pervin, L. A. (1985). Personality: Current controversies, issues, and directions. *Annual Review of Psychology, 36,* 83–114.

Peterson, C., Bettes, B. A., & Seligman, M. E. P. (1985). Depressive symptoms and unprompted causal attributions: Content analysis. *Behavior Research and Therapy, 23,* 379–382.

Peterson, C., Luborsky, L., & Seligman, M. E. P. (1983). Attributions and depressive mood shifts. *Journal of Abnormal Psychology, 92,* 96–103.

Peterson, C., & Seligman, M. E. P. (1987). Explanatory style and illness. *Journal of Personality, 55,* 237–265.

Peterson, C., Seligman, M. E. P., & Vaillant, G. E. (1988). Pessimistic explanatory style is a risk factor for physical illness: A thirty-five year longitudinal study. *Journal of Personality and Social Psychology, 55,* 23–27.

Rogers, C. R., & Skinner, B. F. (1956). Some issues concerning the control of human behavior: A symposium. *Science, 124,* 1057–1066.

Rorer, L. G., & Widiger, T. A. (1983). Personality structure and assessment. *Annual Review of Psychology, 34,* 431–463.

Rosenman, R. H., & Friedman, M. (1974). Neurogenic factors in pathogenesis of coronary heart disease. *Medical Clinics of North America, 58,* 269–279.

Sanford, N. (1965). Will psychologists study human problems? *American Psychologist, 20,* 192–202.

Sears, R. R., Maccoby, E. E., & Levin, H. (1957). *Patterns of child rearing.* Evanston, IL: Row, Peterson.

Shedler, J., & Block, J. (1990). Adolescent drug use and psychological health: A longitudinal inquiry. *American Psychologist, 45,* 612–630.

Shneidman, E. S. (1971). Suicide among the gifted. *Suicide and Life-Threatening Behavior, 1,* 23–45.

Sieber, J. E. (Ed.). (1991). *Sharing social science data: Advantages and challenges.* Newbury Park, CA: Sage.

Stewart, A. J., & Healy, J. M., Jr. (1989). Linking individual development and social changes. *American Psychologist, 44,* 30–42.

Stewart, A. J., Lykes, M. B., & LaFrance, M. (1982). Educated women's career patterns: Separating developmental and social changes. *Journal of Social Issues, 38,* 97–118.

Stewart, A. J., & Platt, M. B. (1982). Studying women in a changing world: An introduction. *Journal of Social Issues, 38,* 1–16.

Stewart, A. J., & Salt, P. (1983). Changing sex roles: College graduates of the sixties and seventies. In M. S. Horner, C. Nadelson, & M. Notman (Eds.), *The challenge of change* (pp. 275–296). New York: Plenum Press.

Terman, L. M. (1925). *Genetic studies of genius: Vol. 1. Mental and physical traits of a thousand gifted children.* Stanford, CA: Stanford University Press.

Tomlinson-Keasey, C., & Little, T. D. (1990). Predicting educational attainment, occupational achievement, intellectual skill, and personal adjustment among gifted men and women. *Journal of Educational Psychology, 82,* 442–455.

Tomlinson-Keasey, C., Warren, L. W., & Elliott, J. E. (1986). Suicide among gifted women: A prospective study. *Journal of Abnormal Psychology, 95,* 123–130.

Vaillant, G. E. (1977). *Adaptation to life.* Boston: Little, Brown.

Vaillant, G. E. (1983). *The natural history of alcoholism.* Cambridge, MA: Harvard University Press.

Winter, D. G. (1982). *Manual for scoring motive imagery in running text.* Unpublished manuscript, University of Michigan, Department of Psychology.

Winter, D. G. (1987). Leader appeal, leader performance, and the motive profiles of leaders and followers: A study of American presidents and elections. *Journal of Personality and Social Psychology, 52,* 196–202.

Winter, D. G. (1988, July). What makes Jesse run? *Psychology Today,* pp. 20–24.

Young, C. H., Savola, K. L., & Phelps, E. (1991). *Inventory of longitudinal studies in the social sciences.* Newbury Park, CA: Sage.

CHAPTER 4

Opportunities and Challenges Posed by Archival Data Sets

Carol Tomlinson-Keasey

The Power of Longitudinal Data Sets

Describing the life paths of individuals provides a singular challenge, for embedded in descriptions of lives are patterns and commonalities that could allow psychologists to predict, and perhaps intervene, in the trajectory of lives. Tracing lives is an ambitious goal, perhaps even a foolhardy one, because predicting self-worth or competence, or for that matter any personal dimension, requires several kinds of knowledge that psychologists have sought diligently and have not always found. This goal assumes that psychologists have a corpus of data that traces the lives of individuals over the decades of childhood, adolescence, and adulthood. Although such studies do exist, they are scarce, and studies that span decades, rather than months or years, are so unique that they constitute a professional treasure in the field of psychology (Brooks-Gunn, Phelps,

& Elder, 1991; Phelps, 1987). The recognition that longitudinal studies provide a critical methodology for scrutinizing characteristics as diverse as temperament, achievement, aggressiveness, alcoholism, and health has sent investigators scurrying to longitudinal data sets that already exist. Conducting secondary analyses of these archival data sets hold the promise of providing investigators with information that will speak eloquently to a variety of contemporary questions. As psychologists rush to embrace such data sets, they need to pause and consider carefully the advantages afforded by secondary analysis of archival data sets, strategies that will enhance the value of these data sets, cautions about hazards that await those who embark on secondary analyses, and encouragement to proceed.

What Sorts of Archival Data Sets Exist?

Two primary categories of archival data sets exist. The first are national longitudinal studies that are broad in scope and have large samples. Examples include the National Longitudinal Survey of Youth (Baker & Mott, 1989; Chase-Lansdale, Mott, Brooks-Gunn, & Phillips, 1991), the Panel Study of Income Dynamics (Duncan & Morgan, 1985), and the National Longitudinal Study of the Class of 1992 (National Center for Education Statistics, 1972). These studies are designed to address a particular issue, such as health, finances, or educational outcomes, and have often lacked data that could address the psychological mechanisms underlying change. Such large-scale survey studies have been a mainstay of sociological and economic research for decades, but until recently their usefulness to psychology has been more limited. The very scope of these studies, involving thousands of subjects seen repeatedly, meant that the depth of the information obtained on a single subject was reduced. However, as Chase-Lansdale et al. (1991) pointed out, the researchers in the National Longitudinal Survey of Youth have recently sought the advice of psychologists and incorporated standardized instruments in their assessments. Data from a similar study in Britain, the National Child Development Study, suggested that national surveys can incorporate more standardized and detailed information on individual subjects (Cherlin et al., 1991).

These large-scale studies are still not well designed to illuminate the mechanisms underlying a particular aspect of development. Intensive studies of psychologically relevant variables compose a second category of archival data available to researchers. These data sets, now available for secondary analysis, were initiated to address a particular question. The Terman data (Terman, 1926), for example, were initially collected to repudiate the notion that giftedness was associated with physical weakness and mental health problems. Despite the focus on gifted children, the 70-year course of the study and the thousands of variables collected over the subjects' lifetimes have made this data set a rich source of information on a diverse set of topics (Elder, Pavalko, & Clipp, 1993; Friedman et al., in press; Shneidman, 1971; Tomlinson-Keasey & Little, 1990).

Categorizing archival data sets as either surveys or intensive psychological studies is bound to misrepresent the range of studies available to help investigators. Within these two broad categories, studies vary enormously on the sorts of variables investigated, the form or existence of the raw data, the time period of the studies, and the completeness of the information on the study. Each of these indexes is critical in an investigator's decision to try to conduct a secondary analysis.

Thanks to the efforts of organizations whose goal is to enhance the study of lives, catalogs now exist that describe longitudinal data sets available for secondary analysis. The Henry A. Murray Research Center at Radcliffe has been at the forefront of the effort to encourage investigators to use longitudinal methodology and to conduct secondary analyses. As part of their mission, they archive data for use by other investigators, provide seminars that introduce investigators to the available data sets, train investigators in secondary analysis, and publicize catalogs describing the longitudinal data sets that are available. In addition to a catalog of the archival data sets actually located at the Murray Center, the staff have been instrumental in organizing and publicizing a comprehensive volume of longitudinal studies that might be accessed by investigators (Young, Savola, & Phelps, 1991). This book builds on the earlier catalogs published by the Social Science Research Council.

Opportunities Offered by Archival Data

Archival Data Sets Provide Complete Descriptions

Archival data sets often contribute complete and complex descriptions of a particular variable: intellectual development, changes in self-esteem, drug use, relationships between the sexes, and life transitions. Although many studies could be mentioned as illustrations, description is a particular strong point of several national surveys (Baydar & Brooks-Gunn, 1991; Cherlin, 1991; Duncan, 1991). The well-known Study of Income Dynamics (Duncan et al., 1984) chronicles the changing economic conditions that have influenced American workers since 1968. Approximately 5,000 families have participated yearly since 1968, and as the years have passed, the researchers have asked broader and more complex questions of their participants. The detailed and variegated descriptions of families in poverty have opened the eyes of social scientists and policymakers.

Archival Data Sets Enhance Prediction

Typically, variegated descriptions of traits or lives serve as a prologue to the larger challenge, predicting those traits or lives from earlier events. Because prediction is central to the mission of developmental psychologists, it must be approached objectively, and maybe even suspiciously. Freud, after all, based life-long predictions on an analysis of the mother–child relationship. He did so without the benefit of any longitudinal data. The questions to be posed are empirical ones. Do psychologically meaningful events and variables in childhood presage adult development? Do losses in childhood continue to exert an influence on the adult? Does the influence of the family of origin linger in an adult's actions long after he or she has left his or her parents' home? Can attributes that shape an adult's personality be spotted in childhood and traced into adulthood (Robins & Rutter, 1990; Rutter, 1989)?

The use of archival data can help psychologists separate the real predictive power of variables from the chaff of developmental inquiry. There are many milestones of infancy, but which particular milestones are useful predictors of similar behaviors 6 months, 1 year, 5 years, or 10 years later? Werner and Smith's (1992) longitudinal study of children in Kauai, Hawaii, documented the ability of infant temperamental characteristics and supportive environments to predict later adjustment while showing the limited predictive power of perinatal complications. Longitudinal data have shown both the power and the frailty of early indicators of intelligence (McCall, 1981). The attainment of physical milestones bears little relation to mental or emotional development in later years. Measures such as attention and response to novelty (Fagan, Shepherd, & Knevel, 1991) are more likely to be predictors of intellectual performance years later. Archival data sets, especially ones that permit researchers to examine development over major life transitions, will help pinpoint meaningful predictors.

Many negative life outcomes are, thankfully, statistically infrequent. Archival data offer the possibility of studying the precursors of such infrequent life events (Brooks-Gunn et al., 1991). Although the suicide rate in the general population is approximately 12 per 100,000 people (Vital Statistics, 1986), archival data have been used to predict this infrequent behavior. Shneidman (1971) examined the Terman Genetic Studies of Genius (Terman, 1926; Terman & Oden, 1959) for precursors of suicide among the men. By immersing himself in the file of each subject, Shneidman reconstructed their lives from their youths until their deaths, all the time looking for "signatures" of suicide. His success in predicting suicide from life events that occurred years before the subject's death documented the power of prospective longitudinal information. The Terman data set offered an unparalleled opportunity to obtain unbiased prospective information about the subjects' lives prior to their self-inflicted deaths (Shneidman, 1971; Tomlinson-Keasey, Warren, & Elliott, 1986).

Vaillant (1983) used the Harvard Medical School's Study of Adult Development to trace the early indicators of alcoholism. More than 600 men from two vastly different social strata were followed from adolescence into their middle years. A third clinical sample of 100 alcoholics was added to the archival sample and followed for 8 years after detoxification. The longitudinal data amassed over the years meant that precursors of alcohol abuse could be examined without fear of retrospective biases. Furthermore, the clinical population's ability to cope with their alcohol problems over a period of years provided critical information for helping alcoholic adults.

Archival Data Sets Evaluate Interventions

The judicious use of archival data may show investigators how to intervene to help shape lives in more productive directions. The effects of preschool programs for disadvantaged youths were documented only after long and careful studies that spanned the school years (Lazar & Darlington, 1982). How these programs altered the children's language, their attitudes toward school, and their interactions with their mothers were all unexpected by-products that lingered long after the preschool years. Initial analyses focused primarily on IQ as an outcome variable. The results indicated that over a short period, IQ scores of participants increased significantly compared with the IQ scores of children who did not participate; however, the long-term results indicated that these early differences in IQ were not maintained throughout the school years (Clarke & Clarke, 1989). What was required to understand the full range of long-term outcomes was an analysis of the data focusing on social and motivational patterns that altered the child's achievement (Consortium for Longitudinal Studies, 1983; Haskins, 1989; Lee, Brooks-Gunn, & Schnur, 1988; McKey et al., 1985; Ramey & Landesman Ramey, 1990).

Archival Data Sets Illuminate Mechanisms

A unique challenge to developmental psychologists that goes beyond description and prediction is to understand the mechanisms by which earlier factors affect later behaviors. A biological analogy is helpful here. A child may develop optimally regardless of whether the carbohydrate base in the diet is rice, beans, potatos, or bread. The critical mechanism is the metabolism of carbohydrates for use by the child's developing body. A focus on the individual carbohydrate base might well tend to mislead investigators.

Transforming this analogy into the psychological realm, one can see that psychologists have been waylaid by comparisons of breast-feeding or bottle-feeding, harsh or permissive toilet training, and the presence or absence of a bonding period at birth. What is more important than the presence or absence of these different factors is the understanding of the process by which their presence or absence affects the child's personality, intellect, or social skills. Harsh toilet training may be just one indicator of a parent–child relationship that degrades the child. As a result, the child may decide that he or she is incompetent and carry this estimation of self-worth throughout the years. The national surveys prized by sociologists and economists (Duncan, 1991) have been less useful to psychologists because the information on each subject lacked the depth necessary to investigate mechanisms. Nevertheless, developmental psychologists recognize that empirical evidence detailing mechanisms that drive development must come from longitudinal studies (Garmezy, 1988; Rutter, 1988). In addition, as Chase-Lansdale et al. (1991) pointed out, studies using national surveys may document important predictors of specific outcomes. Knowing these associations, developmental psychologists can tailor further investigations toward the goal of illuminating mechanisms.

Thomas and Chess (1984), in their seminal longitudinal study of temperament, have demonstrated the force of longitudinal studies in delineating process. Their study described temperamental variables as they exist across infancy, childhood, adolescence, and young adulthood. Just this description constitutes a significant contribution to the field because Chess and Thomas grappled with the changing form of a trait through the transitions of childhood, adolescence, and young adulthood. A difficult child at 6 months may spit food in the investigator's face. At 6 years, the same child may refuse to ride the school bus. At 16, he may have difficulty joining in the social activities of his or her high school.

In addition to these valuable descriptions of temperament, Thomas and Chess (1984) cataloged a range of variables that impinge on an individual throughout development to allay or exaggerate the temperamental characteristics seen during the first year. The resulting view of the development of temperamental characteristics looks for a "goodness of fit" between the temperament and environment. This interactive view identifies and acknowledges the importance of a variety of developmental processes in the formation of a child's temperament. Similarly, archival data sets that contain broad assessments of individuals at several ages allow researchers to examine the mechanisms and processes that give form to development.

Archival Data Clarify Life Transitions

At times, in the cycle of life, development proceeds at a particularly brisk pace. Adolescence is widely recognized as a time of multiple, rapid changes in every sphere of development, and longitudinal data have helped define both the positive and negative poles of this transition (Baumrind, 1992; Cairns, Cairns, & Neckerman, 1989; Shedler & Block, 1990). Marriage, as a life transition, has produced archival data (Kelly, 1955) and secondary analysis of that data (Caspi, Herbener, & Ozer, 1992). Menopause is another, less studied transition. Woodruff (1992) examined several archival data sets, evaluating the life transitions that accompany menopause in women. Woodruff was specifically interested in the woman's satisfaction with her life circumstances as a mediator of psychological adjustment to menopause. Investigating this complicated question sent her to four archival data sets containing data on women in the middle years (Atchley, 1985; Baruch & Barnett, 1985; Davidoff & Platt, 1985; Traupmann, 1985). Her study is particularly interesting because of the different cohorts of women who were investigated to understand this universal life transition.

Archival Data Allow Multigenerational Comparisons

The transmission of poverty across second and third generations has been documented by demographic data (Duncan, Hill, & Hoffman, 1988). Understanding the process by which that transmission occurs requires an in-depth examination of the attitudes of parents, their own aspirations, their aspirations for their children, their child-rearing practices as well as information on work attitudes and patterns (Brooks-Gunn et al., 1991; Furstenberg, Levine, & Brooks-Gunn, 1990). Archival data sets allow investigators to record the parenting practices in a family, then follow the children into adulthood and record their parenting practices with the next generation of children. Elder, Caspi, and Downey (1986) conducted a multigenerational study using the Berkeley Growth archive, investigating the proposition that unstable personalities and unstable family relations persist from one generation to the next. Using four generations, they found that intergenerational continuity of unstable behavior was the most pronounced among women and seemed to flow from families characterized by hostility and discord. They cited a causal path from unstable personalities to unstable family relations (Caspi, Elder, & Bem, 1987).

Archival Data Suggest Causal Directionality

Longitudinal archival data may also help to answer questions concerning the causal direction of correlational data. Developmental researchers are often forced to rely on correlational data. Although theoretical frameworks and the past literature in an area may suggest a particular causal direction, the documentation that one event precedes another requires longitudinal information. In more than one instance, such longitudinal information has suggested that an inferred causal direction could not be substantiated, that the reverse was true, or that mediating variables were responsible for the correlation (Brooks-Gunn et al., 1991). J. H. Block, Block, and Gjerde (1986) demonstrated that boys who experienced divorce were comparatively undercontrolled, aggressive, energetic, and generally troublesome well before the divorce actually occurred. The differences between their behavior and the behavior of boys whose families remained intact were not a consequence of the divorce. Instead, the conflict and distancing that occurred as the marriage deteriorated might have changed the boys' behavior. These findings were recently replicated in studies in the United States and England using large national surveys (Cherlin et al., 1991).

A corollary to determining causal direction is the possibility of using archival data sets to independently replicate a particularly interesting or surprising result. Cross-sectional studies typically report sex differences among adults in the frequency of depression (Neuringer, 1982). Mood disorders such as depression are seldom related to personality in early childhood. Yet, J. Block, Gjerde, and Block (1991) have used their carefully collected longitudinal data to identify a set of coherent personal attributes as early as age 7 that presage depression among male and female adolescents. These precursors of depression among young adults differ substantially by sex.

Archival Data Sets can be Combined

Archival data sets offer the unique possibility of combining several data sets to address a particular question. In a unique midlife research program sponsored jointly by the MacArthur Foundation and the Murray Center, several researchers have combined archival data sets to investigate a particular question (Vandewater & Stewart, 1992; Woodruff, 1992). Vandewater and Stewart (1992) suggested that a change in a woman's commitment to others provides an interpretative framework for personality development and well-being. To evaluate their hypothesis, they investigated three different archival data sets that included college-educated women from different cohorts (Helson, 1967; Stewart, 1985; Tangri & Jenkins, 1986).

Archival Data Sets Provide a Foundation for Further Study

Archival data sets that include variables of interest may offer investigators the opportunity to recontact the subjects. Such follow-ups allow the investigators to design the new wave of data collection to specifically address their question. Franz, McClelland, and Weinberger (1991) provided a recent example of this approach. In 1986, they contacted the children who had participated in a study of child-rearing patterns conducted in the early 1950s (Sears, Maccoby, & Levin, 1957). The initial waves of data collection included ratings made by the parents and teachers of the child's sociability at age 5. Franz et al. (1991) were interested in whether these early indicators of personality would predict the subjects' social accomplishments in middle age. Their findings, that the warmth and affection of fathers played a particularly critical role in social accomplishment, replicated the emerging view that fathers play a pivotal role in families. The force of the father's warmth was still evident 35 years later. By contrast, Franz et al. (1991) were unable to find a relation between difficult childhoods and lower levels of social accomplishment at midlife. This lack of a relation raises some question about the long-term significance of some childhood stressors. Recontacting adult subjects who have supplied detailed information about their childhoods and families of origin is an infrequently used strategy but one that promises to yield valuable information about development.

Archival Data Address Contemporary Questions

Finally, archival data allow investigators who have spent their professional careers gathering richly textured information on individual lives to pass their legacy on to the field. Although the sharing of data has been a canon of the scientific enterprise, in practice few investigators have made their raw data available to others. Lack of resources to prepare the data properly rather than scientific selfishness can be blamed. Preparing data sets for use by other investigators is a time-consuming, altruistic act. Robert Sears spent the last 20 years of his life coding the Terman Genetic Studies of Genius (Terman, 1926) so that other investigators could tap the wealth of information amassed on those 1,500 subjects. His vision, of course, was to assure that the lifetime of data would be useful to future generations of researchers. As testimony to the power of his vision, studies describing gifted children (Feldman, 1984; Janos, 1986), investigating signatures of suicide (Shneidman, 1971), evaluating the effects of acceleration in school (Janos, 1987), detailing precursors of life satisfaction (Sears, 1977), marital attitudes (Holahan, 1984), creativity (Vaillant & Vaillant, 1990), and health (Friedman et al., in press) have been published or are in press.

Similarly, Jack Block has coded and amalgamated the information from his and Jeanne Block's (J. H. Block & Block, 1980) longitudinal study so that other investigators can ask a variety of questions of the information gathered. The scores of papers that have already emerged from the Block and Block study have redefined the parameters of personality development (J. H. Block & Block, 1980), adolescence (J. Block, Block, & Keyes, 1988; Shedler & Block, 1990), family functioning (J. H. Block et al., 1986), mental health (J. Block et al., 1991), and sex differences (J. H. Block, 1983).

The time and resources necessary to prepare longitudinal data for use by other investigators often prohibits researchers from undertaking the task. Three central archives that have taken on the mission of preparing archival data and housing it so that it is available for other re-searchers are the Inter-University Consortium for Political and Social Research at the University of Michigan, the Henry A. Murray Center for the Study of Lives at Radcliffe College, and the Sociometrics Corporation in Los Altos, California, which houses the Data Archive on Adolescent Pregnancy and Pregnancy Prevention as well as the archive for all the recent studies of families that have been funded by National Institute of Child Health and Human Development (NICHD). These organizations work diligently to obtain appropriate data sets, to make sure they are coded coherently, to make code books available to investigators, and to provide the raw data and the code books to other investigators. Cherlin (1991) also pointed out that since the 1960s, the government has been sponsoring large surveys designed for use by social scientists. Computer tapes and CD-ROMs of the data from these surveys are available to re-searchers soon after the interviews are complete.

Challenges Posed by Archival Data Sets

Methodological Issues

Although developmental psychologists often tout the value of longitudinal studies, the difficulty of conducting sound longitudinal studies and ar-chiving the data have frequently deterred investigators from even con-sidering the use of archival data. Such hesitancies are often well grounded. James Morgan offered the following evaluation of the Michigan Panel Study of Income Dynamics: "If we had known we were going to live so long, we would have taken better care of ourselves" (Elder, 1985, p. 16).

When viewed from the 1990s, data collected in the 1930s and 1940s are often regarded as simplistic, unsystematic, and parametrically ques-tionable. Using such data to try to answer important psychological ques-tions posed in the 1990s may seem naive or even disingenuous. However, the difficulties associated with using such data may be balanced by the value of the data to answer a particular question. It is important, then, to recognize the methodological problems of secondary analysis and suggest approaches that will yield meaningful conclusions. Many of the methodological complaints are familiar to psychologists who have dealt with longitudinal data. Some are unique to archival data.

Capitalization on Chance

Whenever data are available before the question under investigation is formulated, an investigator runs the risk of capitalizing on chance considerations. The general rule for avoiding this misstep is that investigators must not use the actual data values to suggest hypotheses or to specify the analyses to be performed (McCall & Appelbaum, 1991, p. 911).

Missing Data

Missing data constitute a serious problem for investigators using archival data sets. Although not limited to longitudinal or archival data, the problem of missing data is exacerbated in such studies because of the multiple waves of data collection. Archival data sets frequently have to be recoded, requiring the concatenation of identical variables across waves of data collection, or the combining of differing indexes of a trait being studied. The computer rejects such concatenations if any of the data are missing.

The most conservative way to handle missing data is to drop individuals who do not have complete data. If the remaining sample has not been biased by eliminating the subjects who have missing data, this strategy is satisfactory from a statistical viewpoint. However, the loss of information may alter the power of the conclusions that can be drawn.

Replacing missing values with mean values may be satisfactory only if a few data points here and there are missing. Unfortunately, this strategy, imposed on all missing data points in a large data set, may artificially constrain the variance and produce spurious tests of significance (McCall & Appelbaum, 1991). One solution to this sticky problem involves setting a standard concerning the amount of data that must be present in each subject's record in order for that subject to be included in the analysis. A cutoff of 60%–75% of the data would guarantee that subjects with large amounts of missing data would be dropped from the analysis. Using such a cutoff typically means that the remaining subjects will have more than 85% of the information to be used in the analyses. Substituting values for those subjects who are still lacking a specific score may not seriously alter the variance of a particular measure.

LaGrangian linear interpolation–extrapolation (McCall, Appelbaum, & Hogarty, 1973) provides an entirely different strategy for replacing missing data that is particularly well suited to longitudinal data. This method requires that the same variable be assessed over several waves of data collection. Missing data points are generated by evaluating the data trend for the individual subject. For example, if a subject's IQ scores for the first, second, fourth, and fifth waves of data collection hovered around 105, the computer might substitute an IQ score of 105 for the individual's score on Wave 3. In their classic article examining developmental changes in mental performance, McCall et al. (1973) traced IQ changes over 14 childhood assessments, replacing missing data points with this technique.

Rubin (1987) suggested a technique called *multiple imputation* for replacing missing data points in survey data. This technique replaces each missing value with two or more acceptable values, thereby acknowledging an investigator's uncertainty about the correct value to substitute for missing data. Multiple imputation relies on the flexibility of the computer and is particularly suited to large surveys. This technique assumes that missing data do not occur randomly and allows the researcher to adjust for the differences between subjects who responded and those who did not.

Other statistical refinements and alternative ways of estimating missing data have been offered by Little and Rubin (1987). A variety of strategies exist to help investigators solve their problems with missing data. The choice of strategy depends on (a) whether there are differences between those who responded and those who did not, (b) whether there are multiple waves of data collection, (c) the size of the sample, and (d) the amount of data present in each subject's protocol.

Attrition

Whenever data collection has multiple waves, some subjects will not be available after the initial testing. Whether such attrition is selective is critical to an evaluation of the study. Selective attrition may alter the data so dramatically that their value is seriously compromised. Hence, an evaluation of attrition must be conducted by investigators after framing their research question and identifying the critical variables for their study. For investigators who find that attrition has introduced selection bias, a technique developed by Heckman (1979) may be helpful. By creating information that evaluates the attrition process, investigators can examine and control for the effects of attrition. A study examining the consequences of divorce illustrates this technique nicely (Glass, McLanahan, & Sørensen, 1985).

Because attrition poses such a problem for longitudinal studies, researchers have devised a number of strategies to keep their subjects actively involved. Newsletters and birthday cards maintain the subjects' interest and help ensure an accurate address. Despite these measures, when a new wave of data collection is contemplated, a certain percentage of subjects is lost. To cope with this problem, investigators have turned into private detectives who trace their subjects (Farrington, Gallagher, Morley, St. Ledger, & West, 1990). In one of the few available discussions of this subject, Farrington et al. (1990) examined voter registration lists, telephone directories throughout England, the Criminal Records Office, and the National Health Service Central Register. In addition, they contacted neighbors and the new occupants at addresses previously listed. The combination of these search strategies allowed them to trace and interview 94% of their original subjects. A case history of their search for one individual is included to highlight the strategies they used.

Case 481 took the investigators 37 days to locate. The last known address was 14 years old. Voter registration lists indicated that the whole family had moved. The London telephone directory had no listing. The man's father owned a printing business in another town, and inquiries were made in that town, to no avail. Professional directories listing printers and computerized records of printers who were members of the union were searched, again to no avail. The occupants of the subject's former address and the neighbors were questioned, but they had no information about the subject's current address. An earlier interview indicated that the subject was planning to attend college. The local registrar could find no trace. A former friend was contacted and was able to provide a more recent address. Voter registration lists, telephone directories, and interviews of neighbors at that address were not successful in locating the individual. Finally, the interviewer examined crime records and found that one of the subject's brothers had been convicted of a crime in another town. The man's father was listed in the telephone directory, and he arranged contact between the son and the investigators (Farrington et al., 1990).

Investigators wishing to recontact subjects from an archival data set are embarking on a difficult and time-consuming task, which becomes more difficult as the years pass. Relocating subjects is made easier if social security numbers or drivers' license numbers are part of the initial records. In the United States, efforts to relocate subjects are often hampered by recent court rulings about access to information. Despite this, voter registration lists, college alumni lists, telephone directories, military records, phone directories arranged by address, postal records, and professional directories can often help reduce attrition.

Cohort Effects

The cohort effect confounds longitudinal data. When individual subjects are followed over time, their cohort experiences a particular culture and a unique set of world events. The effect of these cohort specific experiences cannot be untangled from other developmentally important events. Elder and Caspi (1990) expressed dismay at the lack of attention to cohort effects that accompanied the early longitudinal studies. The Terman study (Terman & Oden, 1959)

> almost succeeded in *not* collecting any systematic information on life experience through the Great Depression and World War II, two of the most encompassing social disruptions of this century. The 1950 follow-up was completely silent on the Second World War, much to the apparent disbelief of the nearly 500 men who served. Some insisted on communicating their sense of neglect on the edges of their questionnaire. (Elder & Caspi, 1990, p. 202)

The distinctive flavor of each cohort can be conveyed by an insistence on a contextual study of lives, a method that Elder (1985) extended into "life-course analysis." Life-course analyses go beyond identifying a particular cohort in history and actually ask questions that link specific changes in the cohort to the life course.

The cohort effect, so often seen as a confound of longitudinal research, can actually be turned into a methodological advantage. By comparing cohorts over time, as Elder (1974) had done so elegantly, one can examine the differential impact of societal forces on individual development.

Approaching Archival Data Sets

Start With a Theoretical Question

Archival data sets yield the most valuable information when investigators approach them with a guiding theoretical issue or question. Obviously, the question posed requires that particular kinds of data be available. To the extent that the data do not exactly address the hypothesis and must be shaped or modified, the data can begin to drive the study. This reverses the normal scientific process and has several methodological and statistical liabilities. Beginning with a question and maintaining that question as the focus of the study will help ensure the study's validity (McCall & Appelbaum, 1991). Furthermore, starting with a particular question means that certain data sets are appropriate and others are not. For example, the Children of the National Longitudinal Survey of Youth project was originally developed by labor force economists, thereby making it ideal for studies of maternal employment and child development but not well suited to questions about the schooling (Chase-Lansdale et al., 1991).

Get to Know the Data Set

Plunging into another investigator's longitudinal data may seem like an effortless way to answer a particular question. After all, one has eliminated the time-consuming activity of data collection; the information is literally sitting on a shelf waiting. In effect, there is the irony of an instant longitudinal study (Janson, 1990). The seeming ease of conducting research using archival data sets is, however, illusory for several reasons. First, in order to understand the data set at both a conceptual and pragmatic level, one must be aware of the questions guiding the original research. These questions dictated the collection of particular data and, importantly, meant that other data were not collected. In the Terman Genetic Studies of Genius (Terman, 1926; Terman & Oden, 1959), there were only a few references to abuse of illicit drugs and virtually no indications of abuse. Such information was never sought and only rarely volunteered. The lack of information on such variables is often as important as the presence of particular information.

Depending on when the data in a particular archive were collected, new investigators must take the time to become aware of both the psychological and cultural contexts operating. To understand the men and women who participated in the Berkeley Growth Studies, one needs to be able to transport oneself into the culture of the Bay Area in the 1930s and to understand the surrounding national and international context. The men and women in the study lived in a pastoral university community during an era when global depression was followed by increasing international tensions and the eruption of a world war. Elder (1974) examined the impact of the Great Depression on differing cohorts from the Berkeley Growth Studies. In the process, he demonstrated compellingly the importance of understanding the contextual variables that impinge on the subjects in the study.

Perhaps less obvious is the necessity of understanding ways in which the culture constrains the information available on a topic. For example, alcohol abuse during Prohibition might have been defined much differently from alcohol abuse in the 1960s. What was regarded as abusive behavior in the former context may be defined as moderate or even social drinking in the latter context. To maintain objectivity, an investigator needs to know how much a person drank at each of those times rather than a subjective assessment of whether the person abused alcohol.

Understanding both the question guiding the investigator and the culture in which the data were collected sets the stage for evaluating the actual data. How were the data collected? Is the documentation available sufficient to check, at every step of the way, whether the data one is analyzing are correct? Stories of investigators who were unaware that a particular variable was coded in a reverse direction or that missing IQ data received a score of zero and were not recoded are reminders that researchers conducting secondary analyses must obtain frequency tables and compare them, one by one, with the codebook. Getting to know the data at this fundamental level takes a great deal of time if one has not been involved with the data collection for the study. Brooks-Gunn et al. (1991) pointed out that few researchers are trained in secondary analysis. Hence, researchers wanting to perform a secondary analysis typically train themselves, with all of the incumbent inefficiencies.

Are the data that were collected relevant to the question one wishes to ask? Many longitudinal studies launched prior to 1950 did not use psychometrically sound instruments, often because none were available. Instead, researchers have questions, interviews, ratings, institutional data, letters, holiday cards, and personal reminiscences that have to be turned into data.

In *Lives Through Time*, J. Block (1971) confronted this problem by constructing case assemblies that included a whole variety of disparate data available in the Berkeley Growth Studies. Trained clinicians evaluated the data and constructed a Q-sort of each individual at various stages in their lives. This procedure yielded a set of psychometrically sound personality ratings on each subject that could be subjected to further analysis.

A similar but perhaps less dramatic approach to recasting the data has been discussed by Elder et al. (1993). Because they wanted to investigate the impact of health changes on day-to-day functioning, they began by evaluating the health measures included in the Terman (1926; Terman & Oden, 1959) studies. After several detours, they discovered that the original codes for health problems did not consider the severity of the diagnosis. One man reported mild ulcer symptoms that were completely controlled by dietary regulation. A second man, also reporting ulcers, required extensive surgery. Both of their surveys were coded as "ulcer." Therefore, the coding scheme was useless and the investigators were forced to recast the original data in terms of "health trajectories" (Elder et al., 1993).

Another approach to handling the disparate data often encountered in longitudinal studies is for researchers to construct their own scale, on the basis of the items included in the study, and then to subject these scales to parametric analyses (McCall & Applebaum, 1991). For example, social support is currently a variable of interest to health investigators. Although no scale specifically designed to tap social support was ever administered to Terman's (1926; Terman & Oden, 1959) subjects, many questions have been asked over the years from which one can derive both quantitative and qualitative measures of social support and loss (Friedman et al., in press). Variables that tap the measure can be factor analyzed or examined through principal-components analysis. Factor scores can then be used to predict a variety of outcomes.

All of these data-reduction strategies repudiate the misconception that secondary analyses involve a simple recombination of existing variables. The most exciting use of archival data occurs when investigators recode, reformulate, or extract new data from the information that exists. An important lesson to all researchers whose data might be of value to future generations is to always code the data in its simplest form. A corollary is to save the original questionnaires, interviews, or answers to items. In this way, the data can be recoded, recast, and reanalyzed in the future to address particular issues.

Validation Samples

Data sets used in secondary analyses are often selected because they have a large number of subjects. Randomly dividing the total pool of subjects into two samples—one for the original analyses and a second to serve as a validation sample—will allow investigators to test hypotheses on two samples independently (McCall & Applebaum, 1991). This procedure offers several advantages. From a statistical viewpoint, it minimizes the risks of Type I and Type II errors. Second, it offers the singular possibility of replicating a longitudinal study. Many archival data sets include multiple waves of data collection conducted over decades. It is extremely unlikely that anyone would undertake or fund a replication. Using secondary analyses and retaining a portion of the sample to validate one's findings offers the possibility of an immediate replication (Tomlinson-Keasey & Little, 1990).

Address Ethical Issues

The significance of a whole range of ethical issues is magnified in archival data sets because as lives are followed, the individuality of each life becomes more prominent. Furthermore, when data are archived to enable other investigators to use them, maintaining the subjects' anonymity and assuring that one has the subjects' consent become extremely important. The Murray Center at Radcliffe has grappled with the ethical issues surrounding archival data as effectively as anyone (Colby & Phelps, 1990). They have identified several areas of concern.

The first focuses on who has access to the data. If the data are anonymous and have been turned over to the public domain, then the issue is simply one of evaluating the credentials of investigators who request access to the data. If, however, the data belong to a particular researcher, that investigator may exercise some control over who gains access. Often, a particular investigator has turned data over to an archive so that other researchers can use it but is still working actively with the data. In such an instance, the researcher who initiated the study may stipulate that certain variables not be used or that analyses by new investigators be limited to those the original researchers are not intending to conduct. Other common controls requested by contributors include careful screening of individuals who wish to use the data. This prevents superficial analyses or misleading findings. The contributors of the data set do not, however, have the right to review or restrict findings emerging from the data set.

A second ethical issue Colby and Phelps (1990) identified concerns a subject's informed consent. On a typical consent form, subjects are told that the data collected will be anonymous and will only be used by the researchers and their graduate students. What does this mean? Does this agreement mean that tapes of individuals may be shown in graduate seminars? How about undergraduate classes? If a researcher decides to turn data over to an archive, does the subject have to be contacted again to sign a new release? Colby and Phelps concluded that as the risk of identification increases, the researcher is obligated to make sure that subjects understand how the data will be used. In the case of videotapes, the current stance of the Murray Center is to renew the consent for each request for access. As more individuals avail themselves of archived data to answer research questions, the consent forms used in research will become more explicit about the possible uses of the data. Studies conducted under the auspices of the Center for Marital and Family Studies, for example, use consent forms specifically addressing the multiple uses of videotapes. Their consent forms specifically request permission to use the data under increasing levels of exposure, from research purposes to use at conferences or training sessions to use in documentaries (Markham, Floyd, Stanley, & Storaasli, 1988).

The third and perhaps most important ethical issue—anonymity—is tied inextricably to the second. Although subject numbers are substituted for names, and identifying material is routinely omitted from archived data, the risk of subject identification is not limited to video-taped data. Although Lewis Terman was fully aware of the importance of confidentiality, one of his books indicated that a particular family had a large number of siblings, all of whom attended the same undergraduate institution. The sex and number of siblings combined with the name of the undergraduate institution provided enough information to enable several readers to identify the subjects. Even occupational information may compromise anonymity, especially if that occupation is an atypical one for a particular sex.

The burgeoning use of video-taped information complicates the issue of anonymity. The most recent technology allows investigators to scramble the faces of subjects who are being interviewed to prevent recognition. In the process of scrambling an infant's face in the Strange Situation procedure, one may lose valuable information. Altering voices is similarly problematic because the tone used is often essential in establishing the nature of the communication. Over the past two decades, the issues of informed consent and confidentiality have resulted in specific policies guiding researchers. Over the next few years, researchers can expect similar discussions to shape new policies concerning appropriate safeguards for video-taped information.

The ethical issues involved in conducting secondary analyses of an archived data set can complicate the use of the data. To some extent, these can be solved by the organization archiving the data. The intent is not to erect obstacles to the use of the data but to make sure that the interests of all involved have been considered and protected.

Conclusions

For decades, archival data have been the backbone of sociological, economic, and historic research. Psychologists have only recently realized that such data, properly collected and archived, offer unparalleled opportunities to answer critical questions of development. Although the call for longitudinal research grows stronger, the ability of contemporary researchers to respond to that call does not. The time commitment and the financial requirements of prospective longitudinal research deter all but the most stalwart from embarking on a study that may span decades. Archival data sets offer an alternative means of responding to that call. Adding to an already existing database by collecting another wave of data can turn cross-sectional studies into prospective longitudinal studies (Franz et al., 1990). Broad-based longitudinal studies in which researchers ask a wide range of questions can also be used to address contemporary issues (Friedman et al., in press). Survey research that documents personal characteristics and records behavior can provide key prospective, longitudinal information for psychologists (Chase-Lansdale et al., 1991). Finally, smaller longitudinal studies addressing specific questions can examine a psychological problem in depth (Caspi et al., 1992; Vaillant, 1983). Although secondary analysis of archival data sets is not without problems, many of the problems are solvable and the value of the resulting information renders the difficulties trivial.

"How then may we obtain truth about the adult life cycle? Clearly, it must be studied prospectively. It is all too common for caterpillars to become butterflies and then maintain that in their youth they had been little butterflies" (Vaillant, 1977, p. 197). Archival data offer psychologists the chance to contemplate the caterpillars and chronicle their transformation into butterflies.

References

Atchley, R. (1985). The impact of retirement on aging and adaptation. In A. Colby (Ed.), *A guide to the data resources* (p. 2). Cambridge, MA: Henry A. Murray Research Center.

Baker, P. C., & Mott, F. L. (1989). *NLSY child handbook, 1989*. Columbus: Ohio State University, Center for Human Resource Research.

Baruch, G. K., & Barnett, R. C. (1985). Women in the middle years. In A. Colby (Ed.), *A guide to the data resources* (p. 13). Cambridge, MA: Henry A. Murray Research Center.

Baumrind, D. (1992). Adolescent exploratory behavior: Precursors and consequences. In L. P. Lipsitt & L. L. Mitnick (Eds.), *Self-regulation and risk taking* (pp. 109–142). Norwood, NJ: Ablex.

Baydar, N., & Brooks-Gunn, J. (1991). Effects of maternal employment and child-care arrangements on preschoolers' cognitive and behavioral outcomes: Evidence from the Children of the National Longitudinal Survey of Youth. *Developmental Psychology, 27,* 932–945.

Block, J. (1971). *Lives through time.* Berkeley, CA: Bancroft Books.

Block, J., Block, J. H., & Keyes, S. (1988). Longitudinally foretelling drug usage in adolescence: Early childhood personality and environmental precursors. *Child Development, 59,* 336–355.

Block, J., Gjerde, P. F., & Block, J. H. (1991). Personality antecedents of depressive tendencies in 18-year-olds: A prospective study. *Journal of Personality and Social Psychology, 60,* 726–738.

Block, J. H. (1983). Differential premises arising from differential socialization of the sexes: Some conjectures. *Child Development, 54,* 1335–1354.

Block, J. H., & Block, J. (1980). The role of ego-control and ego-resiliency in the organization of behaviour. In W. A. Collins (Ed.), *Development of cognition, affect, and social relations. The Minnesota Symposia on Child Psychology* (Vol. 13, pp. 39–101). Hillsdale, NJ: Erlbaum.

Block, J. H., Block, J., & Gjerde, P. F. (1986). The personality of children prior to divorce: A prospective study. *Child Development, 57,* 827–840.

Brooks-Gunn, J., Phelps, E., & Elder, G. H., Jr. (1991). Studying lives through time: Secondary data analyses in developmental psychology. *Developmental Psychology, 27,* 899–910.

Cairns, R. B., Cairns, B. D., & Neckerman, H. J. (1989). Early school dropout: Configurations and determinants. *Child Development, 60,* 1437–1452.

Caspi, A., Elder, G., & Bem, D. (1987). Moving against the world: Life-course patterns of explosive children. *Developmental Psychology, 23,* 308–313.

Caspi, A., Herbener, E. S., & Ozer, D. J. (1992). Shared experiences and the similarity of personalities: A longitudinal study of married couples. *Journal of Personality and Social Psychology, 62,* 281–291.

Chase-Lansdale, P. L., Mott, F. L., Brooks-Gunn, J., & Phillips, D. A. (1991). Children of the National Longitudinal Survey of Youth: A unique research opportunity. *Developmental Psychology, 27*, 918–931.

Cherlin, A. (1991). On analyzing other people's data. *Developmental Psychology, 27*, 946–948.

Cherlin, A. J., Furstenberg, F. F., Jr., Chase-Lansdale, P. L., Kiernan, K. E., Robins, P. K., Morrison, D. R., & Teitler, J. O. (1991). Longitudinal studies of effects of divorce on children in Great Britain and the United States. *Science, 252*, 1386–1389.

Clarke, A. M., & Clarke, A. D. B. (1989). The later cognitive effects of early intervention. *Intelligence, 13*, 289–297.

Colby, A., & Phelps, E. (1990). Archiving longitudinal data. In D. Magnusson & L. R. Bergman (Eds.), *Data quality in longitudinal research* (pp. 249–262). Cambridge, England: Cambridge University Press.

Consortium for Longitudinal Studies. (1983). *As the twig is bent . . . Lasting effects of preschool programs.* Hillsdale, NJ: Erlbaum.

Davidoff, I., & Platt, M. (1985). Two generations of college-educated women: The postparental phase of the life cycle. In A. Colby (Ed.), *A guide to the data resources* (p. 36). Cambridge, MA: Henry A. Murray Research Center.

Duncan, G. J. (1991). Made in heaven: Secondary data analysis and interdisciplinary collaborators. *Developmental Psychology, 27*, 949–951.

Duncan, G. J., Coe, R. D., Corcoran, M. E., Hill, M. S., Hoffman, S. D., & Morgan, J. N. (1984). *Years of poverty, years of plenty: The changing economic fortunes of American workers and families.* Ann Arbor, MI: Institute for Social Research.

Duncan, G. J., Hill, M. S., & Hoffman, S. D. (1988). Welfare dependence within and across generations. *Science, 239*, 467–471.

Duncan, G. J., & Morgan, N. J. (1985). The Panel Study of Income Dynamics. In G. H. Elder, Jr. (Ed.), *Life course dynamics* (pp. 50–71). Ithaca, NY: Cornell University Press.

Elder, G. H., Jr. (1974). *Children of the Great Depression.* Chicago: University of Chicago Press.

Elder, G. H., Jr. (Ed.). (1985). *Life course dynamics.* Ithaca, NY: Cornell University Press.

Elder, G. H., Jr., & Caspi, A. (1990). Studying lives in a changing society. In A. I. Rabin, R. A. Zucker, R. Emmons, & S. Frank (Eds.), *Study in persons and lives* (pp. 201–247). New York: Springer.

Elder, G. H., Jr., Caspi, A., & Downey, G. (1986). Problem behavior and family relationships. Life course and intergenerational themes. In A. Sørensen, F. Weinert, & L. Sherrod (Eds.), *Life-course research on human development* (pp. 293–340). Hillsdale, NJ: Erlbaum.

Elder, G. H., Jr., Pavalko, E. K., & Clipp, E. C. (1993). *Working with archival data: Studying lives.* Newbury Park, CA: Sage.

Fagan, J. F., III, & Shepard, P. A., & Knevel, C. R. (1991, April). *Predictive validity of the Fagan Test of Infant Intelligence.* Paper presented at the Society for Research in Child Development, Seattle, WA.

Farrington, D. P., Gallagher, B., Morley, L., St. Ledger, R. J., & West, D. J. (1990). Minimizing attrition in longitudinal research: Methods of tracing and securing cooperation in a 24 year follow-up study. In D. Magnusson & L. R. Bergman (Eds.), *Data quality in longitudinal research* (pp. 122–147). Cambridge, England: Cambridge University Press.

Feldman, D. H. (1984). A follow-up of subjects scoring above 180 IQ in Terman's Genetic Studies of Genius. *Exceptional Children, 50,* 518–523.

Franz, C. E., McClelland, D. C., & Weinberger, J. (1991). Childhood antecedents of conventional social accomplishment in midlife adults: A 36-year prospective study. *Journal of Personality and Social Psychology, 60,* 586–595.

Friedman, H. S., Tucker, J. S., Tomlinson-Keasey, C., Schwartz, J. E., Wingard, D. L., & Criqui, M. (in press). Does childhood personality predict longevity? *Journal of Personality and Social Psychology.*

Furstenberg, F. F., Jr., Levine, J. A., & Brooks-Gunn, J. (1990). The daughters of teenage mothers: Patterns of early childbearing in two generations. *Family Planning Perspectives, 22,* 54–61.

Garmezy, N. (1988). Longitudinal strategies, causal reasoning and risk research: A commentary. In M. Rutter (Ed.), *Studies of psychosocial risk* (pp. 29–44). New York: Cambridge University Press.

Glass, J., McLanahan, S. S., & Sørensen, A. (1985). The consequences of divorce: Effects of sample selection bias. In G. H. Elder, Jr. (Ed.), *Life course dynamics* (pp. 267–281). Ithaca, NY: Cornell University Press.

Haskins, R. (1989). Beyond metaphor: The efficacy of early childhood education. *American Psychologist, 44,* 274–282.

Heckman, J. (1979). Sample selection bias as a specification error. *Econometrica, 47,* 153–161.

Helson, R. (1967). Personality characteristics and developmental history of creative college women. *Genetic Psychology Monographs, 76,* 205–256.

Holahan, C. K. (1984). Marital attitudes over 40 years: A longitudinal and cohort analysis. *Journal of Gerontology, 39,* 49–57.

Janos, P. M. (1986). The socialization of highly intelligent boys: Case material from Terman's correspondence. *Journal of Counseling and Development, 65,* 193–195.

Janos, P. M. (1987). A fifty-year follow-up of Terman's youngest college students and IQ-matched agemates. *Gifted Child Quarterly, 31*(2), 55–58.

Janson, C. (1990). Retrospective data, undesirable behavior, and the longitudinal perspective. In D. Magnusson & L. R. Bergman (Eds.), *Data quality in longitudinal research* (pp. 100–121). Cambridge, England: Cambridge University Press.

Kelly, E. L. (1955). Consistency of the adult personality. *American Psychologist, 10,* 659–681.

Lazar, I., & Darlington, R. (1982). Lasting effects of early education: A report from the consortium for longitudinal studies. *Monographs of the Society for Research in Child Development, 47*(Serial No. 195).

Lee, V. E., Brooks-Gunn, J., & Schnur, E. (1988). Does Head Start work? A one-year follow-up comparison of disadvantages children attending Head Start, no preschool, and other preschool programs. *Developmental Psychology, 24*, 210–222.

Little, R. J. A., & Rubin, D. B. (1987). *Statistical analysis with missing data.* New York: Wiley.

Markham, H. J., Floyd, F. J., Stanley, S. M., & Storaasli, D. (1988). Prevention of marital distress: A longitudinal investigation. *Journal of Consulting and Clinical Psychology, 56*, 210–217.

McCall, R. B. (1981). Early predictors of later IQ: The search continues. *Intelligence, 5*, 141–148.

McCall, R. B., & Appelbaum, M. I. (1991). Some issues of conducting secondary analyses. *Developmental Psychology, 27*, 911–917.

McCall, R. B., Appelbaum, M. I., & Hogarty, P. S. (1973). Developmental changes in mental performance. *Monographs of the Society for Research in Child Development, 38* (3, Serial No. 150).

McKey, R. H., Condelli, L., Granson, H., Barrett, B., McConkey, C., & Plantz, M. (1985). *The impact of Head Start on children, families and communities.* Final report of the Head Start Evaluation, Synthesis, and Utilization Project (DHHS Publication No. 90–31193). Washington, DC: U.S. Government Printing Office.

National Center for Education Statistics. (1972). *National longitudinal study of the class of 1972* [Machine-readable data file]. Washington, DC: National Center for Education Statistics.

Neuringer, C. (1982). Affect configurations and changes in women who threaten suicide following a crisis. *Journal of Consulting and Clinical Psychology, 50*, 182–186.

Phelps, E. (1987, April). *Recycling data: Why not?* Symposium presented at the biennial meetings of the Society for Research in Child Development, Baltimore, MD.

Ramey, C. T., & Landesman Ramey, S. (1990). Intensive educational intervention for children of poverty. *Intelligence, 14*, 1–9.

Robins, L. N., & Rutter, M. (1990). *Straight and devious pathways from childhood to adulthood.* Cambridge, England: Cambridge University Press.

Rubin, D. B. (1987). *Multiple imputation for nonresponse in surveys.* New York: Wiley.

Rutter, M. (1988). Longitudinal data in the study of causal processes: Some uses and some pitfalls. In M. Rutter (Ed.), *Studies of psychosocial risk* (pp. 1–28). New York: Cambridge University Press.

Rutter, M. (1989). Pathways from childhood to adult life. *Journal of Child Psychology and Psychiatry, 30*, 23–51.

Sears, R. R. (1977). Sources of life satisfaction of the Terman gifted men. *American Psychologist, 32*, 119–128.

Sears, R. R., Maccoby, E. E., & Levin, H. (1957). *Patterns of child rearing.* Evanston, IL: Row, Peterson.

Shedler, J., & Block, J. (1990). Adolescent drug use and psychological health: A longitudinal inquiry. *American Psychologist, 45,* 612–620.

Shneidman, E. S. (1971). Suicide among the gifted. *Suicide and Life-Threatening Behavior, 1,* 23–45.

Stewart, A. J. (1985). Longitudinal study of the life patterns of college-educated women. In A. Colby (Ed.), *A guide to the data resources* (p. 179). Cambridge, MA: Henry A. Murray Research Center.

Tangri, S. S., & Jenkins, S. R. (1986). Stability and change in role innovation and life plans. *Sex Roles, 14,* 647–662.

Terman, L. M. (1926). *Genetic studies of genius: Vol. 1. Mental and physical traits of a thousand gifted children.* Stanford, CA: Stanford University Press.

Terman, L. M., & Oden, M. H. (1959). *Genetic studies of genius: Vol. 5. The gifted group at mid-life.* Stanford, CA: Stanford University Press.

Thomas, A., & Chess, S. (1984). *Origins and evolution of behavior disorders.* New York: Brunner/Mazel.

Tomlinson-Keasey, C., Warren, L. W., & Elliott, J. E. (1986). Suicide among gifted women: A prospective study. *Journal of Abnormal Psychology, 95,* 123–130.

Tomlinson-Keasey, C., & Little, T. D. (1990). Predicting educational attainment, occupational achievement, intellectual skills, and personal adjustment among gifted men and women. *Journal of Educational Psychology, 82,* 442–455.

Traupmann, J. (1985). McBeath Institute Aging Women Project. In A. Colby (Ed.), *A guide to the data resources* (p. 193). Cambridge, MA: Henry A. Murray Research Center.

Vaillant, G. E. (1977). *Adaptation to life.* Boston: Little, Brown.

Vaillant, G. E. (1983). *The natural history of alcoholism.* Cambridge, MA: Harvard University Press.

Vaillant, G. E., & Vaillant, C. O. (1990). Determinants and consequences of creativity in a cohort of gifted women [Special issue]. *Psychology of Women Quarterly, 14,* 607–616.

Vandewater, E., & Stewart, A. J. (1992). *Changes in commitment as an interpretive framework for understanding women's personality development and well-being at mid-life.* Manuscript in preparation.

Vital Statistics. (1986). Advance report of final mortality statistics, 1984. *National Center for Health Statistics, 35,* No. 6. Washington, DC: U.S. Government Printing Office.

Werner, E. E., & Smith, R. S. (1992). *Overcoming the odds: High risk children from birth to adulthood.* Ithaca, NY: Cornell University Press.

Woodruff, W. J. (1992). *Transitions in midlife: Implications for women's health and development.* Manuscript in preparation.

Young, C. H., Savola, K., & Phelps, E. (1991). *Inventory of longitudinal studies in the social sciences.* Newbury Park, CA: Sage.

CHAPTER 5

Comparing Longitudinal Studies of Adult Development: Toward a Paradigm of Tension Between Stability and Change

Ravenna Helson

This chapter has two related objectives. The first is to argue that even though assumptions and designs in the field of longitudinal personality research bias findings in the direction of an overemphasis on stability of personality, the evidence for personality change is substantial enough to justify efforts of researchers to study both stability and change. The second objective is to encourage attempts to compare longitudinal studies, both to show generality of the findings about personality stability and change and to evaluate the influence of social climate and cohort.

What do longitudinal personality researchers have to say about change in adulthood? The emphasis of the field is certainly not on change but on consistency of personality, and the main contributions to the question of change have been reactive: to contradict claims of inconsis-

This work was supported by National Institute of Mental Health Grant 43948.

tency in personality that were based on flawed scholarship or to contradict incorrect conclusions about change that were based on cross-sectional research. These contributions have been of first importance. One thinks of the work of J. Block (1971, 1981), and later of Conley (1984) and Costa and McCrae (1980), to contradict the claim of Mischel (1968) and his followers that personality is largely an illusion, that behavioral outcomes depend on particularities of situations. Studies from the "Block project" on personality of children prior to divorce (J. H. Block, Block, & Gjerde, 1986) and on the childhood antecedents of drug use in adolescence (J. Block, Block, & Keyes, 1988) have demonstrated that longitudinal research is necessary for the assessment of situational or environmental influence, whether to show that such influence changes personality or—more commonly—that it does not.

Personality is defined in terms of characteristics that endure over time. The instruments of personality psychologists are developed to measure characteristics that show rank order stability in individual differences. More than 20 years ago, in *Lives Through Time*, J. Block (1971) discussed this focus on stability to the neglect of change:

> The dominant conceptualizations of the basis and laws of personality development—psychoanalysis, reinforcement theory, and the constitutional-genetic viewpoint—concur in construing later personality as the result primarily of an orderly unfolding of capacities and qualities intrinsic to an individual or laid down earlier. (p. 11)

Thus, change over time

> disappoints the investigator, for he is prevented from the visible accomplishment of predicting the future .... Inconstancy over time is viewed as indicative of poor psychological measurement or as due to an unanalyzable, irreducible, random component in human behavior or as evidence of the unimportance of the variable involved. (J. Block, 1971, p. 11)

The prejudice against finding change could reflect an identification with the biological sciences and a lack of interest in sociology, cultural anthropology, and history. If so, it might be a hopeful sign that researchers have begun to study the relation between personality and environmental variables over time. However, there is a surprise here: Investigators continue to demonstrate the stability or consistency of personality. In *Personality and Adulthood*, McCrae and Costa (1990) asserted that adult personality does not change in more than trivial ways after age 30. Personality shapes lives, but life experiences do not influence personality. Caspi (1987) has outlined an impressive research framework that would seem to give more influence to age-graded roles and other societal variables. However, although Caspi, Bem, and Elder (1989) used such variables, their work shows the continuity of personality characteristics, such as shyness and explosiveness, from early childhood to middle age. They chose to study how explosiveness, for example, is maintained by self-selection into or out of roles and by persisting patterns of interaction with others, not why some people (and, in fact, most people) become less explosive over time. A review essay by Caspi and Bem (1990) was called "Personality Continuity and Change Across the Life Course," but the authors ended with an apology for not having addressed the question of change. "A claim of systematic change," they said, "requires a theory that specifies in what way the observed absence of continuity is systematic" (Caspi & Bem, 1990, p. 569). However, when the term *change* appears in the literature, they continued, it most frequently denotes merely the absence of continuity.

How surprising and puzzling that hypotheses about change are not tested. I agree with Kogan (1990) that researchers have demonstrated stability in personality and that they need to go on to questions about the nature and amount of change in personality at different periods of the life course and in different life contexts. Of course, the demonstration of change is complicated. Schaie (1965) advocated the use of cross-sequential and time-sequential research designs to separate change attributable to age, cohort, and time of measurement. He used his ideas in original and important ways: to show that the increasing educational level of successive cohorts was largely responsible for what had previously been considered a marked maturational decline in intelligence with age (Schaie, 1979). Nevertheless, his model is seldom used in personality research and is unrealistic for the study of lives. More recent treatments of methods in the study of change (Nesselroade, 1991) have emphasized careful sampling of measures, occasions and subjects, and the inevitability of compromises and trade-offs.

Therefore, I advocate that researchers look for both systematic change and continuity in longitudinal research and compare their findings with those of other samples in which there are different patterns of life span influence. Although far short of perfection, what researchers learn in attempting such evaluations will advance them toward a more adequate understanding of lives in society through time.

It is difficult to compare longitudinal studies. Hulbert and Schuster (1993) have gathered accounts of 14 longitudinal studies of educated American women in the United States. Even with a common focus on educated women, those studies did not use the same instruments, did not cover the same topic areas, had different kinds of samples, and tested subjects at different ages. Nevertheless, important questions about personality coherence and change require cross-sample comparisons, and techniques for making these comparisons need to be developed.

What Factors Affect the Finding of Personality Change in Adulthood?

The first question I want to discuss is why one longitudinal study shows evidence of personality change in adulthood when another does not. A critical factor is how personality and change in personality are conceptualized.

How Personality Is Conceptualized

According to one conception, personality consists of basic components that generate dimensions of individual differences in tendencies to show consistent patterns of thoughts, feelings, and actions. To fill out this conception, trait theorists try to identify and measure these basic components and to demonstrate high rank order stability over time. Costa and McCrae have shown particular enterprise in this endeavor, and I return to their work shortly.

A different conception of personality treats it largely in terms of the experiential self. The self reflects identities that depend importantly on social roles and relationships that do, of course, change over time. Although some scholars (Gergen, 1980) emphasize discontinuities in the self, others, such as Cantor and Kihlstrom (1987), Greenwald (1980), Swann (1987), and Wells and Stryker (1988), have been impressed by the high degree of stability despite environmental and role changes. To account for the fact that the self does not seem to change as much as might be expected from this viewpoint, it is conceived of as having a regulating function that maintains stability. Social psychologists interested in the self tend to advance complex theories about its structure and functioning, and deductions from these theories may be tested in experiments, but only in a narrow or brief kind of longitudinal research. It will be worthwhile to select from or modify their ideas for the study of lives through time.

According to a third view, which is mine, personality is the relatively enduring organization of motivations and resources that a person manifests in structured and unstructured, implicit and explicit, individual activities and interpersonal interactions over the life course. A definition such as this encourages one to consider a variety of fairly stable motivational and resource patterns, to take into account the social world through which the individual moves, and to try to show when and why the organization of motivations and resources changes. It is framed at a level that is intended to be useful for longitudinal research and for showing both stability and change over time.

How Change Is Conceptualized

If one's goal is to show the stability of personality, change tends to be treated as error variance. It is packaged in big empty envelopes such as biases attributable to practice effects, sample biases, and effects attributable to period or cohort. There is no attempt to gather the kind of data about the social world or the individual's life experience that would enable one to evaluate differentiated hypotheses about change. To the contrary, the investigator may cleave nature every 6 inches rather than at the joints and combine different kinds of people, environments, ages, and time intervals so that factors that produce change cancel each other out.

On the other hand, if one wants to find out whether and why personality changes in a longitudinal study, one musters some ideas about what might produce change of different kinds and one selects measures and conducts analyses with these ideas in mind. In a broad-band study, one would be interested in the ideas of stage theorists about patterns of personality change that take place generally throughout the seasons of life, in psychodynamic theories about change associated with particular personality patterns, and in ideas of age-status theorists about changes related to the tasks and reward patterns along specific life paths. One might be interested in how change results from conscious evaluative processes (Stewart, Vandewater, Landman, & Malley, 1992); in what actually changes when change occurs (e.g., which "basic beliefs" change after catastrophe; Epstein, 1990); and in trying to understand what is involved in cohort, social climate, and period effects. Researchers need a framework to help them remember the many kinds and contexts of change and structural models of personality and life structure in which change can be discussed (Conley, 1985; Kimmel, 1974).

I now examine how the conceptualization of personality and personality change accounts for the highly different conclusions about personality change of the Baltimore Longitudinal Study (McCrae & Costa, 1990) and the Mills Longitudinal Study (Helson, Mitchell, & Moane, 1984; Helson & Wink, 1992; and other work cited).

Comparison of the Baltimore and Mills Longitudinal Studies

Baltimore Longitudinal Study

McCrae and Costa (1990) have based their minimization of personality change in adulthood on a number of research investigations, but particularly on their own Baltimore study and the NEO Personality Inventory. Participants in the Baltimore study are approximately 1,000 predominantly White, college-educated men and women (aged 20–96) who agreed to take biomedical and psychological tests in return for physical examinations. Recruitment to the study is continuous, and some nonmember spouses and peers have also contributed. The first testing was in 1980, and the longest interval between testings so far has been 6–7 years.

In what is their most ambitious article on personality change to date, Costa and McCrae (1988) reported the results of cross-sectional, longitudinal, cross-sequential, and time-sequential analyses of NEO Personality

Inventory data gathered in 1980 and 1986 (assessing neuroticism, extraversion, and openness,) or, for the more recently developed Agreeableness and Conscientious scales, in 1983 and 1986. NEO spouse–observer data were also included. Table 1 shows many "age effects," but there were actually even more because Table 1 is a condensation of the original findings as presented later by McCrae and Costa (1990). It is easier to understand, but it omits the subscales (facets) under each major scale. The complete longitudinal findings were that this large heterogeneous cross-sectional sample, retested after 6 years, had lower scores in neuroticism and two of its facets, hostility and impulsivity. The sample had also changed in several but opposite ways on different facets of extraversion and openness, yielding no overall change on these two dimensions. Over a period of 3 years, the sample had lower scores on a preliminary version of agreeableness and conscientiousness. Despite the apparent evidence for change, Costa and McCrae (1988) dismissed all of the longitudinal findings on the grounds that none of them was consistently supported by cross-sectional analyses, cross-sequential analyses, and spouse–observer data.

TABLE 1

Age Effects From Analyses of NEO–PI Domain Scales

	Cross-sectional		Longitudinal		Cross-sequential
NEO–PI Scale	Self-report	Spouse rating	Self-report	Spouse rating	Self-report
Neuroticism	– –	– – –	–	+	0
Extraversion	– – –	– – –	0	0	+
Openness	– – –	– –	0	0	+
Agreeableness	+	0	– – –		– – –
Conscientiousness	0	+ + +	–		–

Note. NEO–PI = NEO Personality Inventory. Minus signs indicate a negative association of the variable with age; plus signs indicate a positive association. Effects accounting for less than 2% of the variance are marked with one sign; those accounting for 2% to 5% are marked with two signs; and those accounting for more than 5% are marked with three signs. Zeros indicate nonsignificant effects. Longitudinal analyses of Agreeableness and Conscientiousness were conducted only for self-reports. From *Personality in Adulthood* (p. 70) by R. R. McCrae and P. T. Costa, Jr., 1990. New York: Guilford Press. Copyright © 1990 by Guilford Press. Reprinted by permission.

Thus, when McCrae and Costa (1990) claimed that there is only trivial personality change after age 30, they meant that there is no "maturational" change, no linear change with age from the 20s to the 90s found after a mere 3–6 years across sex, educational level, cohort, time of testing, and reports from both self and others. They meant that there was no change strong enough to overcome repetition effects and differences that were almost certain to exist between the original sample that was retested and the second sample that was constituted for cross-sequential and time-sequential analyses. They considered all of these factors, producing in the reader admiration for their rigor and resourcefulness, along with confusion and dismay at the chaos of assessing change. They concluded that personality does not change in any important way on the grounds that half a dozen factors treated as sources of error variance could account for what might appear to be change. They believed that it is much more reasonable to build around the stability of personality. They showed extremely high correlations demonstrating longitudinal stability.

Mills Longitudinal Study
In the Mills Longitudinal Study (Helson, 1967; Helson & Wink, 1992; and other work cited), the original sample consisted of 140 members of the Mills College classes of 1958 and 1960. My colleagues and I have studied them at average ages 21, 27, 43, and 52, using at each time a mixture of ratings and open-ended questions about various areas of life, along with the California Psychological Inventory (CPI; Gough, 1957/1987) at all four times of testing, the Adjective Check List (ACL; Gough & Heilbrun, 1983) at three times, and other instruments once or twice.

My colleagues and I have found considerable rank order and mean-level stability in adult personality, but we have also found several kinds of personality change. Here, I describe some of our work on three kinds: change observed for the entire sample (normative change), change associated with different personality types or syndromes, and change associated with roles and role trajectories.

Figure 1 shows mean scores on the CPI Femininity/Masculinity (F/M) scale for 79 women who completed it at all four times of testing. Results are virtually identical if one uses means based on all women who

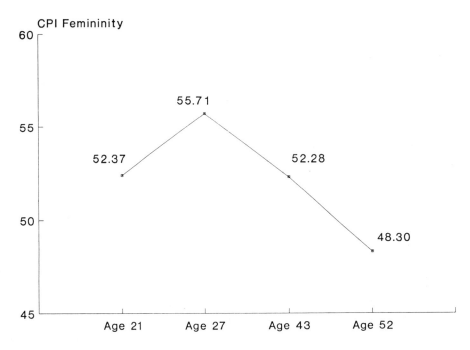

FIGURE 1. Change with age on the California Psychological Inventory (CPI) Femininity/Masculinity scale. (Subjects were 79 women who completed the CPI at all four of the ages shown. Figure is from R. Helson, "Women's Difficult Times and the Rewriting of the Life Story," *Psychology of Women Quarterly, 14,* p. 342. Copyright © 1990 by Division 35, American Psychological Association. Reprinted by permission.)

completed the CPI at any given time of testing: 140 at age 21, 94 at age 27, 107 at age 43, and 106 at age 52. Note that there is change, it is curvilinear, and it continues well beyond age 30. The sign test evaluating the direction of change at each time of measurement showed that most women changed in the same direction. The F/M scale showed good longitudinal stability: .51 was the lowest coefficient for the first interval shown, and the other two were higher than .60. However, the CPI scales do not aim to measure hard-wired traits but a pattern of motivations and resources. High scorers on the F/M scale are sympathetic and compassionate but feel vulnerable, self-critical, and lacking in confidence and initiative. The pattern of change on this scale, up and then down and down again, is consistent with the idea that young adult roles increase women's femininity but that women become more confident and assertive around midlife, which is what life span theorists such as Jung (1931/1960), Neugarten and Gutmann (1958), and Gutmann (1987) have been saying over many decades. Role theorists would also find this pattern reasonable. Therefore, we doubt that it is attributable to the random unanalyzable particularities of the Mills sample.

Figure 1 illustrates what we call *normative personality change*, meaning that most women in the sample changed in the same way. The word *normative* also has the connotations of being a standard to be achieved. In an advantaged sample, personality change that is normative can often be understood to indicate that the individual is actualizing his or her potential. We have conducted several studies of normative change in which this seems to be the case (Helson & Moane, 1987; Helson & Wink, 1992; Mitchell & Helson, 1990; Wink & Helson, in press).

In a recent study, Wink & Helson (in press) compared ACL scores of the Mills women and their partners in the early parental and postparental periods. In the early parental period, the women had an average age of 27 years, and their partner's average age was 31. In the postparental period, the women had an average age of 52 years, and the partners— not necessarily the same partners—had an average age of 56 years. Figure 2 shows that at the first period, the women scored (significantly) higher than their partners on the ACL Succorance scale but that at the second period, they scored about the same as their partners. We were able to compare the postparental ACL scores with those obtained for a subsample of the Mills women's own mothers and fathers who had filled out the ACL in 1961, also at average ages 52 and 56. At the age when the Mills women and their partners no longer showed the gender-traditional difference, the mothers of the Mills women scored significantly higher on the Succorance scale than did their husbands. They also scored significantly higher than their daughters at the same age. These mothers and fathers lived through a conservative era of sex roles. Fewer mothers than fathers had completed 4 years of college, there was virtually no divorce, and few mothers were employed after they married. This difference between cohorts on Succorance scores illustrates why we prefer the concept of normative change to that of maturational change. Women do not always

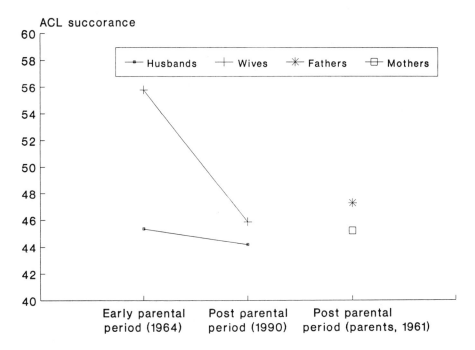

FIGURE 2.   Means on the Succorance scale of the Adjective Check List (ACL) for women and their partners at the early parental (n = 65) and postparental (n = 48) periods and for a subsample of the women's parents (n = 29) at the postparental period. From Wink & Helson (in press). Reprinted by permission.

become less dependent over time. Whether they do depends on their social world.

A second kind of change that interested us was pioneered by J. Block (1971); change associated with particular personality syndromes. In the Mills study, Wink (1991, 1992) studied a dimension he called *self- versus object-directedness.* Using a Q-sort prototype technique that he learned from Block, Wink identified three subtypes among the self-directed (narcissistic) women: hypersensitive, willful, and autonomous. Each group showed a different pattern of change between ages 21–43 (Wink, 1992). The willful subtype (n = 12), which was closest to our usual concept of narcissist, scored consistently lower than the rest of the sample on the CPI Self-Control scale, and its change pattern showed features in common with Block's (1971) dominating narcissists. In the Mills study, the CPI showed that from ages 21 to 27, the willful women increased in effective functioning and well-being and became more sociable and confident. However, in accord with psychoanalytic theory predicting worsened adjustment of narcissistic individuals by midlife, from ages 27 to 43, these women showed insignificant declines rather than the positive changes that characterized the sample as a whole. Life data showed that over this period, they tended to have problems in relationships, to use drugs, and to start promising careers that they could not maintain. Thus, Wink's work showed systematic personality change, different over different periods of adulthood, that was not normative but related to a particular psychodynamic pattern.

A third kind of change my colleagues and I have studied is that associated with role patterns and trajectories. Valory Mitchell, Geraldine Moane, and I wanted to describe adult development in terms that would take into account conditions of social life yet be applicable across cohort. We took Neugarten's (1977) concept of a system of age norms, a social clock. The social clock is superimposed on a biological clock and regulates sequential changes in behavior and self-perception over time. We focused on norms about behaviors related to the big endeavors of young and middle adulthood, which we called "social clock projects," and to the implications for the individual of her choice of projects and of succeeding or failing in these at various points in time (Helson, Mitchell, & Moane, 1984).

The Mills sample belonged to a cohort in which women expected to marry and start a family in early adulthood and knew that others expected them to accomplish these things. We called this schedule part of the "feminine social clock" (FSC) that regulated their behavior. We found that women who followed the FSC had tended in college to have a desire to do well, to like a clear structure, and to be optimistic, trusting, confident, and sensible. Between ages 21 and 27, women who had become mothers had increased self-control, responsibility, and tolerance, but they had decreased sociability and confidence. In a later study, we found that by age 43, women who had maintained the traditional FSC path, unlike all other groups in the sample, had not gained in dominance or independence but had become increasingly overcontrolled (Helson & Picano, 1990). This pattern of change is consistent with theoretical statements about the effects of the homemaker role in which women subordinate their own needs to those of others. Clausen and Gilens (1990) have described the older cohorts of women in longitudinal samples studied at the Institute of Human Development (IHD) as predominantly followers of the FSC; they reported some of the same findings that we did about personality change associated with adherence to this life pattern.

Although I have followed the homemaker trajectory in my examples, we have been equally interested in women who chose what we called the "masculine occupational clock," or other life paths (Helson et al., 1984).

Besides the social clock studies, my colleagues and I have examined the influence on personality of variables such as multiple roles and the kind of work in which women have been engaged (Helson, Elliott, & Leigh, 1990). Sometimes we found change and sometimes we did not. Our graduate students today know that there are bodies of sociological theory and research on these topics. One does not have to assume that change is either maturational or caused by error variance.

There is exciting work to be done in conceptualizing when and why change occurs and the forms that it takes. Of course, the Mills study is not alone in this enterprise. Among longitudinal investigations that have shown personality change in adulthood, there is a wonderful study by Howard and Bray (1988), who followed 200 AT&T male managerial candidates from the late 1950s, when the men were in their 20s, to the late 1970s, when they were in their 40s. Howard and Bray paid careful attention to cultural and institutional contexts, and they reported examples of the same kinds of personality change that I described in the Mills study: normative change, change related to personality patterns, and change related to role sequences. In addition, they presented first results from the study of a later cohort, more heterogeneous in sex and ethnicity.

So far, I have been primarily discussing differences between the Baltimore and Mills studies in the conceptions of personality and in the kind of analyses that are conducted to assess change. It would be easier to compare actual findings in the two studies if one could use the same constructs. This point leads me to a second topic: tools for comparing longitudinal samples.

Tools for Comparing Longitudinal Samples

Versatile Instruments (the ACL)

Sometimes, one instrument can be used to construct scales from another. One cannot compare the Mills and Baltimore findings perfectly, but Oliver John and Brent Roberts plan to score the Mills sample on "Big Five" scales (Neuroticism, Extraversion, Openness, Agreeableness, and Conscientousness) that they have developed from the ACL, a checklist of 300 adjectives descriptive of personality. John and Roberts plan to make hypotheses on the basis of previous studies that have reported normative personality change on ACL measures in the Mills sample (Helson & Moane, 1987; Helson & Wink, 1992; Wink & Helson, in press). John anticipates that from the early parental to the postparental period, conscientiousness will be found to increase and neuroticism to decrease but that within a broad factor, such as extraversion, different facets may change in different ways. Assertiveness may increase, whereas sociability and activity level may stay the same or decline. This would mean that a level of analysis less inclusive than the Big Five is needed for tracking personality change.

Measuring Secular Trends

It would be fascinating to know how personality has changed over the last 300 years. This is a fantasy, but Gough (1991) has developed a scale of items that show increasing or decreasing endorsement by young people who have taken the CPI over 30 years. Correlates of this Secular Trends Scale indicate that since the 1950s, students have become increasingly tolerant and sophisticated but also increasingly cynical and self-centered, at least until the mid-1980s.

Brent Roberts examined secular trends in the Mills sample. His unpublished data show that the women increased significantly on the Secular Trends Scale from ages 21 to 27 and again from 27 to 43, then declined slightly from 43 to 52, nicely paralleling Gough's (1991) results. Furthermore, Roberts found a tendency ($p < .08$) for the Mills class of 1960 to show more influence of secular trends than the class of 1958. This is interesting because the class of 1960 grew up in larger communities than the class of 1958, went to church less often, and entered Mills College when a curriculum that explicitly emphasized women's traditional interests was being replaced by a modern liberal arts program. I hope that Gough's (1991) scale and perhaps others like it can be used to calibrate the influence of secular trends on samples over recent decades and to help researchers understand the spread and concentration of these effects.

Making Sets of Open-Ended Data Comparable: The California Adult Q-Set (CAQ)

The Q-sort is a superlative tool for comparing longitudinal studies that lack common personality measures but have in common abundant open-ended data. Block (1961/1978, 1971) has shown how the Q-sort can render such data quantifiable so that one can compare and even combine samples.

The Four Faces of Eve

Here is an example of a Q-sort study that demonstrated general features of personality across samples and cohorts. York and John (1992) used 100-item CAQs, which, through the efforts of Wink and others, had been completed on the basis of extensive questionnaire data available for the Mills sample at age 43. They did an inverse factor analysis of these data for 51 women of the Mills class of 1958, replicating it among the 52 women of the class of 1960. On the basis of conceptual analyses of the items most and least descriptive of the different factors, they labeled their types *individuated, conflicted, traditional,* and *assured* because they resembled the types that Rank (1945) conceived as modes of coping with separation and individuation problems. They scored the Mills sample in terms of the empirical types that Block (1971) described among women in the older IHD sample and were able to show a surprising level of congruence between their types and four of Block's six. They took the classifications that Block provided and compared the percentages of matched types in the IHD and Mills samples. IHD had more adapted and conflicted women and fewer individuated women than the later-born and better educated Mills sample.

In the Mills sample, York and John (1992) found a strong relation between their Q-sort types and measures derived from personality inventories. These relationships supported their Rankian hypotheses and also the validity of Q-sorts based on abundant open-ended questionnaire material. York and John are now making a more intensive comparison of the types and their life correlates in the Mills and IHD samples.

More Data, Shorter Instruments

The CAQ requires a considerable amount of diverse data. Observers have to see and preferably interact with the subjects, interviewers have to spend time with them, or there has to be much open-ended material from them in questionnaires. Each Q-sort takes time to do, and there need to be several Q-sorts for each subject to ascertain reliability. These Q-sorts provide marvelous, comprehensive, versatile measures, but there is no quick and easy way to get them. I think many investigators should get more data than they do, but for some purposes researchers need some simpler procedures and perhaps shorter, theoretically derived instruments. For example, there are sets of good questionnaires or delimited interviews available from previous cohorts that do not provide sufficient material for the 100-item Q-sort, but they could be used with appropriate simpler tools.

Q-Sort Prototypes

Jack Block has done a great service in showing how judges can use the Q-sort to describe exemplars (prototypes) of complex personality patterns (such as the narcissist or the individual with achieved or foreclosed identity) in a way that lends itself to quantitative analyses. The use of Q-sort prototypes to study change patterns in longitudinal samples is just beginning (Helson, 1992; Helson & McCabe, in press; Mallory, 1984; Wink, 1992), and its use in comparisons of longitudinal samples is still ahead.

Education, occupation, and a few other demographic variables are the usual means for showing whether it is appropriate to compare samples, or they provide the basis for stratifying samples. Block (1971) objected to the crudity of social class indicators for inferring psychological characteristics, but what else can be used? The idea of the social clock project that I described earlier was one attempt to meet this problem, and the types identified by York and John (1992) is another. The following is a third idea that uses a Q-sort prototype.

Ego-Identity Prototypes

Marcia (1966) derived the concept of ego-identity status from Erikson (1963). He developed an interview to assess four identity statuses: achieved, in moratorium, foreclosed, and diffuse. Classification was based on the patterning of active search and commitment by adolescents, especially in the areas of occupation and values. Marcia's interview was somewhat awkward to use with adults, but Mallory (1984), working with Block, enlisted the aid of researchers who had worked with the concept of ego-identity status to develop Q-sort prototypes for each of the four. Mallory correlated the Q-sorts of individual members of the IHD Oakland Growth and Berkeley Guidance samples with the four ego-identity Q-sort prototypes and used the correlations as scores. She did this for the samples at several different ages and reported patterns of change in ego-identity status over time. Block made these prototypes available to the Mills Study, and similar scores were obtained for the Mills women at age 43.

Although Erikson (1963, 1968) discussed the formation of identity as occurring mainly in adolescence, J. Block (personal communication, August 18, 1992) conceptualizes these identity statuses in terms of a fairly enduring pattern of ego-resilience and ego-control, mixed with a little introspectiveness. One can think of them even more generally as aspects of a self-system that affects the ability to change. In an examination of changes women made in their social clock projects during middle age, Laurel McCabe and I found that in three groups of women (traditionals, singles, and women divorced in early middle age), women classified as achieved or as in moratorium on the basis of file-rater Q-sorts at age 43 made more successful changes in their lives across middle age than did women classified as foreclosed or diffuse (Helson & McCabe, in press). On the basis of the women's accounts of their experiences, we speculated that women who were achieved or in moratorium had more freedom in imagining new possible selves (Markus & Nurius, 1986) than foreclosed women, who leaned toward conformity, or diffuse women, who tended to lack the structure to maintain goals.

In the Mills sample, the largest number of women was classified as achieved, the foreclosed and moratorium groups were about the same, and the diffuse group was much smaller. In the IHD sample, studied by Mallory (1984), the largest group at a comparable age was achieved, but the next largest was foreclosed, and the moratorium and diffuse groups were much smaller. Stratifying on the basis of ego-identity status might improve one's chances of findings similar relationships and meaningful differences across samples.

Different Kinds of Samples to Compare

Ingenious tools can help researchers to make comparisons among longitudinal samples, which are required for showing generality of findings and for addressing questions of cohort, climate, and period. However, good tools can accomplish only so much. Another important consideration is finding appropriate samples to compare.

Sometimes there are two longitudinal samples available for one's purposes. The best known comparison of longitudinal studies is Elder's (1979) use of the Oakland Growth and Berkeley Guidance samples to study the influence of the Great Depression on the lives of individuals who experienced these events at different points in their development. However, one does not always have two longitudinal studies, or not of the type one would like. How else can one study such questions?

Splitting One Longitudinal Sample

Sometimes it is possible to split one longitudinal sample. There is usually the advantage that the same measures are available for all subjects. Stewart and Healy (1989) partitioned the Ginzberg and Associates (1966) and Yohalem (1979) sample of women graduate students who attended Columbia University in the years after World War II. These women, who varied considerably in age, all saw opportunities for women in the labor force during the war, followed by the era of "feminine mystique." Stewart and Healy considered young adulthood to be a particularly important time for the influence of social and political events on lives. They tested some ingenious hypotheses about the different ways that women of three age strata within the sample would combine family and career in the face of apparently contradictory social influences.

Combining Cross-Sectional and Longitudinal Samples

Another substitute for two longitudinal samples is one longitudinal sample and one or more cross-sectional samples. In the Mills study, my colleagues and I (Helson, Mitchell, & Moane, 1984) were aware of the particular cohort of our longitudinal sample, and we wanted to know more about women older and younger. Therefore, in 1983, we inserted a centerfold questionnaire in the Mills alumnae magazine and obtained returns from about 700 alumnae of all ages. These data afford an interesting perspective on some of the topics we have studied. For example, Figure 3 shows what women of various ages remembered as their ideas about future employment when they were in college.

Valory Mitchell and I used the cross-sectional and longitudinal data together in a study of the concept of "prime of life." We began our article (Mitchell & Helson, 1990) by discussing what the prime of life is, whether women have a prime of life, and then bringing forth various arguments that it might be the early 50s. (Note that this study can be considered an attempt to show the characteristics of a period of life.)

Figure 4, based on the large cross-sectional sample, shows our basic finding. The question was, Is this time of your life first-rate, good, fair, or not so good? Women in their early 50s rated their lives more favorably than did other women. We then made two kinds of comparisons. We compared the early 50s (or prime) women with older and younger middle-aged groups on demographic indexes and various measures of interests, problems, and satisfactions. Next, we compared women of the longitudinal sample in their early 50s with themselves in their early 40s.

In the course of those analyses, we were frustrated by the fact that the questionnaire used with the large cross-sectional sample produced measures that were not entirely the same as those available in the lon-

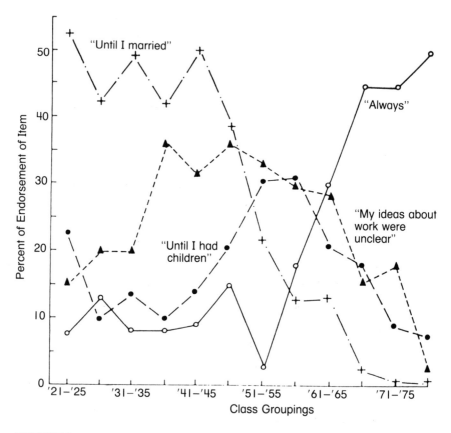

FIGURE 3. Plans for paid work after college as recollected by Mills alumnae of 12 age groups. (Figure is from R. Helson, T. Elliott, & J. Leigh, "Adolescent Personality and Women's Work Patterns." In D. Stern & D. Eichorn (Eds.), *Adolescence and work* (p. 266), 1989, Hillsdale, NJ: Erlbaum. Copyright ©1989 by Lawrence Erlbaum Associates, Inc. Reprinted by permission.)

gitudinal study and that even in the longitudinal study, the measures available for the women in their early 40s were not all the same as those available for them in their early 50s. Nevertheless, women in their early 50s in each sample—cross-sectional and longitudinal—were characterized by the demographic characteristics of living with partners in "empty nests," good health, and high income. Other data showed that they felt fully engaged in life and were more contented and freer of negative affect than women in their early 40s.

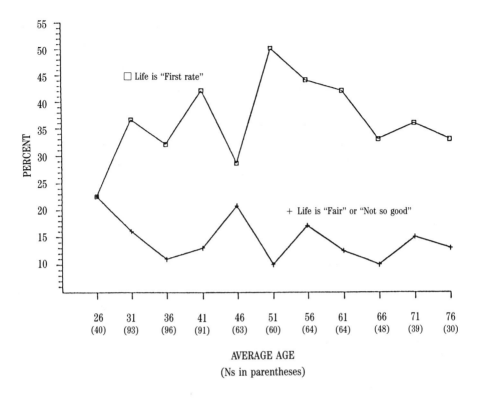

FIGURE 4. Percentages of 688 college alumnae, by age, who rated life as "first-rate," "fair," or "not so good." (Percentages who rated life as "good" are omitted. Figure is from V. Mitchell & R. Helson, "Women's Prime of Life," 1990, *Psychology of Women Quarterly, 14,* p. 456. Copyright ©1990 by Division 35, American Psychological Association. Reprinted by permission.)

Although we faced a deadline that limited our time to digest these data, the study had some nice features. The women in their early 50s in the cross-sectional study were born in the early 1930s and those in the longitudinal study in the late 1930s, about 7 years apart. We offered evidence that the two samples were different enough in their college expectations and in the importance of paid work in their lives to be considered different cohorts. This added impact to our demonstration of a similar prime of life in each.

In the longitudinal sample we were able to show that the CPI Well-Being scale at age 43 predicted quality of life at age 52 but that the multiple correlation rose from .35 to .67 when we also took into account the rating of health at age 52, whether or not the woman lived in a household with her partner only and, to a lesser extent, the status level of her work. Therefore, we conceptualized prime of life as depending on both personality characteristics and a facilitating environment.

There are less elaborate ways to combine cross-sectional and longitudinal samples advantageously. Donahue, Robins, Roberts, and John (in press) were interested in comparing people who described themselves as different in different situations with people who saw themselves as similar across situations. This is a problem that Jack Block investigated in 1961. Donahue et al. did their first study with University of California undergraduates, as Block had done, and then used the Mills sample at age 52 to replicate their strong finding that describing oneself as different in different situations is associated with maladjustment. They showed that self-differentiation (or fragmentation) at age 52 had significant personality correlates back to age 21. Problems in personality and social psychology that researchers study with a short-term focus on the present can take on whole new dimensions of meaning when examined in a longitudinal context.

Ingenuity in the recruitment of contemporary cross-sectional samples can help the older longitudinal studies address contemporary dilemmas. Tomlinson-Keasey and Blurton (1992) found a match for Terman's gifted women at midlife (Terman & Oden, 1959) among members of a local Mensa chapter and parents of gifted children. They also found a sample of nongifted women. The contemporary women were asked some of the same questions that the Terman sample had answered in the 1950s. Contemporary women had achieved more, especially the gifted, and the modern-day gifted were more confident and energetic (well adjusted), but Terman women expressed more satisfaction with their families, marriages, and avocational activities.

Concluding Remarks

I have argued that for the study of lives, personality should be defined, contextualized, and analytically appraised so that stability, continuity, and change in personality can all be evaluated. I have argued that researchers need to compare their longitudinal findings with results in other samples to demonstrate their generality and to understand the influence on personality of factors such as cohort and climate that they now prefer to ignore. I have given illustrations of studies that demonstrate different kinds of personality change and discussed tools and strategies for comparing findings across samples. At several points I have expressed the wish for conceptualizations, measures, and techniques that are lacking. Stewart and Healy (1989) stated that the reason psychologists do not incorporate the individual's social–historical experience into their research is that they lack a conceptual model of how to do it. Stewart and Healy offered several good ideas. One can find other good ideas from the self psychologists, cognitive developmentalists, and those who study personality in situations, as well as from survey researchers, sociologists, anthropologists, historians, and psychobiographers. The need to study subjects in life context argues for interdisciplinary receptiveness (Featherman & Lerner, 1985).

There are many ambiguities and frustrations in measuring change and in comparing samples. There could be nothing less appropriate than offering a tribute to Jack Block that would encourage loose and incompetent research. As Jack Block says in Chapter 2 of this book, "If a line is cast only into the shallow waters of a nearby pond, only little fish will be caught. For the big fish, it is necessary to venture out into deep water." There is certainly a lot of mud and old tires around this place where we researchers are, and we cannot forget them, but maybe they can handle a bigger pond.

References

Block, J. (1961). Ego-identity, role variability, and adjustment. *Journal of Consulting and Clinical Psychology, 25,* 392–397.

Block, J. (1971). *Lives through time.* Berkeley, CA: Bancroft Books.

Block, J. (1978). *The Q-sort method in personality assessment and psychiatric research.* Palo Alto, CA: Consulting Psychologists Press. (Original work published 1961)

Block, J. (1981). Some enduring and consequential structures of personality. In A. I. Rabin, J. Aronoff, A. M. Barclay, & R. A. Zucker (Eds.), *Further explorations in personality* (pp. 27–43). New York: Wiley.

Block, J., Block, J. H., & Keyes, S. (1988). Longitudinally foretelling drug usage in adolescence: Early childhood personality and environmental precursors. *Child Development, 59,* 336–355.

Block, J. H., Block, J., & Gjerde, P. F. (1986). The personality of children prior to divorce: A prospective study. *Child Development, 57,* 827–840.

Cantor, N., & Kihlstrom, J. (1987). *Personality and social intelligence.* Englewood Cliffs, NJ: Prentice-Hall.

Caspi, A. (1987). Personality and the life course. *Journal of Personality and Social Psychology, 53,* 1203–1213.

Caspi, A., & Bem, D. J. (1990). Personality continuity and change across the life course. In L. A. Pervin (Ed.), *Handbook of personality theory and research* (pp. 549–575). New York: Guilford Press.

Caspi, A., Bem, D. J., & Elder, G. H., Jr. (1989). Continuities and consequences of interactional styles across the life course. *Journal of Personality, 57,* 375–406.

Clausen, J. A., & Gilens, M. (1990). Personality and labor force participation across the life course: A longitudinal study of women's careers. *Sociological Forum, 5,* 595–618.

Conley, J. J. (1984). Longitudinal consistency of personality: Self-reported psychological characteristics across 45 years. *Journal of Personality and Social Psychology, 47,* 1325–1333.

Conley, J. J. (1985). A personality theory of adulthood and aging. In R. Hogan & W. H. Jones (Eds.), *Perspectives in personality* (Vol. 1, pp. 81–116). Greenwich, CT: JAI Press.

Costa, P. T., & McCrae, R. R. (1980). Still stable after all these years: Personality as a key to some issues in aging. In P. B. Baltes & O. G. Brim (Eds.), *Life-span development and behavior* (Vol. 3, pp. 65–102). San Diego, CA: Academic Press.

Costa, P. T., & McCrae, R. R. (1988). Personality in adulthood: A six-year longitudinal study of self-reports and spouse ratings on the NEO Personality Inventory. *Journal of Personality and Social Psychology, 54,* 853–863.

Donahue, E. M., Robins, R. W., Roberts, B. W., & John, O. P. (in press). Divided we fall: Self-concept differentiation, personality, and psychological adjustment. *Journal of Personality and Social Psychology.*

Elder, G. H. (1979). Historical change in life patterns and in personality. In P. B. Baltes & O. G. Brim (Eds.), *Life-span development and behavior* (Vol. 2, pp. 117–159). San Diego, CA: Academic Press.

Epstein, S. (1990). Cognitive-experiential self-theory. In L. A. Pervin (Ed.), *Handbook of personality theory and research* (pp. 165–192). New York: Guilford Press.

Erikson, E. (1963). *Childhood and society.* New York: Norton.

Erikson, E. (1968). *Identity: Youth and crisis.* New York: Norton.

Featherman, D. L., & Lerner, R. M. (1985). Ontogenesis and sociogenesis: Problematics for theory and research about development and socialization across the lifespan. *American Sociological Review, 50,* 659–676.

Gergen, K. J. (1980). The emerging crisis in life-span developmental theory. In P. B. Baltes & O. G. Brim, Jr. (Eds.), *Life-span development and behavior* (Vol. 3, pp. 32–63). San Diego, CA: Academic Press.

Ginzberg, E., & Associates. (1966). *Lifestyles of educated American women.* New York: Columbia University Press.

Gough, H. G. (1987). *Manual for the California Psychological Inventory.* Palo Alto, CA: Consulting Psychologists Press. (Original work published 1957)

Gough, H. G. (1991, August). *Scales and combinations of scales: What do they tell us, what do they mean?* Paper presented at the 99th Annual Convention of the American Psychological Association, San Francisco.

Gough, H. G., & Heilbrun, A. B., Jr. (1983). *The Adjective Check List manual: 1980 edition.* Palo Alto, CA: Consulting Psychologists Press.

Greenwald, A. G. (1980). The totalitarian ego: Fabrication and revision of personal history. *American Psychologist, 35,* 603–618.

Gutmann, D. L. (1987). *Reclaimed powers: Toward a new psychology of men and women in later life.* New York: Basic Books.

Helson, R. (1967). Personality characteristics and developmental history of creative college women. *Genetic Psychology Monographs, 76,* 205–256.

Helson, R. (1992). Women's difficult times and the rewriting of the life story. *Psychology of Women Quarterly, 16,* 331–347.

Helson, R., Elliott, T., & Leigh, J. (1990). Number and quality of roles: A longitudinal personality view. *Psychology of Women Quarterly, 14,* 83–101.

Helson, R., & McCabe, L. (in press). The social clock in middle age. In B. Turner & L. Troll (Eds.), *Growing older female: Theoretical perspectives in the psychology of aging.* Newbury Park, CA: Sage.

Helson, R., Mitchell, V., & Moane, G. (1984). Personality and patterns of adherence and nonadherence to the social clock. *Journal of Personality and Social Psychology, 46,* 1079–1096.

Helson, R., & Moane, G. (1987). Personality change in women from college to midlife. *Journal of Personality and Social Psychology, 53,* 176–186.

Helson, R., & Picano, J. (1990). Is the traditional role bad for women? *Journal of Personality and Social Psychology, 59,* 311–320.

Helson, R., & Wink, P. (1992). Personality change in women from the early 40s to the early 50s. *Psychology and Aging, 7,* 46–55.

Howard, A., & Bray, D. (1988). *Managerial lives in transition: Advancing age and changing times.* New York: Guilford Press.

Hulbert, K. D., & Schuster, D. T. (1993). *Women's lives through time: Educated American women of the twentieth century.* San Francisco: Jossey-Bass.

Jung, C. G. (1960). The stages of life. In H. Read, M. Fordham, & G. Adler (Eds.), *Collected works* (Vol. 8, pp. 387–403). Princeton, NJ: Princeton University Press. (Original work published 1931)

Kimmel, D. C. (1974). Personality processes and psychopathology. In *Adulthood and aging* (pp. 289–314). New York: Wiley.

Kogan, N. (1990). Personality and aging. In J. E. Birren & S. W. Schaie (Eds.), *Handbook of the psychology of aging* (pp. 330–346). San Diego, CA: Academic Press.

Mallory, M. E. (1984). Longitudinal analysis of ego-identity status (Doctoral dissertation, University of California, Davis, 1983). *Dissertation Abstracts International, 44,* 3955-B.

Marcia, J. E. (1966). Development and validation of ego-identity status. *Journal of Personality and Social Psychology, 3,* 551–558.

Markus, H., & Nurius, P. (1986). Possible selves. *American Psychologist, 41,* 954–969.

McCrae, R. R., & Costa, P. T., Jr. (1990). *Personality in adulthood.* New York: Guilford Press.

Mischel, W. (1968). *Personality and assessment.* New York: Wiley.

Mitchell, V., & Helson, R. (1990). Women's prime of life: Is it the 50s? *Psychology of Women Quarterly, 14,* 451–470.

Nesselroade, J. R. (1991). Interindividual differences in intraindividual change. In L. M. Collins & J. L. Horn (Eds.), *Best methods for the analysis of change* (pp. 92–105). Washington, DC: American Psychological Association.

Neugarten, B. L. (1977). Personality and aging. In J. E. Birren & K. W. Schaie (Eds.), *Handbook of the psychology of aging* (pp. 626–649). New York: Van Nostrand Reinhold.

Neugarten, B. L., & Gutmann, D. L. (1958). Age–sex roles and personality in middle age: A thematic apperception study. *Psychological Monographs, 72* (Whole No. 470).

Rank, O. (1945). *Will therapy and truth and reality.* New York: Knopf.

Roberts, B. (1992). [Secular trends in the Mills sample]. Unpublished raw data.

Schaie, K. W. (1965). A general model for the study of developmental problems. *Psychological Bulletin, 64,* 92–107.

Schaie, K. W. (1979). The primary mental abilities in adulthood: An exploration in the development of psychometric intelligence. In P. B. Baltes & O. G. Brim (Eds.), *Life-span development and behavior* (Vol. 2, pp. 68–115). San Diego, CA: Academic Press.

Stewart, A. J., & Healy, J. M., Jr. (1989). Linking individual development and social changes. *American Psychologist, 44,* 30–42.

Stewart, A. J., Vandewater, E. A., Landman, J., & Malley, J. E. (1992). *Recognizing the limitations of one's own past: Motivations for change in women's lives.* Unpublished manuscript.

Swann, W. B. (1987). Identity negotiations: Where two roads meet. *Journal of Personality and Social Psychology, 53,* 1038–1051.

Terman, L. M., & Oden, M. H. (1959). *Genetic studies of genius: Vol. 5. The gifted group at midlife.* Stanford, CA: Stanford University Press.

Tomlinson-Keasy, C., & Blurton, E. U. (1992). *Aspirations, achievements, satisfaction and personal adjustment of women in the 1950s and 1980s.* Unpublished manuscript.

Wells, L. E., & Stryker, S. (1988). Stability and change in self over the life course. In P. B. Baltes, D. Featherman, & R. Lerner (Eds.), *Life-span development and behavior* (Vol. 8, pp. 192–224). Hillsdale, NJ: Erlbaum.

Wink, P. (1991). Self- and object-directedness in adult women. *Journal of Personality, 59,* 769–791.

Wink, P. (1992). Three types of narcissism in women from college to midlife. *Journal of Personality, 60,* 7–30.

Wink, P., & Helson, R. (in press). Personality change in women and their partners. *Journal of Personality and Social Psychology.*

Yohalem, A. M. (1979). *The careers of professional women: Commitment and conflict.* Montclair, NJ: Allanheld, Osmun.

York, K., & John, O. P. (1992). The four faces of Eve: A typological analysis of women's personality at midlife. *Journal of Personality and Social Psychology, 63,* 494–508.

CHAPTER 6

Judgments as Data for Personality and Developmental Psychology: Error Versus Accuracy

David C. Funder

Introduction: Judgments as Data

If data are no good, then theorizing based on those data cannot be any good either. For this reason, an important part of every science is the invention, construction, and validation of data-gathering tools. In many fields of research, these are instruments such as scales, electron microscopes, or sonographs. In all fields, the construction of these instruments must be meticulous and the process of validating the relationship between the data they provide and the underlying reality they seek to measure must be ongoing.

This research was supported by National Institute of Mental Health Grant R01-MH42427. Steve Reise provided valuable statistical advice. A reviewer of a draft of this chapter provided other helpful advice.

The human judge has long been an important data-gathering tool for personality psychology in general and longitudinal research on personality development in particular. In the typical application, a judge becomes acquainted with a subject, watches a subject's behavior, or peruses a file of information about the subject and then renders judgments of various personality attributes. A widely used technique, the California Q-Sort, requires the judge to rate 100 attributes such as "Is critical, skeptical, not easily impressed," "Has a wide range of interests," and "Is a genuinely dependable and responsible person" (J. Block, 1961/1978). Judgments such as these have contributed greatly to the landmark longitudinal data set of Jack and Jeanne Block (e.g., J. Block, 1971; J. H. Block & Block, 1980) and the numerous related research endeavors of the Blocks and their collaborators, discussed elsewhere in this book.

As an instrument for gathering data, the human judge has some attributes that are peculiar and other attributes that are not peculiar at all. Peculiar attributes of the human judge include the way the distinction between the source of data and the person who reads the data can become blurred and the way that many sources of bias possible with a human judge are different from those associated with more mechanical measurement devices. A nonpeculiar attribute is that the same considerations of precision, calibration, and fidelity to underlying reality come into play for human judgments of personality as for the output of any measuring device. A cardinal rule prevails: If the data are not valid, then the science built on those data is in deep trouble.

It is no wonder, then, that many personality and developmental psychologists have spent much of the past 25 years casting frequent anxious glances over their shoulders. Their fundamental source of data has been under strong and unrelenting attack for at least that long. A major theme of the psychological literature for 25 years or so has been that human judgment is fundamentally flawed and that judgments of *personality* are especially flawed (for a prototypical example of this point of view, see Ross, 1977).

It was into this unencouraging *zeitgeist* that I launched my own research career as a graduate student at Stanford about 15 years ago. Its influence was not slow to reach me. One of the first studies I ever conducted was an examination of correlations between parents' assessments of their children's personalities (rendered through the California Child Q-Set, or CCQ) and an experimental measure of the children's delay of gratification. The study yielded a good number of sizable correlations, and these correlations seemed to provide important information about the psychological properties of our experimental situation (see Bem & Funder, 1978, Study 1).

In some quarters, these findings were greeted with skepticism if not outright incredulity. The basis of this not-uncommon reaction was the source of my data: How could one possibly find out anything valid about one's subjects using mere judgments, some colleagues wished to know, when just down the hall at Stanford, Lee Ross, and elsewhere in the country luminaries such as Richard Nisbett, Daniel Kahneman, and Amos Tversky were so successfully demonstrating the numerous (and I quote) "shortcomings" of the intuitive psychologist (Ross, 1977)?

Over time I have managed to generate two answers to this question. The first is that the numerous meaningful and converging psychological findings yielded by research that uses personality judgments provide ample, albeit indirect, testimony to what must be their validity (Kenrick & Funder, 1988).

The second answer confronts the accuracy issue a little more directly. I have sometimes argued that despite its discouraging tone, the vast literature on error in human judgment says nothing, or next to nothing, about accuracy and in particular *cannot* be taken to indicate that, as a general rule, judgments of personality are inaccurate (Funder, 1987). Moreover, in more recent years, I have come to the conclusion that judgmental accuracy can be meaningfully addressed through research but that the appropriate paradigm is fundamentally different from the one typically used to study error.

The purpose of this chapter is to elaborate and update this second argument—to describe why the study of error is not relevant to evaluations of judgmental accuracy and to describe the kind of research that is relevant to accuracy concerns. In this chapter I summarize some recent results of my own research on accuracy in personality judgment, make suggestions for the future, and discuss some implications of current research for the use of human judgment in personality and developmental psychology.

DAVID C. FUNDER

Accuracy Versus Error

There is something ironic about the way that research on error in personality judgment became widely influential at just about the time that social psychologists had largely given up on studying accuracy. Consider this quote from an authoritative textbook published in 1979:

> The accuracy issue has all but faded from view in recent years, at least for personality judgments. There is not much present interest in questions about whether people are accurate or about what kinds of people are accurate. There is, in short, almost no concern with normative questions of accuracy. On the other hand, in recent years there has been renewed interest in how, why, and in what circumstances people are inaccurate. (Schneider, Hastorf, & Ellsworth, 1979, p. 224)

Two observations can be made about this historically important paragraph. The first is that it quite correctly reflects an attitude about accuracy research that was widespread at the time and that remains held by some psychologists to this day. The attitude is that there is something fishy about the whole topic of accuracy and maybe even the very word: Everybody knows accuracy in personality judgment does not exist and that, at best, there are no criteria by which one could ever show that it does; therefore, nothing useful can be said about accuracy and social psychologists are much better off concentrating on studies of the *process* of judgment that, as Jones (1985) has pointed out, "[solve] the accuracy problem by bypassing it" (p. 87).

The second observation is that the last two sentences of the paragraph just quoted can reasonably strike one as being mutually contradictory. Years ago, a bright undergraduate asked me to explain how research could possibly "ignore normative questions of accuracy" at the same time it showed "renewed interest in how ... people are inaccurate." I am sure my answer was incoherent and unconvincing; in truth, I did not understand that passage either.

In the years since, however, I think I have come to understand and now believe that Schneider et al. (1979) were exactly correct (albeit somewhat cryptic). The student's question goes to the heart of a fundamental limitation of the paradigm on which research on error is based.

Schneider et al. were *correct* to imply that research on judgmental error is largely irrelevant to evaluations of judgmental accuracy, despite the seeming paradox. The reason is that there is a large middle ground between perfect accuracy and complete error. Although the literature on error indeed shows human judgment to be *imperfect*, it falls far short of establishing that human judgment is *usually* or even *often* incorrect. In the next section of this chapter, I attempt to explain why.

The Error Paradigm

The term *error paradigm* refers to a style of research that dominated the study of judgment in general and personality judgment in particular during most of the 1980s and remains prominent, although (perhaps) dwindling slowly in influence, to this day. Daniel Kahneman and Amos Tversky (e.g., 1973) published a large amount of influential research intended to document general errors in judgment and decision making. Richard Nisbett and Lee Ross soon translated this work, rather directly, into research more specifically aimed at errors in interpersonal judgment (e.g., Nisbett & Ross, 1980; Ross & Nisbett, 1991). Both sets of investigators inspired a sizable cadre of other researchers, and the psychological literature on judgmental error became quite large.

For more than a decade, this research on error enjoyed what could only be described as wild success. As just one indication, Lee Ross's (1977) chapter on the shortcomings of the intuitive psychologist was the most widely cited article in social psychology during the 1980s (Ross & Nisbett, 1991). Moreover, the influence of this literature can easily be found throughout psychology. For instance, in a recent review of a book on cognitive science, a reviewer stated the following:

> Considering what we know about the foibles of human judgment, how will the hapless judge be able to differentiate between communicative patterns of a real person and even a poor imitation? . . . The last four decades of research in cognitive psychology suggest that a human judge could be easily fooled. (Shaklee, 1991, p. 941)

One could find equivalent comments in many issues of many journals. I use this one only as a typical illustration of the way psychologists in fields removed from research on error have incorporated that research into their thinking—in this case, into a belief that most people would be unable to distinguish the speech production of a human being from that of a computer simulation, even a "poor" simulation. This seems a remarkable (and dubious) conclusion, but it stems naturally from the widespread habit of describing human judgment as being beset by numerous "foibles," as being "easily fooled" or even "hapless," and so forth (Lopes, 1991). Research on error has been amazingly influential and has led psychologists across the entire field to draw conclusions that—like the one presented earlier—seem otherwise unlikely yet are potentially consequential.

Other psychologists, perhaps those with a contrarious bent and including myself, are slower to draw these sorts of conclusions. Personality dispositions (such as contrariousness) aside, there are three reasons for being less than completely persuaded by the fundamental message of research on error: the evidence, the implications, and the tone.

The Evidence

Of course, it would be beyond the scope of this chapter to even begin to review the thousands of studies generated by the error paradigm. Instead, I attempt to characterize these studies with a demonstration and two examples.

Count the Fingers

The demonstration can be a Gedanken experiment, or you can try it on your friends (or students). I first saw it done by Robert Zajonc. It goes like this: Ask your audience to tell you how many fingers you are holding up, and then raise one finger at a time, slowly, while your audience counts to 10. When you are holding out all 10 fingers, ask, "Quickly now, how many fingers in *10* hands?" In my experience, about 80% of any audience (even one primed to expect a trick) will call out "100." Only about 20% will give the alternative (and putatively correct) answer, which is 50.

What can be made of this little demonstration? I would argue that if this trick were an experiment on error in judgment, it would probably be used to show that people cannot multiply 5×10. Of course, this demonstration actually shows something else entirely: Communication between trickster and tricked, or (in many cases a close analogy) between experimenter and subject, proceeds on multiple channels. Subjects can seem to be misled when, in violation of conversational ethics, the messages on different channels are contradictory. (It also demonstrates the fun to be had in fooling one's audience, perhaps a nontrivial attraction of the error paradigm; see Crandall, 1984).

In the demonstration just described, *two* messages, not one, were actually sent. The auditory channel asked, "How many fingers in 10 hands?" The correct answer here is indeed 50. But the nonverbal channel, an important manner of communication in its own right, asked, "How many fingers in 10 of these?" (two hands being held up). Now, the correct answer is 100. Therefore, I always tell those few in the audience who answered 50 not to be so smug. The minority is right, and the majority wrong, only if one presumes for some reason that the verbal channel has precedence over the nonverbal channel. And why should it?

This demonstration encapsulates much of my critique of the error paradigm. It illustrates the way experimenters often draw inappropriate conclusions from subjects' responses to situations that were deliberately designed to fool them. It illustrates how experimenters often send contradictory messages on different channels, then claim that it is right to respond to one channel and wrong to respond to the other. It also illustrates the way experimenters often violate conversational ethics (Grice, 1975): by sending contradictory instead of complementary messages on different channels and by providing information that is "uncooperative" in the sense of being irrelevant if not deliberately misleading.

Overattribution

Now consider two actual examples from the judgment literature (for others, see Funder, 1987). The first is one of the pioneer studies of error in social judgment and perhaps still the most widely cited, the demonstration of "overattribution" by Jones and Harris (1967). In that study, subjects were given essays to read that either favored or opposed the regime of Fidel Castro. Some subjects were told that the essays were written by individuals who had free choice as to what position to take (the "choice" condition). Other subjects were told that the position expressed in the essays had been assigned to the writers (the "no-choice" condition). Subjects were then asked to estimate the writer's "true attitude toward Castro" (Jones & Harris, 1967, p. 5) on a scale in which higher numbers reflected a more pro-Castro position. The results are reproduced in Table 1.

The result that has been emphasized over the years is that the two numbers in the right-hand column of this table are not exactly equal. As Jones and Harris (1967) put it, "perhaps the most striking result of the first experiment was the tendency to attribute correspondence between behavior and private attitude even when the direction of the essay was assigned ... their tendency ... would seem to reflect incomplete or distorted reasoning" (p. 7).

A couple of other aspects of this study have received less attention over the years. The first is that *all* of the pairwise comparisons in Table 1 were in fact statistically significant; in particular, stronger attitudes were attributed in the choice than the no-choice conditions for both the pro- and anti-Castro essays (59.6 was significantly greater than 44.1 and 17.4 was significantly less than 22.9, both at the .01 level). Thus, it was *not* the case that subjects ignored the choice information; they moderated their judgments substantially when told of the duress under which the essay writers performed.

This observation leads to a finer recognition of what the subjects were guilty of, exactly. As just shown, they were not guilty of ignoring the choice manipulation; it affected their judgments to a significant degree.

TABLE 1

Imputed Attitudes Toward Castro in Jones and Harris (1967)

	Condition	
Attitude expressed	Choice	No choice
Pro-Castro	59.6	44.1
Anti-Castro	17.4	22.9

Note. Higher numbers reflect a more "pro-Castro" position imputed to the essay writer. All pairwise comparisons are statistically significant ($p < .01$). This table was adapted from Jones and Harris (1967).

What they were guilty of was of *not* ignoring the attitude manipulation. That is, the two numbers in the right-hand column of Table 1 would have had to be exactly equal for Jones and Harris (and two decades of secondary referencers) to impute anything but error to the subjects' judgments. To achieve this equality, subjects would have had to ignore the most prominent stimulus in the experiment, the essay whose writer they were asked (based on little other information) to judge. In which case, the subjects could well have asked, Why was this essay provided in the first place?

Here is the sense in which this experiment, like so many others that came later in the error paradigm, sends two messages to subjects at the same time and is a little like the finger-counting demonstration. Subjects are provided a prominent and vivid stimulus—like the essay, or like the two hands being held up—and are asked to make a judgment. Subjects are then judged to be in error to the degree their judgments fail to ignore this stimulus.

Behavioral Prediction

To avoid being accused of picking on research that is nearly 25 years old, I offer as a second example a more recent study by Kunda and Nisbett (1986), which was summarized in some detail by Ross and Nisbett (1991). In that study, subjects were asked questions such as the following:

> Suppose you observed Jane and Jill in a particular situation and found that Jane was more honest than Jill. What do you suppose is the probability that in the next situation in which you observe them you would also find Jane to be more honest than Jill? (Kunda & Nisbett, 1986, p. 210)

It turns out that the average answer subjects gave to this sort of question was "78%," an answer the authors calculated was equivalent to predicting a behavioral consistency correlation of .80. This result, according to Ross and Nisbett (1991, p. 124), shows how people "dramatically overestimate" behavioral consistency because empirical research obtains consistency correlations that are much lower (they specifically cited Hartshorne & May, 1928, as the source of their authoritative estimate of actual consistency). This is a fairly routine example of the kind of evidence used in recent years to demonstrate flawed human judgment, particularly as it involves dispositional inference.

There are a number of problems with this evidence. First, a relatively technical point: Kunda and Nisbett's (1986) claim that the 78% figure corresponds to a subject-estimated cross-situational consistency correlation of .80 stems from a complex derivation that goes from probability to Kendall's tau to Spearman's *rho*. A simpler calculation yields a different figure. One can chart the situation described in the previous paragraph in the manner shown in Table 2.

Table 2 illustrates subjects' predictions that 78 out of 100 "Janes" who were more honest than "Jill" at Time 1 would also be more honest at Time 2. This setup is equivalent to Rosenthal and Rubin's (1982) binominal effect size display, and a simple calculation using the formula for the phi coefficient yields a correlation of .56 rather than .80, a substantial difference.[1]

Even this correlation is one that Ross and Nisbett (1991) would surely claim is much too high given what they claim is an established empirical limit of .30 for behavioral consistency. However, the .30 estimate is derived from studies of single behavioral acts and not particularly modern studies at that (e.g., Hartshorne & May, 1928). A more recent study by Funder and Colvin (1991) examined the cross-situational consistency of behaviors at a more general level of analysis, a level similar to that of the (otherwise unspecified) "honesty" in Kunda and Nisbett's (1986) stimulus paragraph. Funder and Colvin found that numerous behaviors at that level of analysis could manifest cross-situational corre-

---

[1] The difference between these two figures hinges on whether one prefers to translate the subjects' average subjective probability of 78% into Kendall's tau or Spearman's *rho*, with the former yielding .56 and the latter, preferred by Kunda and Nisbett (1986), yielding .80. Hayes (1973, pp. 788–794) presented a detailed discussion of the difference between these two statistics, describing them as highly correlated with each other but "not identical" (p. 792). The crux of the difference is that as a measure of correlation "Spearman's *rho* places somewhat different weights on *particular* inversions in order, whereas in *tau* all inversions are weighted equally by a simple frequency count" (Hayes, 1973, p. 793). This difference may be arcane at best, although the conversion from lay probability judgments to tau (or its equivalent via the binomial effect size display) seems the more straightforward. It is interesting that Kunda and Nisbett (1986) preferred the more complex statistic that yields a higher estimate of association and therefore a larger imputed error.

TABLE 2

Binomial Conversion of Kunda and Nisbett's (1986) Prediction Problem

Time 1	Time 2		Total
	More honest	Less honest	
More honest	78	22	100
Less honest	22	78	100
Total	100	100	200

Note. This is a tabular representation of subjects' responses to the prediction problem posed by Kunda and Nisbett (1986). Although Kunda and Nisbett claimed that these responses yielded an implied correlation coefficient of .80, by the method of Rosenthal and Rubin (1982), they yielded a correlation of .56.

lations of .60 and even higher. Thus, it is not at all clear that, compared with recent and relevant research, a .56 estimate for the consistency of a general behavior such as honesty is in fact excessively high.

Moreover, the alternative calculation shown in Table 2 exemplifies a more general point, which is that in many demonstrations of judgmental error, a great deal depends on exactly how one construes the problem that is posed to subjects and even exactly how one calculates the statistics used to reflect and evaluate their judgments. In the present case, highly different correct answers can be derived depending on exactly how one interprets vague terms such as *behavior, situation,* and *probability* (and depending even on the specific formula used to calculate this last term). What error researchers typically do, however, is choose one particular interpretation of the stimulus problem and therefore one particular answer, and then chastise subjects for being wrong to the extent that their answers do not exactly match.

A final observation is that studies of error, like the one just described, typically restrict subjects' responses. Wright and Mischel (1988) have shown that when given the opportunity, subjects were eager to qualify behavioral predictions with conditional hedges that specified the particular circumstances under which they would and would not expect a person to manifest the behavior in question. Kunda and Nisbett's (1986) subjects were not afforded this opportunity; they could mark only a Likert scale, remain otherwise silent, and then be criticized for making too strong and unqualified of a prediction.[2]

Of course, the demonstration and two studies just reviewed far from exhaust the literature on judgmental error. However, I claim that they are reasonably representative of the literature as a whole and are sufficient to lead one to conclude that the many studies that claim to have detected flaws in human judgment themselves deserve to be examined with a critical eye.

The Implications

Some of the implications of the error paradigm seem as disturbing as the evidence. The most obvious implication, and the one that has been most widely influential, is that people are poor judges of much of anything. This widely publicized and highly influential conclusion yields a depressing view of human nature that some might find counterintuitive, offensive, or even dangerous.

Even if one does not share those negative reactions, it is still important to note that the widespread characterization of human judgment as being generally "poor" (or even "hapless"; see Shaklee, 1991) is vague at best. Any characterization of the general quality of human judgment (or of anything else) requires a standard of comparison, and within the error paradigm a standard is seldom explicitly stated. Its typical characterization of judgment as poor would seem to imply that judgment fails to attain even some basic (although unspecified) level of functioning. But, ironically, the actual standard that research on error typically uses is *perfection:* To the degree any experimentally rendered judgment fails to match a normative prescription *exactly*, it will be dubbed *erroneous*. (The Jones & Harris, 1967, study discussed earlier provides just one example.) In this light, characterizations of judgment as poor or hapless lose much of their force. Perhaps one should eschew the insults for a while and get on with the business of ascertaining when judgment is and is not likely to be accurate. I return to this point later.

[2]Reid Hastie first brought this point to my attention.

A more particular implication of research on error is that the way to improve human judgment is to train human judges to make fewer errors. This implication will be untrue to the extent that laboratory-based errors demonstrate processes that are adaptive in real life. In an earlier article (Funder, 1987), I discussed as an analogy the study of errors in visual perception. Visual illusions are numerous and often quite striking, but they seldom are taken as evidence that people cannot see. Instead, they are used to demonstrate the workings of general processes of vision that under normal, nonexperimental circumstances produce valid perceptions. Certainly, nobody seriously suggests that if airline pilots could be trained out of susceptibility to the visual "Ponzo" illusion, for instance, air travel would become safer. Indeed, pilots with such training would be likely to fly their planes into the ground! Similarly, it is far from clear that training subjects not to make the kind of errors demonstrated in laboratory settings will make their judgments in real life more accurate. The few studies that have tried have generally obtained the reverse effect (e.g., Borman, 1975).

The problem here is that researchers understand too little about how subjects make judgments that are *accurate* to the extent that they are. This is more than a matter of emphasis. If researchers do not understand how something works, they are ill-prepared and perhaps ill-advised to try to improve it. Training people not to commit the kinds of errors demonstrated in laboratory experiments may be about as likely to improve the quality of their judgments as moving wires around at random inside one's television set is to improve the quality of its picture.

Another problematic implication of error research is the way that it "blames the victim," to borrow a phrase from sociology. Repeatedly in the error literature one sees the assumption, sometimes explicit and sometimes implicit, that errors happen because subjects (people) are inept, not because the information provided for their judgments was insufficient, ambiguous, misleading, or deliberately deceptive. Indeed, with regard to the last point, it is remarkable how many demonstrations of error are deception experiments: Subjects often are told outright lies (e.g., "This pro-Castro essay was written by a North Carolina high school student" or "This real subject was observed to be honest"), and then their naive judgments of these deliberately deceptive stimuli are adjudged to be erroneous.

The problem with this implication goes beyond the injustice of the accusation. By blaming subjects for making errors, the error paradigm implies that the way to improve human judgment is to improve the judge. What about improving the information to the judge? In the error paradigm, this alternative possibility remains unexamined.

A final implication of error research is that extraordinary efforts should be made to inform judges that they are likely to be wrong. As Evans (1984) claimed, "it is much more important to know when they [decision makers] are not [accurate].... Surely, the imperative message for us to impart to decision makers is that of their proneness to error" (pp. 1500–1501).

The idea seems to be that such a message at least cannot hurt; making people doubtful will get them to slow down and consider their decisions more deliberately, leading them to be more accurate. However, Bandura (1989) pointed out how such a strategy has its own dangers; too little confidence can be as harmful as too much:

> People who believe strongly in their problem-solving capabilities remain highly efficient in their analytic thinking in complex decision-making situations, whereas those who are plagued by self doubts are erratic in their analytic thinking. Quality of analytic thinking, in turn, affects performance accomplishments. (p. 1176)

The average human judge, Bandura (1989) seemed to imply, should be prevented from reading the error literature.

The Tone

This last aspect of the error paradigm is the most subjective but possibly important nonetheless. The tone of much research on error is captured in a string of direct quotes from the Ross and Nisbett (1991) book that I recently reviewed (Funder, 1992, p. 319):

> "Laypeople" are "guilty" of being "naive" (p. 119), "oblivious" (p. 124), and "insensitive." They also suffer from "ignorance" (p. 69), "lack of awareness" (p. 82), "dramatic ... overconfidence," "general misconcep-

tions," and a "whole range" of other "shortcomings and biases" (p. 86), so it is no wonder they "fail to recognize" (p. 85) the real causes of behavior. The only question left: "How could people be so wrong?" (p. 139)

This is remarkable language for psychologists to use in scientific writing. Moreover, this language expresses a view of the human judge that is fundamentally misleading because it ignores the many accomplishments (e.g., pattern recognition) that psychologists do not understand and cannot duplicate with any sort of formal model, let alone a "normative" formal model.

It is revealing to note that psychologists who work in the field of computerized artificial intelligence (AI) never use the pejorative language of error. AI psychologists have set themselves the task of setting up artificial, formal systems that can duplicate the achievements of human perception and thought. Most have found their work to be profoundly humbling. They have come to be deeply impressed by the human mind's massively parallel systems for pattern recognition and judgment that can function under ambiguous and shifting circumstances, and the last thing they are tempted to do is to insult these systems (see Lopes & Oden, in press). Rather, they are attempting to understand, a piece at a time, how these systems manage to function at all.

My own research on accuracy in human social judgment is far different from the AI tradition. However, it shares the same goal: to try to understand what people *can* do, when they can do it, and, ultimately, how they can do it.

The Accuracy Paradigm

The study of accuracy differs from the study of error in several fundamental ways. Instead of asking subjects to judge stimuli that are artificial and arbitrary, accuracy research asks subjects to make judgments of real individuals, often close acquaintances. Instead of deliberately deceiving subjects, accuracy research provides subjects information in a direct and honest manner. In addition, instead of searching for instances of what people *cannot* do, accuracy research tries to show what people *can* accomplish with their judgmental abilities.

The model that underlies my own research is fundamentally simple. First, a group of real people (typically undergraduate, real people), who usually are actually acquainted, make judgments of each other's personalities. Then, I and the others in my laboratory gather the best evidence we can to help us decide the degree to which these judgments are right or wrong. The evidence is of two types. The first type is interjudge agreement, either among acquaintances or between acquaintances and the subjects they judge. The assumption is that judgments that agree with each other are more likely to be accurate than judgments that disagree (Funder & Colvin, 1988; Funder & Dobroth, 1987). The second type of evidence is behavioral prediction. We observe subjects' behavior in laboratory situations, have them complete diary and "beeper" measures of behavior, and then attempt to predict these behavioral measures from personality descriptions provided by the subjects' acquaintances (as well as by the subjects themselves;) (Colvin & Funder, 1991; Funder & Colvin, 1991; Funder, Kolar, & Colvin, 1992). The presumption here is that personality judgments that can be used to predict behavior are more likely to be accurate than judgments that fail to demonstrate predictive validity.

A Brunswikian Framework

The research on accuracy can be located within a Brunswikian framework (see Figure 1). According to Egon Brunswik's "lens model" (Brunswik, 1956; see also Hammond, 1966), the study of judgmental accuracy can be

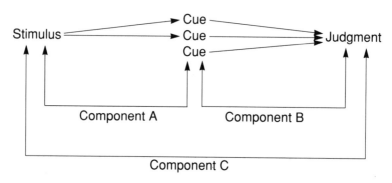

FIGURE 1.   Components of the Brunswik "lens model" applied to person perception. From E. Brunswik (1956). Reprinted with permission.

organized in terms of three components or relationships. The first component (labeled *A* in the figure) is the relationship between actual properties of the stimulus that is judged and the cues that it gives off. For example, an object of visual perception gives off various cues in the light array that are informative as to its physical structure, and an object of social perception (a person) may act in certain ways or give off nonverbal cues as to his or her personality. The second component (*B*) is the relationship between the various cues in the environment, whether diagnostic of the stimulus or not, and the judgments that subjects ultimately render. The third component (*C*), which is in a sense the sum of the first two, is the relationship between attributes of stimulus objects or people, on the one hand, and judgments made of those objects or people, on the other hand.

Historically, the psychological study of interpersonal judgment (sometimes called "person perception") has focused nearly exclusively on Component B. The typical social psychological study of person perception provides subjects with *artificial* stimuli (e.g., a list of trait terms, a paragraph about a hypothetical person) that are manipulated experimentally and arbitrarily. Error research falls in this category, but so does the mass of other studies surveyed in classic texts such as the one by Schneider et al. (1979).

Such research does show how people would, could, or might respond to certain stimuli, but it does not provide information about either the frequency of those stimuli in the real-world environment or the relationship between those stimuli and actual objects of perception. The real-world relevance of this kind of research depends on how faithful the experiment's model of social reality is to real life. When evidence on this sort of verisimilitude of the experimental context and stimuli is lacking, as it often is, then experimental research on interpersonal judgment can say little about accuracy in real life.

The relationship between actual attributes of stimuli and the cues the stimuli give off (Component A) translates, in the social domain, to the study of personality. That is, personality psychology (at its best) focuses on individual differences between people and the way these differences are reflected or revealed in behavior. Unfortunately, tradition and history have produced a vast gulf between this area of research and the usual concerns of social psychology that has only recently begun to be bridged. Indeed, an explicit intention of my and my colleagues' research program is to serve as such a bridge, by beginning an intensive examination of what kinds of cues different kinds of people give off, integrated with an examination of how judges use behavioral cues to conclude that stimulus people are of different kinds. Research that ties Component A together with Component B is complex and only recently begun, with a study from our lab that shows that the same behaviors laypeople believe to be diagnostic of extraversion indeed do seem to be shown, in videotaped episodes, by people diagnosed otherwise (e.g., by self-report) as extraverts (Funder & Sneed, 1992; see also Borkenau & Liebler, 1992; Gangestad, Simpson, DiGeronimo, & Biek, 1992; Kenny, Horner, Kashy, & Chu, 1992).

Most of our research to date has focused on a third aspect of interpersonal judgment, labeled *Component C* in the figure. That component is the relationship between a judgment and the attribute that is judged. Although, as mentioned, *C* is in a sense the sum of *A* and *B*, it can also be studied independently. Personality judgments of real people can be gathered, and one can then obtain as much information as possible that might help determine the degree to which these judgments are accurate. In our research, the criteria we use for accuracy are interjudge agreement and behavioral prediction. We are cognizant that neither can serve as an *absolute* criterion for accuracy and that, in fact, no such absolute criterion exists (Funder, 1987). However, we do believe that such criteria remain *reasonable* and can be used to assess the relative likelihood that judgments are more and less accurate.

Goals of the Research Program

At first, the research program concentrated on the task of demonstrating that lay judgments of personality could have any validity at all. I sometimes fantasize that future generations of psychologists, if they happen to encounter these early publications deep in library stacks (or on CD-ROM or whatever) 100 or more years from now, will read them with astonishment and amusement. Nonetheless, they were probably necessary at the time.

In the *zeitgeist* of the 1980s, the idea that human judgment in general, and social judgment in particular, was flawed to the point of almost complete invalidity had a near-stranglehold on large sectors of psychological thought. So, I hope colleagues yet unborn will understand that it was *necessary* to show that two close acquaintances can judge somebody with a fair amount of agreement between each other and with the person who is judged and that this agreement is not just some statistical artifact (Funder, 1980; Funder & Dobroth, 1987). It was also necessary to show that what people will do in one situation has important connections to what they will do in other situations (Funder & Colvin, 1991) and that assessments of personality traits are correlated with these behavioral consistencies (e.g., Funder & Colvin, 1991; Funder & Harris, 1986). I hasten to add that the self-citations generously sprinkled in this paragraph constitute just a small part of a large research effort by many investigators on these issues (for a review, and one more self-citation, see Kenrick & Funder, 1988).

The skepticism about personality and human judgment that dominated psychology for so long now seems to be slowly abating. Although pockets of resistance remain (see Ross & Nisbett, 1991), I think it is safe to say that most psychologists now are willing to acknowledge that (a) human behavior exhibits an important degree of consistency across diverse situations; (b) such consistencies are captured to an important (if incomplete and subject-to-improvement) degree by assessments of personality; and (c) one useful method to gather such assessments is to obtain judgments of personality from people who know the person to be judged.

That settled (finally), research on accuracy in personality judgment can now turn to more interesting and important matters. Two general, interrelated questions provide a focus for the next generation of research. The first question is, What are the moderators of accuracy? Under what circumstances are personality judgments more and less likely to be accurate? The second question is, By what processes are accurate (and inaccurate) judgments possible? Answers to the second question will be informed to an important degree by the answers, as they are gathered, to the first. Moreover, I believe the most promising general framework for examining these questions together is the Brunswikian approach diagramed in Figure 1.

Moderators of Accuracy

My colleagues and I have organized our research around four potential moderators of accuracy in interpersonal judgment. These moderators go by the labels *good judge, good target, good trait,* and *good information.* The following summary presents the current state of research on these topics in our lab; for a more complete review of the literature on these topics, to which many other researchers have also contributed, see the chapter by Funder and Colvin (in press).

Good Judge

Historically, this is the moderator of accuracy that has received the most attention: Is there such a thing as a good judge of personality and, if so, what are the properties of the good judge? An early wave of research on this question, conducted before about the mid-1950s, managed to reach no clear answer to this question (Taft, 1955). The analytic and substantive difficulties are daunting (Cronbach, 1955), but a future goal of our research project is to use modern methods in studying it anew.

Good Target

This moderator of accuracy is the flip side of the good judge: Perhaps some individuals are more easily judged than others. In a recent study from our project, Colvin (in press) found that certain individuals yielded better interjudge agreement about their personalities *and* manifested behavior that was more predictable from these personality judgments. Such individuals, according to Colvin, tended to be psychologically well adjusted. Other research in our lab is continuing the examination of the good target to assess whether this property is partly a function of the contexts in which the target is judged or the contexts to which behavior is predicted.

Good Trait

Recent research has shown clearly that some traits are judged more accurately than others. Funder and Dobroth (1987), for instance, found that more "visible" traits, especially those relevant to extraversion, were judged with much higher interjudge agreement than were less visible traits, such as cognitive and ruminative styles and habits.

This finding has a more general implication as well. Some psychologists, reluctant to concede that peer judgments of personality can be accurate, have maintained that interjudge agreement is a result of conversations judges have had with each other, or with the subjects, about the subjects' personalities, and not on observations of actual behavior. If this were true, then there would be no particular reason for observable traits to yield better agreement than unobservable ones. Both kinds of traits are equally susceptible to being talked about, but unobservable traits are harder actually to *observe*. Thus, the nature of differences between traits in interjudge agreement is an important indication that trait judgments are based more on direct behavioral observation than on reputational considerations.

Good Information

This may be the most promising research direction of all. One conclusion of the analysis of the error literature presented earlier in this chapter was that demonstrations of error may put too much blame on shortcomings of the judge and too little blame on shortcomings in the information that is available to the judge. This conclusion implies that the best way to improve human judgment might be to improve the information with which judges must work and that research on the information that judges do or could use will be highly important.

One aspect of our research has documented the simple point that, in interpersonal judgment, more information is better than less information for most purposes. Close acquaintances provide judgments of personality that agree with each other and with the person judged much better than do judgments of relative "strangers," who have viewed the subject in only one brief situation (Funder & Colvin, 1988). Additional research has shown that judgments rendered by these strangers had nearly equivalent validity for predicting behavior in a future, similar situation as judgments rendered by close acquaintances (Colvin & Funder, 1991).

This latter finding demonstrates a specific boundary on the acquaintanceship effect. Current research in our lab is examining whether the same limitation holds when the predictive criterion is not behavior in a single situation similar to the one strangers observed, but behavior in other, more different situations, or the aggregate of behavior across multiple situations. We expect that when the behavioral criterion is general rather than specific, the judgments of close acquaintances will regain their predictive advantage over the judgments of strangers. Moreover, Stinson and Ickes (in press) found that close acquaintances were much more accurate at evaluating each other's thoughts and feelings in face-to-face interaction than were strangers and that an important basis of their advantage is information accumulated over the course of their acquaintanceship.

Another topic for future research is how different specific kinds of information, including different kinds of acquaintanceship, contribute differentially to judgmental accuracy. So far, acquaintanceship as an independent variable has been operationalized crudely—typically strangers are compared with close acquaintances or judges rate "how well do you know" the subject on a simple 7- or 9-point scale. The time has come to be more specific about the kinds of experience and information that accumulate differentially over time in different relationships and contexts, and how this all contributes to the enhancement or detriment of judgmental accuracy (cf. Andersen, 1984).

Other recent studies in our lab have examined other facets of the informational factor in social judgment. Funder et al. (1992) examined the degree to which personality descriptions provided by others can yield as good or better predictions of behavior than descriptions rendered by the subjects themselves. They considered their findings in light of the differing informational perspectives on behavior held by "actors" and "observers."

Funder and Sneed (1992) have examined the process by which judges go from observation of behavior to general personality judgment. They found that judges were generally highly skilled and knowledgable; they seemed to know much about which behaviors were more positively and negatively diagnostic of several aspects of personality. However, there were some behavioral cues that judges used that were not valid, and there were other behavioral cues that were valid but that judges did not use, which opens the possibility of specific training programs that could improve the accuracy of interpersonal judgment.

Conclusions

It is possible to regard "error" research as a paradigm that treats the glass as being half (or maybe more than half) empty, whereas the "accuracy" paradigm treats the glass as being more nearly half full (see Figure 2). Similarly, research on error is sometimes regarded as pessimistic, whereas research on accuracy is regarded as optimistic.

However, perhaps the time has come for psychologists to become more like the character in the fourth panel of the cartoon (the one who

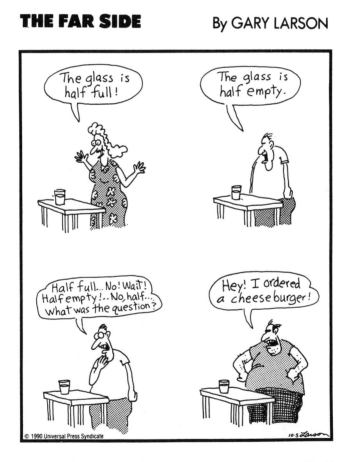

FIGURE 2. The four basic personality types. The Far Side ©1990, Far Works, Inc. Reprinted with permission of Universal Press Syndicate. All rights reserved.

wants a cheeseburger). That is, rather than play the game of accuracy evaluation in terms of how much, or how bad, or half full, or half empty, psychologists need a new game. The basis of this new research game will be to find out *when* judgments of personality are most and least likely to be accurate as well as *why*.

For social psychology, the payoff of this research will be an enhanced understanding of the relationship between social judgment and social reality. For personality psychology and research on personality development, the payoff will be more concrete: an enhanced understanding of the basis of one of the most important data-gathering tools in psychology and a deeper appreciation of both the capabilities and the limits of human judgment as a personality assessment device.

References

Andersen, S. M. (1984). Self-knowledge and social inference: II. The diagnosticity of cognitive/affective and behavioral data. *Journal of Personality and Social Psychology, 46*, 294–307.

Bandura, A. (1989). Human agency in social cognitive theory. *American Psychologist, 44*, 1175–1184.

Bem, D. J., & Funder, D. C. (1978). Predicting more of the people more of the time: Assessing the personality of situations. *Psychological Review, 85*, 485–501.

Block, J. (1971). *Lives through time.* Berkeley, CA: Bancroft Books.

Block, J. (1978). *The Q-sort method in personality assessment and psychiatric research.* Palo Alto, CA: Consulting Psychologists Press. (Original work published 1961)

Block, J. H., & Block, J. (1980). The role of ego-control and ego-resiliency in the organization of behavior. In W. A. Collins (Ed.), *Minnesota Symposium on Child Psychology* (Vol. 13, pp. 39–101). Hillsdale, NJ: Erlbaum.

Borkenau, P., & Liebler, A. (1992). Trait inferences: Sources of validity at zero acquaintance. *Journal of Personality and Social Psychology, 62*, 645–657.

Borman, W. C. (1975). Effects of instructions to avoid halo error on reliability and validity of performance ratings. *Journal of Applied Psychology, 62*, 64–69.

Brunswik, E. (1956). *Perception and the representative design of experiments.* Berkeley: University of California Press.

Colvin, C. R. (in press). Judgable people: Personality, behavior, and competing explanations. *Journal of Personality and Social Psychology.*

Colvin, C. R., & Funder, D. C. (1991). Predicting personality and behavior: A boundary on the acquaintanceship effect. *Journal of Personality and Social Psychology, 60*, 884–894.

Crandall, C. S. (1984). The overcitation of examples of poor performance: Fad, fashion, or fun? [Comment]. *American Psychologist, 39,* 1499–1500.

Cronbach, L. J. (1955). Processes affecting scores on "understanding of others" and "assumed similarity." *Psychological Bulletin, 52,* 177–193.

Evans, J. St. B. T. (1984). In defense of the citation bias in the judgment literature [Comment]. *American Psychologist, 39,* 1500–1501.

Funder, D. C. (1980). On seeing ourselves as others see us: Self-other agreement and discrepancy in personality ratings. *Journal of Personality, 48,* 473–493.

Funder, D. C. (1987). Errors and mistakes: Evaluating the accuracy of social judgment. *Psychological Bulletin, 101,* 75–90.

Funder, D. C. (1992). Everything you know is wrong [Review of *The person and the situation*]. *Contemporary Psychology, 37,* 319–320.

Funder, D. C., & Colvin, C. R. (1988). Friends and strangers: Acquaintanceship, agreement, and the accuracy of personality judgment. *Journal of Personality and Social Psychology, 55,* 149–158.

Funder, D. C., & Colvin, C. R. (1991). Explorations in behavioral consistency: Properties of persons, situations, and behaviors. *Journal of Personality and Social Psychology, 60,* 773–794.

Funder, D. C., & Colvin, C. R. (in press). Congruence of self and others' judgments of personality. In S. Briggs, R. Hogan, & W. Jones (Eds.), *Handbook of personality psychology.* San Diego, CA: Academic Press.

Funder, D. C., & Dobroth, K. M. (1987). Differences between traits: Properties associated with interjudge agreement. *Journal of Personality and Social Psychology, 52,* 409–418.

Funder, D. C., & Harris, M. J. (1986). On the several facets of personality assessment: The case of social acuity. *Journal of Personality, 54,* 528–550.

Funder, D. C., Kolar, D. W., & Colvin, C. R. (1992). *When do others know us as well as we know ourselves? Perspectives on personality by the self and by others.* Manuscript submitted for publication.

Funder, D. C., & Sneed, C. (in press). Behavioral manifestations of personality: An ecological approach to judgmental accuracy. *Journal of Personality and Social Psychology.*

Gangestad, S. W., Simpson, J. A., DiGeronimo, K., & Biek, M. (1992). Differential accuracy in person perception across traits: Examination of a functional hypothesis. *Journal of Personality and Social Psychology, 62,* 688–698.

Grice, H. P. (1975). Logic in conversation. In P. Cole & J. L. Morgan (Eds.), *Syntax and semantics* (Vol. 3, pp. 41–58). San Diego, CA: Academic Press.

Hartshone, H., & May, M. A. (1928). *Studies in deceit.* New York: Macmillan.

Hammond, K. R. (1966). Probabilistic functionalism: Egon Brunswik's integration of the history, theory, and method of psychology. In K. R. Hammond (Ed.), *The psychology of Egon Brunswik* (pp. 15–80). New York: Holt, Rinehart & Winston.

Hayes, W. L. (1973). *Statistics for the social sciences* (2nd ed.). New York: Holt, Rinehart & Winston.

Jones, E. E. (1985). Major developments in social psychology during the past five decades. In G. Lindzey & E. Aronson (Eds.), *The handbook of social psychology* (Vol. 2, pp. 219–266). San Diego, CA: Academic Press.

Jones, E. E., & Harris, V. A. (1967). The attribution of attitudes. *Journal of Experimental Social Psychology, 3,* 1–24.

Kahneman, D. T., & Tversky, A. (1973). On the psychology of prediction. *Psychological Review, 80,* 237–251.

Kenny, D. A., Horner, C., Kashy, D. A., & Chu, L. (1992). Consensus at zero acquaintance: Replication, behavioral cues, and stability. *Journal of Personality and Social Psychology, 62,* 88–97.

Kenrick, D. T., & Funder, D. C. (1988). Profiting from controversy: Lessons from the person–situation debate. *American Psychologist, 43,* 23–34.

Kunda, Z., & Nisbett, R. E. (1986). The psychometrics of everyday life. *Cognitive Psychology, 18,* 195–224.

Lopes, L. L. (1991). The rhetoric of irrationality. *Theory and Psychology, 1,* 65–82.

Lopes, L. L., & Oden, G. C. (in press). The rationality of intelligence. In E. Eells & T. Maruszewski (Eds.), *Rationality and reasoning.* Amsterdam: Rodopi.

Nisbett, R. E., & Ross, L. (1980). *Human inference: Strategies and shortcomings of social judgment.* Englewood Cliffs, NJ: Prentice-Hall.

Rosenthal, R., & Rubin, D. B. (1982). A simple, general purpose display of magnitude of experimental effect. *Journal of Educational Psychology, 74,* 166–169.

Ross, L. (1977). The intuitive psychologist and his shortcomings. In L. Berkowitz (Ed.), *Advances in experimental social psychology* (Vol. 10, pp. 174–214). San Diego, CA: Academic Press.

Ross, L., & Nisbett, R. E. (1991). *The person and the situation: Perspectives of social psychology.* New York: McGraw-Hill.

Schneider, D. J., Hastorf, A. H., & Ellsworth, P. C. (1979). *Person perception* (2nd ed.). Reading, MA: Addison-Wesley.

Shaklee, H. (1991). An inviting invitation [Review of *An invitation to cognitive science: Vol. 3. Thinking*). *Contemporary Psychology, 36,* 940–941.

Stinson, L., & Ickes, W. (in press). Empathic accuracy in the interactions of male friends versus male strangers. *Journal of Personality and Social Psychology.*

Taft, R. (1955). The ability to judge people. *Psychological Bulletin, 52,* 1–23.

Wright, J. C., & Mischel, W. (1988). Conditional hedges and the intuitive psychology of traits. *Journal of Personality and Social Psychology, 55,* 454–469.

CHAPTER 7

The Q-Sort Method and the Study of Personality Development

Daniel J. Ozer

C onsider the task of describing an individual's personality: Psychologists might administer a multiscale inventory, have trained observers code behavior as it occurs in some standardized situation, or have peers complete a set of trait ratings. These procedures differ markedly from those that psychologists might use when engaged in the same task in some nonprofessional context. When describing my accountant to my neighbor during a poolside conversation, I hardly refer to Likert scales, but instead provide a character sketch, noting those attributes of the other that are most salient, most unusual, most characteristic, and most differentiating. Such a character sketch is fully individuated, created only for the purpose of describing a single individual. It is not a template that can be reused to describe another by modifying adjectives (*very* to *not at all*), in the way a Minnesota Multiphasic Personality Inventory profile sheet is a constant across assessees, with differences only in scale scores to differentiate one person from another.

There are various ways to characterize the differences between these formal and informal personality assessment procedures (e.g., one is objective and quantitative, the other subjective and qualitative). Allport (1962), the psychologist perhaps the most sensitive to these methodological differences, used the terms *dimensional* and *morphogenic* to summarize and label the variety of procedures available to both lay and professional assessors. Allport (1962) was fully convinced that morphogenic personality assessment is an absolute requirement for capturing the unique qualities of each individual and so he identified and championed the use of morphogenic methods. Allport's labels have become laden with meaning supplied by this larger, metatheoretical value that emphasizes the uniqueness of each individual, a value that need not be necessarily endorsed to find utility in methods that might be described as "person centered" rather than "variable centered." J. Block (1961) used these terms to capture one fundamental methodological difference among personality assessment strategies. An assessor may start with one or many personality variables of interest and then seek to measure one or more individuals on these variables; alternatively, the assessor may start with one or more persons of interest and then seek the variables that characterize each. In the former, the variable-centered approach, the focus is on interindividual differences; in the latter, the person-centered approach, the emphasis is on intraindividual variation.

Note that the contrast between formal and lay methods of personality assessment is aligned with, but certainly not identical to, the distinction between variable- and person-centered methods. When choosing sides for a game by selecting the best athletes first, children use a variable-centered procedure, and some formal methods of personality assessment (e.g., Kelly's Role Construct Repertory Test) are person centered. Although there are important and notable exceptions, both morphogenic and person-centered assessment approaches are used relatively infrequently in psychological research. Q-methodology, initially described by Stephenson (1935, 1953) and subsequently adapted by J. Block (1961) and applied to the longitudinal study of personality (J. Block, 1971), offers a person-centered assessment approach that has characteristics that recommend its use in the study of personality development.

The Q-sort procedure requires judges to sort a set of items into ordered categories, ranging from extremely characteristic or salient to extremely uncharacteristic or negatively salient. This judgment is made with reference to some specified target. The categories into which the items are sorted are given a numerical label that becomes the score of all items placed in that category. The number of items permitted in any category is fixed in advance, so the shape of the distribution of item scores is fixed and constant for all judges. Thus, Q-sorting is a form of rank ordering in which the number and location of ties is specified. Usually, the items consist of a set of verbal statements that are likely to vary in terms of how descriptive they are of the specified target; in the ensuing discussion, items are assumed to be verbal statements. Still, it is useful to recognize that alternative kinds of items may be used (e.g., a set of facial photographs to be sorted in terms of their attractiveness).

The goal of this chapter is to encourage the use of the Q-sort in the study of personality development by providing a primer of Q-sort methods and procedures, especially as applied to the longitudinal study of personality, while also addressing some unresolved issues in the use of the Q-sort method. Existing descriptions of the Q-sort method are often designed as introductions to specific Q-sets such as the California Q-Set (J. Block, 1961) or the Attachment Q-Set (Waters & Deane, 1985) or are textbook discussions designed to provide a breadth of coverage that necessarily leaves much to the imagination of readers with a specific area of interest. Thus, this chapter is designed to address general issues of Q-methodology within the specific domain of longitudinal personality research. Some methodological issues arise as a specific function of the Q-sort method (e.g., what the optimum shape of the forced distribution is), and other, more general issues become especially important in the domain of Q-technique (e.g., the consequences of ipsative measurement), although they may arise elsewhere as well. A surprising number of such issues, some of them basic, have yet to be fully identified and resolved (e.g., how to assess reliability). I discuss a subset of these issues, those either basic to all Q-sort applications and those especially relevant to longitudinal personality research. However, before turning to these matters, I offer some clarifications concerning the designation Q to refer to the methods to be described.

The Meaning of *Q*

Stephenson (1936) described four systems or kinds of data structures and analyses. Two of these, designated R and Q, were seen as basic and independent, whereas the remaining two were seen as derivative of the first pair. Stephenson (1953) denied that his description of Q was equivalent to Cattell's (1946) description of Q-technique. Because Cattell's system has subsequently become better known than Stephenson's, and because the "Q" in Q-sort is inspired by the latter's framework, some understanding of the difference is crucial to avoid confusion.

Cattell (1946) described six correlational techniques (R, Q, P, O, S, and T) derived from the various possible correlations (between rows and between columns) in three types of data matrices: Persons × Variables, Persons × Occasions, and Variables × Occasions. The familiar correlation between variables in a sample of persons is Cattell's R-technique, whereas the transpose of this operation, the correlation between persons in a sample of variables is Cattell's Q-technique. Although Q-sort data may be, and often are, analyzed using Cattell's Q-technique, other types of analyses are often used in the analysis of Q-sort data.

Stephenson (1953) viewed the Q-sort method as encompassing distinct interpretations of sampling, scaling, and data analysis that offer insight into intraindividual variation and structure. Items, not persons, are regarded as samples, and measurement is ipsative rather than normative. These conditions, in Stephenson's view, create a system that has properties not inherent in the simple transpose of R.

As an assessment technique, the Q-sort procedure can be used as either a self- or observer-report method. Although there are important and notable exceptions (e.g., Rogers & Dymond, 1954), the latter approach is more common in personality and developmental psychology. Stephenson (1953), however, emphasized the capacity of the method to render the internal, subjective world of the person open to inspection and quantitative analysis. Indeed, the capacity of the Q-sort method to represent the internal frame of reference of the respondent was seen by Stephenson as an important if not crucial distinction between Q and R, in which the emphasis on individual differences represents the perspective of an external frame of reference. This conception of Q-technique implies that the Q-sort should serve as a self- rather than observer-rating device. McKeown and Thomas (1988) provided a thorough introduction to Q-sort methods from this perspective.

J. Block (1961) presented the case for using the Q-sort method as an observer-based assessment device, and the logic of his viewpoint represents more of an extension of Stephenson's (1953) position rather than a rejection of it. J. Block also noted the individual difference orientation of R and the intraindividual difference orientation of Q, describing the former as variable centered and the latter as person centered. In the domain of observer evaluations, a primary advantage of variable-centered approaches, like trait ratings, is their objectivity of method (so that replication is possible) and their yield of numerical data amenable to quantitative analysis. Person-centered approaches, as exemplified by case histories, permit a more detailed formulation of the rich interrelations among the personality structures of each individual considered within his or her own life context. The case history reflects the subjective yet considered impression of another's personality. J. Block (1961) characterized the Q-sort method of personality assessment as a person-centered approach, reflecting the judges' subjective impressions of the person qua person while also possessing the objective methodology and quantitative yield of trait-rating procedures. Idiosyncracies, biases, and errors of individual judges are overcome through the use of a composite Q-sort based on the average of multiple, independent judges.

The Q-sort method, as used today in personality and developmental psychology, reflects the original formulation of Stephenson (1953) and the extension and elaboration of the technique by J. Block (1961). This brief historical introduction does not do full justice to a variety of issues pertinent to defining Q, and because these issues affect the use of the Q-sort method in the study of personality development, I discuss them shortly. For now, it is sufficient to realize that Q in the context of the Q-sort method means more than Cattell's (1946) Q-technique: An orientation toward intraindividual variation and a method of data collection and measurement is also implied.

Q-Sort Procedures

Developing a set of items, and then using and analyzing Q-sort data, involves a variety of concerns common to all data collection methods; however, various additional, less common concerns become relevant as well.

Q-Sort Judgments

The differences between the Q-sort method and other rating procedures become explicit if one considers in some detail the task faced by the judge in each and the nature of the evaluations required. Imagine a set of adjectives to be used in a self-report task. Subjects might be asked to rate themselves from 1 *(not at all like me)* to 7 *(very much like me)* on each item. The typical subject will consider each item in turn, assign a rating, and be done with the task. Most subjects will proceed without question; those few who ask " 'very much like me' compared with what?" will be encouraged to reread the directions and not make the task more difficult than necessary. A college sophomore, well practiced in such a task, might need as long as 5 minutes to complete 50 such items. Consider the data that emerge: The within-subjects means and standard deviations will vary across subjects, reflecting both various response biases and real differences. The researcher must hope, but has no guarantee or way to verify, that each subject's standards (how "much like me" an item must be to qualify as a 7, a 6 or a 5) remain constant throughout the task.

Now consider the subject's task when completing a 50-item adjective Q-sort, with its forced distribution (e.g., 7 items in each of 7 categories, numbered 1 through 7, with Category 4 to contain 8 items). To conform to the forced distribution, several passes through the items will almost certainly be necessary, making the task more time consuming but also forcing the subject to reconsider many judgments time and time again. The forced distribution also creates a clear basis for each decision, which in its simplest form reduces to which of two items provides a better description. If the equal means and standard deviations of the ratings within subjects lead one to miss some real differences, much error and bias is also eliminated.

When the Q-sort method is used to collect observer judgments, these same advantages accrue: more carefully made judgments against a more explicit standard with reduced error and bias. However, with observer judgments, the effect of these advantages has an additional consequence: The desirability of using a fixed and unchanging panel of judges is greatly reduced. When standard rating scales are used, the different within-judge means and standard deviations can be made to exert a less consequential constant rather than a systematically varying effect if each judge rates all subjects. Such a design holds judge effects constant. The forced distribution of the Q-sort accomplishes this same end: Judge main effects are removed from the data, and so using different judges to assess subjects is considerably less problematic when the Q-sort method is used.

Q-Sort Items

In Q-technique, items are understood as being members of a population, so that Q-set items may be construed as samples. Various kinds of item samples are possible, just as various kinds of samples of persons are possible: random samples, samples of convenience, and stratified samples (called "structured samples" by Stephenson, 1953). It is even possible to use a Q-set that contains the entire population of items, although the only attempt seems to be Stephenson's listing of all of Jung's (1924) statements describing his various personality types. Stephenson explicitly opposed the development of any standardized Q-set to be used over and over again in a series of studies. He believed that this would be akin to using a standard set of subjects in batteries of experiments conducted within the framework of his R-system. If items are in fact samples drawn from a population, then tests of statistical significance would be appropriate because generalization of results to any parent population using methods of statistical inference requires an appropriate sampling technique. Specifying a small sample for continued and regular, even sole, usage undermines the use of standard techniques of statistical inference that Stephenson (1953) hoped to apply within his Q-system.

J. Block (1961) rejected Stephenson's (1953) arguments on this point, and after offering a detailed criticism of Stephenson's views, he opted to use a standard set of items to be used in the several Q-sets he developed.

The use of a standard set of items offers various advantages over the sampling procedures described by Stephenson, advantages that are both pragmatic (it is much more efficient) and scientific (scoring keys, as in the use of criterion or prototypical Q-sorts need not be ad hoc devices, as is the case when the sampling method described by Stephenson is used). Perhaps the only real disadvantage in using standard Q-sets is that statistical analyses based on samples of Q-items (e.g., a correlation between two Q-sorts, as in Cattell's, 1946, Q-technique) cannot be tested for statistical significance in the typical fashion. Statistical inference of this kind is problematic at best and should be avoided.

Constructing a Q-set involves many of the same considerations that come into play in writing items for other kinds of instruments. The domain of interest must be specified, and items descriptive of the domain must be produced and selected. The domain may be broad, encompassing all aspects of personality, as in the California Q-Set (J. Block, 1961), or more narrow, such as the Attachment Q-Set (Waters & Dean, 1985), which includes content clusters relevant to attachment relationships and approximates a one-facet structured sample as described by Stephenson (1953).

Although the forced distribution of the Q-sort controls certain response biases, it also imposes certain kinds of restrictions on the item set. Because the judge is making discriminations among items, the item set must be multidimensional or targets at the extreme tails of the dimension will not be aptly described by the items forced into a symmetric distribution (e.g., if all of the items in a set are descriptive of high sociability, which items could be placed in an "uncharacteristic" category when describing a highly sociable person?). The item content, and the shape of the forced distribution, must be chosen so that most targets can be reasonably described.

Once a pool of items has been assembled and piloted, various statistical criteria can be used to identify poor items. Items with low judge agreement, with low standard deviations, and with undesirable correlations to other items may all be candidates for deletion. These undesirable correlations may be those either too low or too high, depending on intentions. In some instances, nonredundancy is sought, and so items with many large correlations to other items might be deleted. In other instances, the goal may be to form scales of items with similar content, so low correlations to other items on the same putative scale may create a cause for concern.

The Q-Sort Distribution

After identifying a set of items, the next step in constructing and using a Q-sort must be determining the number of categories and the shape of the forced distribution. Although considerable research has examined the properties of forced versus free distributions, the effect of different distribution shapes has received little attention. A forced distribution that permitted no ties (i.e., as many categories as items—a rank ordering) would force the judges to make a maximum number of discriminations among the items. If there are n_i items in $i = 1, \ldots, k$ categories, then Equation 1 specifies the number of discriminations among items required by judges to complete a Q-sort containing a total of Σn items in the k different categories. Thus, for any fixed number of items, as k, the number of categories approaches Σn, the number of discriminations increases; however, for any fixed number of categories, the number of discriminations is maximized if a rectangular distribution is forced:

$$.5 \left(\Sigma\Sigma n_i n_i - \Sigma n_i^2 \right) \tag{1}$$

Although Equation 1 provides a means of calculating the number of discriminations required by a particular distribution, it says little about how many ought to be required. Given maximum resources (i.e., judges have unlimited time), then it would be a straightforward empirical procedure to determine, for any Q-sort, how many discriminations judges could make reliably. However, resources are rarely unlimited, and as the number of discriminations increases, surely the amount of time judges require to complete a Q-sort increases as well. In practice, the California Q-Sort, with its 100 items and 9 categories with a forced quasi-normal distribution (5, 8, 12, 16, 18, 16, 12, 8, and 5 items in Categories 1 through 9, respectively), requires 4,349 discriminations. The number of discriminations increases only slightly (to 4,444) if a rectangular distribution (11 items in 8 categories, 12 items in 1 category) is used. Presumably, judge agreement would increase as the number of discriminations required decreases, but there are no readily identifiable studies systematically examining this question with Q-sort methodology.

Ipsativity and the Q-Sort

The forced distribution of the Q-sort yields ipsative data because item means and standard deviations of each sorter's distribution are all equal. This ipsativity is a distinctive feature of the method, reflecting the intraindividual person-centered focus of the method. Ipsativity also creates a variety of statistical concerns that do not arise with normative data, offering many pitfalls to the unwary.

The forced-distribution of the Q-sort forces the sorter to make comparisons among items to determine which are more or less salient descriptors. In order to fit the distributional constraints, the sorter is often obliged to make distinctions among items that at first glance seem equivalently descriptive. The sorter must work with a degree of care and diligence often dodged when no distributional constraints are imposed. Moreover, the forced distribution controls for certain kinds of rater error, such as the tendency to use extreme ratings. It is, of course, possible that the forced distribution will require distinctions even when the sorter is convinced that they are unwarranted, and so items are placed into categories contrary to the sorter's best considered judgment.

These difficulties are ameliorated when observers, whose judgments will be composited, are the source of the Q-sort. If distinctions forced by the distributional constraints are indeed arbitrary, then judges will, in the long run, not agree in the arbitrary decisions forced on them, and the effect will average out. By some criteria, ratings from forced distributions may be superior to ratings obtained without distributional constraints. J. Block (1956) found that ratings from forced distributions were more replicable and included more discriminations than did ratings from unforced distributions, although these effects were not large. Ipsative and normative ratings are typically correlated with one another to such an extent that they can, for some purposes, be considered equivalent (J. Block, 1957).

There are, however, important nonequivalences between ipsative and normative ratings that must be kept in mind. Analyses of item means is one such problem area. In a longitudinal study in which the same rating variable has been used on multiple occasions, means obtained by the sample on two different occasions may be compared. Given appropriate safeguards (e.g., multiple judges at each age, independent panels of judges), differences in means on a normatively rated variable may be interpreted as an age change. With ipsative data such as Q-sort items, nonindependence among the item means undermines such an interpretation. At best, such an effect obtained with ipsative data reflects a change in salience, not growth or decline. Age changes cannot be inferred from mean differences in Q-sort items. Conversely, normative growth may occur and not be reflected in mean Q-item placements (Ozer & Gjerde, 1989).

There are other consequences of the statistical properties of ipsative data. For example, when item variances are equal, the average correlation between some external variable and the ipsative variables will be zero, and the average interitem correlation will be $-1/(N - 1)$, where N is the number of items (Clemans, 1966; Hicks, 1970). As this latter property implies, the intercorrelation matrix of a set of ipsative variables is singular. As a result, analyses that depend on the calculation of the inverse of a matrix (e.g., factor analysis of the items) are not possible. Although principal-components analysis is mathematically possible, the mean negative intercorrelations will typically lead to components with comparatively low eigenvalues, resulting in having to choose between leaving much variance unexplained or retaining many components that may be unstable unless sample size is very large (Guadagnoli & Velicer, 1988).

Reliability of Q-Sort Data

Replicability of measurement outcomes is a necessary feature for any measurement or assessment procedure if it is to be useful. To evaluate reliability, multiple measurement trials are required, and reliability is then a function of the amount of agreement in measurement outcomes across trials and the number of trials. The Spearman-Brown formula provides a quantitative statement of reliability as a function of amount of agreement and number of measurement trials. When Q-sorts are used by observers, the multiple judges describing each subject provide replications over trials; therefore, the reliability of the Q-sort is a function of interjudge agreement and the number of judges.

It is important to distinguish between reliability and judge agreement. Measurement error, which weakens statistical tests and biases measures of effect size, is a function of reliability. Because interjudge agreement is related to measurement error only through the relation described by the Spearman-Brown formula, reliability may be high even when interjudge agreement is low if there is a relatively large number of judges. In certain circumstances, interjudge agreement is relevant to the evaluation of the validity of Q-sort data independent of reliability considerations, as I discuss shortly. Here, the focus is on the psychometrics of reliability estimation with Q-sort data.

There are two methods that have been widely used to assess the reliability of Q-sorts. One may assess the reliability of each item by obtaining the average interjudge correlation in the Person (Target) × Judge data matrix, estimating the reliability of the composite "correcting" this correlation with the Spearman-Brown formula, and then averaging across items to obtain the average item reliability. Alternatively, the Item × Judge data matrix of each person may be used as the source of the average interjudge correlation, which may be entered into the Spearman-Brown formula and then averaged across persons. This reliability coefficient may be described as the average person reliability. In the former case, each item has a reliability estimate, whereas in the latter case, each person in the sample has a reliability estimate. Sometimes one of these methods is reported and sometimes the other is; in rare instances both are used (e.g., J. Block, 1971). What is the difference between these two procedures, and does this difference lead to any rational basis for preferring one approach over the other for at least some purposes?

Assuming a fully crossed and balanced design of Persons (Targets) × Judges × Items, it is possible to show that the average item reliability can never exceed the average person reliability and that the two will be equal only when the item means, averaged over judges and persons, are all equal, a circumstance that is highly unlikely in real data. To the extent that some items are judged to be more salient than other items by all judges regardless of who they are describing, the average person reliability will be increased, whereas the average item reliability will be unaffected.

This difference between person and item reliability can be demonstrated in two somewhat different but equivalent ways. If one takes the approach of generalizability theory (Cronbach, Gleser, Nanda, & Rajaratnam, 1972) to reliability estimation in this full three-facet (Persons × Judges × Items) design, the generalizability coefficient of interest is that associated with the Person × Item interaction (i.e., the degree to which item means vary as a function of the person being described). Within an analysis of variance framework, this two-way interaction may be decomposed into constituent simple main effects in either of two ways: the person effect in the Person × Judge data matrix for each item (the matrices used to estimate item reliability) and the item effect in the Item × Judge data matrix for each person (the matrices used to estimate person reliability). The sum of these simple main effect sum of squares is related to the sum-of-square terms of the full three-facet design, as shown in Equations 2 and 3:

$$\Sigma SS(\text{Persons}) \text{ at Item}_k = SS(\text{Persons}) + SS(\text{Persons} \times \text{Items}) \qquad (2)$$

$$\Sigma SS(\text{Items}) \text{ at Person}_i = SS(\text{Items}) + SS(\text{Persons} \times \text{Items}). \qquad (3)$$

Equation 2 shows the simple main effects of persons in the Person × Judge matrices as being equal to the sum of two effects in the three-facet model, but the ipsativity of the Q-sort guarantees that there is no variability in person means or totals: $SS(\text{Persons}) = .00$. Reliability analyses based on the Person × Judge matrices are decompositions of only the Person × Item interaction of the three-facet design.

As shown in Equation 3, simple main effect analyses of the item effect at each person also decompose the sum of two effects in the three-facet design, but in this instance, ipsativity restricts the values of neither of these terms. Variability defined as item main effects in the three-facet design is included in reliability analyses based on the Item × Judge matrices.

Equations 2 and 3 show that these two sums of simple main effects (and the item and person reliability coefficients based on the individual simple main effects) will be equal if and only if SS(Items) = .00 in the three-facet design. To the extent that item main effects exist, person reliability will exceed item reliability.

This difference in person and item reliability coefficients can also be understood through a consideration of the Q correlations used to estimate person reliability, and the impact of item main effects on person reliability is perhaps more clearly demonstrated in this way. If the Q-sort descriptions of different judges describing different persons are, on average, positively correlated (a situation that creates the item main effects described earlier), then some portion of the correlation between different judges describing the same target cannot be attributed to the judges' agreement about that target, but would be expected even when describing different individuals.

This item effect is consistent with two interpretations: It may reflect some bias among the judges, which leads them to see individuals as being more similar to each other than they actually are, or it may reflect accurate judgments reflecting some degree of homogeneity among the persons being described. For example, if a sample is of above-average intelligence and a Q-sort item that pertains to intelligence is included, it would not be unexpected if this item was, on average, rated as being relatively more rather than less descriptive of subjects. This tendency would create an item main effect and a positive correlation among descriptions of different individuals.

Which method of estimating reliability is most appropriate? The answer would seem to depend on how the Q-set data will be subsequently used. Analyses of Q items (e.g., correlating some external variable to each Q item) call for the use of the item reliability coefficients, whereas analyses involving Q correlations (e.g., using each subject's Q correlation to some prototypical description as a score in subsequent analyses) should be supported by reporting person reliabilities, despite the impact of item main effects. Distributions of Q correlations are influenced by these same item main effects, and the reliability estimate should be the one most pertinent to the variable under analysis. When the focus is on judge agreement rather than reliability, then the item reliability coefficient is clearly preferable because it reflects agreement on the distinctive features of the subjects.

Validity of Q-Sort Data

The validity of a Q-sort item, or score derived from a Q-sort, is subject to the same considerations applicable to any other psychological measure. However, the difficulties of demonstrating the validity of a Q-sort indicator are geometrically more complex when observers are the source of Q-sort data because generalization over judges as well as subjects is required. Measurement error specific to a Q-set and error attributable to judges are confounded. As a result, there is no "off the shelf" valid Q-sort indicator for any psychological construct, as there are in several other domains of psychological measurement (e.g., self-report scales for screening a population for depression, cognitive tests for measuring intellectual abilities).

For many purposes, judge agreement is relevant to the evaluation of the validity of a set of composite Q-sorts. If judges have access to the same information, then agreement among the judges is a necessary but not sufficient criterion for validity. To the extent that judges have access to different information about the subject, then disagreement among the judges is possible even if all are valid. In some circumstances, in which the characteristics under evaluation are interpersonal and the judges represent important others in the real-life milieu of the subjects, judge agreement may, by itself, constitute prima facie evidence for validity (Ozer, 1989). In other contexts, the validity of Q-sort variables must be developed out of the data by demonstrating that the Q-sort measure relates to other variables in ways predicted by theory. J. H. Block and Block's (1980) description of the development of their Q-sort measures of ego-control and ego-resiliency provides an example of this type of theory-guided construct validation.

Types of Analyses

Q-sort data can be used in various types of analyses. Each item may be considered as a variable of interest to be related to some external variable.

Such analyses elucidate the meaning of the external variable and are a part of what Gough (1965) referred to as a "conceptual analysis." Ozer (1987) used the California Q-Sort in this way to describe the personality implications of scores on a mental rotations task.

For various reasons, ranging from a desire to test theory to sheer convenience, researchers may wish to reduce the number of variables, finding the item-by-item approach unsatisfactory. Reducing the number of variables may proceed in any of several different fashions. J. H. Block and Block (1980) described the development of criterion sorts, descriptions of hypothetical and prototypical targets, for ego-control and ego-resiliency. The Q correlation between the criterion sort and Q-sort descriptions of actual individuals constitute scores on these constructs. Scales of various kinds may be built into the Q-set from the beginning, as in the Attachment Q-Set (Waters & Deane, 1985), or they may be constructed subsequent to data collection. Green (1980) showed the fundamental equivalence of the criterion sort and traditional scale method, demonstrating that correlations to a criterion sort are equivalent to a scale using all items in weighted combination.

When scales have not been built into a Q-set, and when theory offers no guidance as to the appropriate content for developing criterion sorts, submitting the items to an R-type factor analysis may appear appropriate. The ipsative nature of Q data precludes any strong recommendation in favor of this practice (Clemans, 1966). If exploratory factor analysis is desirable, then Q-type factor analysis, based on the matrix of Q correlations among subjects, may be preferable. Factor scores from this Q-type factor analysis provide information about the structure of items. McKeown and Thomas (1988) provided extensive discussion and examples of using Q-type factor analysis for understanding item structure.

Among the more powerful applications of Q-sort methods is obtaining the correlation between Q-sorts of the same individual on multiple occasions. The correlation between these Q-sorts then provides a measure of consistency versus change during the interval bracketed by the measurement occasions. J. Block (1971) and Ozer and Gjerde (1989) used this method for examining consistency and change in personality. As noted earlier, traditional tests of significance should not be applied to Q correlations of this type, but the reasons for this recommendation go beyond the sampling considerations noted earlier. The expected value of such Q correlations is unlikely to be zero, and so demonstrating that such a correlation is significantly different from zero is pointless. Empirical sampling distributions for Q correlations can be derived and used (e.g., Caspi & Herbener, 1990; Ozer & Gjerde, 1989) as a basis for evaluating the magnitude of such correlations.

Advantages of the Q-Sort Method

As a way of summarizing several attributes of the Q-sort method, and linking more general claims about the Q-sort to particular applications in the study of personality development, I present a list of positive attributes of Q-sort methodology. The Q-sort method is certainly not the only assessment procedure to possess these characteristics; indeed, the entire set may not be unique to the Q-sort. One might simply construe this list as six reasons to use the Q-sort method.

1. The Q-sort procedure requires little training of raters, so that the only major limitation on who may appropriately be used as a sorter is the degree of sophistication required to understand the items. Various sources—self, peer acquaintances, graduate student examiners, clinicians, teachers, and parents have been used as sorters (Caspi et al., in press). If the language of a particular Q-set is not appropriate for a particular population of sorters, items may be altered as in Caspi et al., wherein the development of a "common language" version of the California Child Q-Set (J. Block & Block, 1980) is described.

2. The Q-sort can accommodate a variety of information sources. Peers may provide data based on their prolonged acquaintance with a target (e.g., Funder & Colvin, 1988); information may also come from a short videotape, as in Harrington, Block, and Block (1978), in which parental teaching strategies are assessed by observers who viewed parent–child interactions. J. Block (1971) used the California Q-Set to make the diverse records of longitudinally studied subjects commensurate on a common set of variables that then provided a basis for describing different types of developmental trajectories. The Q-sort's capacity to accommodate a diverse and idiosyncratic mix of qualitative information is also apparent in Craik's (1988) use of biographies of U.S. presidents as the data source for sorters. This "transportability" of the Q-sort method is

not merely a means of accommodating to the vagaries of existing data; constructs that are tied to a particular set of measurement operations that prove too limiting for some purposes may be removed from this context dependency by the Q-sort procedure. Waters and Deane's (1985) use of the Q-sort method to assess attachment relationships permits the examination of the theoretically rich attachment construct outside of the laboratory.

3. Many well-constructed rating methods may, at least in principle, be used by a variety of raters in diverse contexts. In actual practice, various forms of rater error (e.g., halo effects) undermine such applications. Control of rater error is among the primary benefits of the Q-sort method because it permits the virtues of both self- and observer evaluations to accrue in the absence of at least some of the usual flaws. As already noted, this advantage arises from the forced distribution of Q-sort ratings. Sorters are required to provide ratings that have identical distributions. Rater bias arising from a tendency to use or avoid extreme ratings are thereby eliminated. Even the operation of response biases such as social desirability are reduced by the Q-sort procedure because the number of highly desirable (and undesirable) items will, in a well-designed Q-sort, far exceed the number of available slots at the extremes, forcing the sorter to decide which desirable items are the most applicable. Although the Q-sort cannot entirely eliminate all forms of systematic rater error, no rating technique has so many built-in safeguards.

4. It is true that assessment in developmental psychology must be age appropriate, but conforming to this imperative is more difficult than recognizing its necessity. Indicators of a construct often do not remain constant over age (e.g., one would not expect irritability to be revealed by identical behaviors in infancy and adolescence); however, using different measures at different ages may defeat the intentions of longitudinal research because there may be no guarantee that the different measures are in fact assessing the same construct. Human observers can do more than tabulate the occurrences of particular behaviors; they may also make inferences about the meaning of behavior. When observers agree in their interpretations, and this consensual interpretation itself corresponds to other, perhaps more objective assessment outcomes, a genuine solution

to the problem is obtained. J. H. Block and Block (1980) used this strategy in their longitudinal examination of ego-control and ego-resiliency. When children were aged 3, 4, 5, and 7 years, various different experimental tasks and the same Q-sort measures were used to assess these constructs. The convergence in results, both within and across methods, solidified the substantive interpretation of their results by ruling out alternative methodological artifacts.

5. Because normative rating methods generally require judges to evaluate an entire sample serially on a set of items, the number of items actually used is often small and with content constrained by the researchers' original interest. By contrast, the Q-sort procedure requires judges to evaluate individuals serially on a set of items, a set usually large in number with wide-ranging content. As a result, a variety of constructs are assessed, and data may be used for many purposes and for analyses far from the original intentions of the research. Constructs may be assessed in a variety of ways: by focusing on single items, by classifying items into content categories, and by forming new scales. For example, Harrington et al. (1978) used 1 of the 100 items of the California Child Q-Set ("Becomes anxious when the environment is unpredictable or poorly structured") as a centerpiece in their analyses of intolerance of ambiguity. J. H. Block (1973) classified Q-sort items used in ideal-self descriptions as indicative of either agency or communion to show cross-cultural generality in sex role stereotypes. In addition, although the California Q-Set was not intended to assess a small number of basic, general traits, McCrae, Costa, and Busch (1986) have shown that the Big Five (Neuroticism, Extraversion, Openness, Agreeableness, and Conscientiousness) may be found there.

Multidimensional and metatheoretical constructs are also accessible through the Q-sort method. Theoretical and empirical analyses of consistency and change constitute a primary emphasis in the study of personality development. Most approaches are variable centered, focusing on consistency and change of single attribute. However, because the same event may change people differently, one must either anticipate and assess the many possible moderators or recognize that many effects may be missed. An alternative approach is to use a person-centered, multiattribute measure of consistency and change, such as an individual's across-time Q correlation (e.g., J. Block, 1971; Ozer & Gjerde, 1989). J. H. Block, Block, and Morrison (1981) used a similar multiattribute strategy to assess parental agreement on child-rearing practices, using the Q correlation between mothers' and fathers' Child-Rearing Practices Report (a Q-sort used by parents to describe values, attitudes, and behaviors relevant to child rearing). This multiattribute measure of parental agreement predicted a variety of outcomes, including the subsequent occurrence of divorce.

6. The Q-sort method invites the consideration of a variety of novel data-analytic strategies. Several of these (e.g., Q correlations as measures of across-time change) have already been noted; others have been described by Caspi et al. (in press). Caspi et al. also provided a demonstration of how the Q-sort may be used to demonstrate convergence among measures. The 100 items of their revised version of the California Child Q-Set completed by caregivers were each correlated with three indicators: self-reported delinquency, caregiver reports of disruptive disorders, and teacher ratings of externalizing problems. These analyses resulted in three vectors, each containing 100 correlations describing the personality implications of each of the three indicators. By obtaining the correlations among these three vectors of correlations (which all exceeded .70), Caspi et al. (in press) demonstrated considerable convergence in the personological implications of these three different measures of antisocial behavior.

Summary and Conclusions

The contributions already made by Q-sort methods in the study of personality development are numerous, yet the potential of the method greatly exceeds existing accomplishments. Lack of familiarity and unsolved technical problems may both contribute to the reluctance of some researchers to use the method. By reviewing some of the basics of Q-sort procedures, by offering examples of successful usage of the technique, and by addressing some of the unsolved problems, in this chapter I have attempted to address these possibilities. Although the Q-sort, like any method, has its limitations, it does offer leverage against a variety of difficulties in the study of personality development.

References

Allport, G. W. (1962). The general and the unique in psychological science. *Journal of Personality, 30*, 405–422.

Block, J. (1956). A comparison of the forced and unforced Q-sorting procedures. *Educational and Psychological Measurement, 16*, 481–493.

Block, J. (1957). A comparison between ipsative and normative ratings of personality. *Journal of Abnormal and Social Psychology, 54*, 50–54.

Block, J. (1961). *The Q-sort method in personality assessment and psychiatric research.* Springfield, IL: Charles C Thomas.

Block, J. (1971). *Lives through time.* Berkeley, CA: Bancroft Books.

Block, J., & Block, J. H. (1980). *The California Child Q-set.* Palo Alto, CA: Consulting Psychologists Press.

Block, J. H. (1973). Conceptions of sex-role: Some cross-cultural and longitudinal perspectives. *American Psychologist, 28*, 512–526.

Block, J. H., & Block, J. (1980). The role of ego-control and ego-resiliency in the organization of behavior. In W. A. Collins (Ed.), *Minnesota Symposia on Child Psychology* (Vol. 13, pp. 39–101). Hillsdale, NJ: Erlbaum.

Block, J. H., Block, J., & Morrison, A. (1981). Parental agreement-disagreement on child-rearing orientations and gender-related personality correlates in children. *Child Development, 52*, 965–974.

Caspi, A., Block, J., Block, J. H., Klopp, B., Lynam, D., Moffitt, T. E., & Stouthamer-Loeber, M. (in press). A "common language" version of the California Child Q-Set for personality assessment. *Psychological Assessment.*

Caspi, A., & Herbener, E. S. (1990). Continuity and change: Assortative marriage and the consistency of personality in adulthood. *Journal of Personality and Social Psychology, 58*, 250–258.

Cattell, R. B. (1946). *The description and measurement of personality.* New York: World Book.

Clemans, W. V. (1966). An analytical and empirical examination of some properties of ipsative measures. *Psychometric Monographs, 14.*

Craik, K. H. (1988). Assessing the personalities of historical figures. In W. M. Runyan (Ed.), *Psychology and historical interpretation* (pp. 196–218). New York: Oxford University Press.

Cronbach, L. J., Gleser, G. C., Nanda, H., & Rajaratnam, N. (1972). *The dependability of behavioral measurements: Theory of generalizability for scores and profiles.* Urbana: University of Illinois Press.

Funder, D. C., & Colvin, C. R. (1988). Friends and strangers: Acquaintanceship, agreement, and the accuracy of personality judgments. *Journal of Personality and Social Psychology, 55*, 149–158.

Gough, H. G. (1965). Conceptual analysis of psychological test scores and other diagnostic variables. *Journal of Abnormal Psychology, 79*, 294–302.

Green, B. F. (1980). Note on Bem and Funder's scheme for scoring Q sorts. *Psychological Review, 87,* 212–214.

Guadagnoli, E., & Velicer, W. F. (1988). Relation of sample size to the stability of component patterns. *Psychological Bulletin, 103,* 265–275.

Harrington, D. M., Block, J. H., & Block, J. (1978). Intolerance of ambiguity in preschool children: Psychometric considerations, behavioral manifestations, and parental correlates. *Developmental Psychology, 14,* 242–256.

Hicks, L. E. (1970). Some properties of ipsative, normative, and forced-choice normative measures. *Psychological Bulletin, 74,* 167–184.

Jung, C. G. (1924). *Psychological types.* New York: Harcourt, Brace.

McKeown, B., & Thomas, D. (1988). *Q methodology.* Newbury Park, CA: Sage.

McCrae, R. R., Costa, P. T., & Busch, C. M. (1986). Evaluating comprehensiveness in personality systems: The California Q-set and the five factor model. *Journal of Personality, 54,* 430–446.

Ozer, D. J. (1987). Personality, intelligence, and spatial visualization: Correlates of mental rotations test performance. *Journal of Personality and Social Psychology, 53,* 129–134.

Ozer, D. J. (1989). Construct validity in personality assessment. In D. M. Buss & N. Cantor (Eds.), *Personality psychology: Recent trends and emerging directions* (pp. 224–234). New York: Springer-Verlag.

Ozer, D. J., & Gjerde, P. F. (1989). Patterns of personality consistency and change from childhood through adolescence. *Journal of Personality, 57,* 483–507.

Rogers, C. R., & Dymond, R. F. (Eds.). (1954). *Psychotherapy and personality change: Coordinated research studies in the client-centered approach.* Chicago: University of Chicago Press.

Stephenson, W. (1935). Correlating persons instead of tests. *Character and Personality, 6,* 17–24.

Stephenson, W. (1936). The foundations of psychometry: Four factor systems. *Psychometrika, 1,* 195–209.

Stephenson, W. (1953). *The study of behavior: Q-technique and its methodology.* Chicago: University of Chicago Press.

Waters, E., & Deane, K. E. (1985). Defining and assessing individual differences in attachment relationships: Q-methodology and the organization of behavior in infancy and early childhood. In I. Bretherton & E. Waters (Eds.), Growing points of attachment theory and research (pp. 41–65). *Monographs of the Society for Research in Child Development, 50*(1–2, Serial No. 209).

CHAPTER 8

The Structure of Personality Traits: Vertical and Horizontal Aspects

Lewis R. Goldberg

I t has taken a long time (at the very least since Aristotle provided a taxonomy of human character traits in his Nichomachean Ethics), but the past decade has witnessed a growing consensus that perceived personality traits can be organized within five orthogonal domains, alternatively referred to as the "Big Five" factor structure or the "five factor" model (e.g., Digman, 1990; John, 1990; McCrae & John, 1992; Wiggins & Pincus, 1992; Wiggins & Trapnell, in press). These broad domains incorporate hundreds, if not thousands, of bipolar traits: Factor I (Surgency) contrasts traits such as extraversion, assertiveness, and activity level with traits such as introversion, passivity, and reserve; Factor II (Agreeableness) contrasts traits such as kindness, trust, and warmth with traits such

This project was supported by Grant MH-39077 from the National Institute of Mental Health. The author is indebted to Paul T. Costa, Jr., Willem K. B. Hofstee, and Robert R. McCrae for stimulating some of the ideas in this chapter and to Peter M. Bentler, John M. Digman, Donald W. Fiske, Robert M. Guion, Henry F. Kaiser, Clarence McCormick, Robert R. McCrae, Warren Norman, Gerard Saucier, Auke Tellegen, Amos Tversky, and Keith Widaman for their thoughtful reactions and suggestions.

as hostility, selfishness, and distrust; Factor III (Conscientiousness) contrasts traits such as organization, thoroughness, and dependability with traits such as carelessness, negligence, and unreliability; Factor IV (Emotional Stability vs. Neuroticism) contrasts traits such as stability and imperturbability with such traits as nervousness, moodiness, and temperamentality; and Factor V (whether labeled *Intellect* or *Openness to Experience*) contrasts traits such as imagination, intelligence, and creativity with traits such as shallowness and imperceptiveness.

Any complete taxonomy of personality traits must include both the vertical and the horizontal features of their meanings. The vertical aspect refers to the hierarchical[1] relations among traits (e.g., reliability is a more abstract and general concept than punctuality), whereas the horizontal aspect refers to the degree of similarity among traits at the same hierarchical level (e.g., wit involves aspects of both intelligence and humor). Scientists who emphasize the vertical aspect of trait structure could use multivariate techniques such as hierarchical cluster analysis, or they could use oblique rotations in factor analysis and then factor the correlations among the primary dimensions, thus constructing a hierarchical structure. Scientists who emphasize the horizontal aspect of trait structure could use discrete cluster solutions or orthogonal factor rotations. In fact, however, there has been no one-to-one relation between the emphasis of investigators and their methodological preferences.

For example, both Eysenck (1970) and Cattell (1947) have developed explicitly hierarchical representations, with Eysenck's leading to three highest level factors and Cattell's to eight or nine. However, whereas Cattell has always advocated and used oblique factor procedures, Eysenck has typically used orthogonal methods. Historically, the five-factor model grew out of exploratory factor analyses by investigators using orthogonal

---

[1]There are two related but logically distinct meanings of the concept of "hierarchy." In its classic definition, a hierarchy refers to a structure that includes subsets strictly nested within larger sets (e.g., "animal" is a more inclusive concept than "dog"). As used in the literature on personality traits, however, the concept of hierarchy accepts the fuzzy relations among traits and indexes the levels of traits that differ in their category breadth; the breadth of trait categories refers to the range of different types of behaviors included in the trait descriptor (e.g., Hampson, John, & Goldberg, 1986; John, Hampson, & Goldberg, 1991).

rotations (e.g., Goldberg, 1990; Norman, 1963; McCrae & Costa, 1985, 1987; Tupes & Christal, 1961). Yet, some of these same investigators construed the model in an expressly hierarchical fashion (e.g., Costa, McCrae, & Dye, 1991; McCrae & Costa, 1992), whereas others emphasized its horizontal aspects (e.g., Hofstee, de Raad, & Goldberg, 1992; Peabody & Goldberg, 1989). Is one point of view more correct or more useful?

Vertical Approaches to Trait Structure

The defining feature of hierarchical models of personality traits is that they emphasize the vertical relations among variables (e.g., from the most specific to the most abstract) to the exclusion of the relations among variables at the same level. Figures 1a and 1b show two of the most famous hierarchical models of individual differences, the first a representation of human abilities and the other of those personality traits that fall in the Extraversion domain. Figure 1a is a schematic presentation of the classic Vernon–Burt hierarchical model of abilities (e.g., Vernon, 1950); specific test items combine to form ability tests, which combine to make up specific factors, which in turn combine to form the minor group factors, which in turn make up the major group factors, which at their apex form the most general factor, g for general intelligence. Figure 1b is a version of Eysenck's (1970) model of extraversion; specific responses in particular situations (e.g., telling a joke, buying a new car) are considered to be subordinate categories to habitual responses (e.g., entertaining strangers, making rapid decisions), which in turn combine to make up traits such as sociability and impulsiveness, which finally form the superordinate attribute of extraversion. What is important to observe in both panels is that for the variables at any one level that are associated with the same higher order factor, no other relations among them are specified, and thus their order in the figure is completely arbitrary.

Figure 2 illustrates this limitation of hierarchical representations even more clearly by presenting Eysenck's complete model of personality traits (H. J. Eysenck & M. W. Eysenck, 1985). Note that each of the superfactors of Psychoticism, Extraversion, and Neuroticism is formed from exactly nine traits and that the relations among the nine traits in

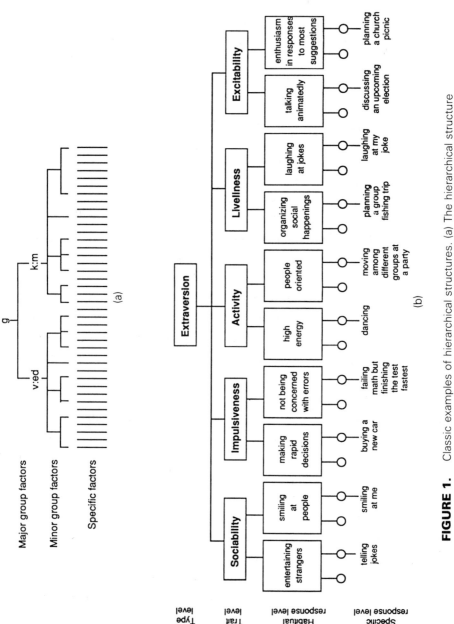

FIGURE 1. Classic examples of hierarchical structures. (a) The hierarchical structure of human abilities (Vernon, 1950). (b) Eysenck's (1970) model of Extraversion. Reprinted with permission.

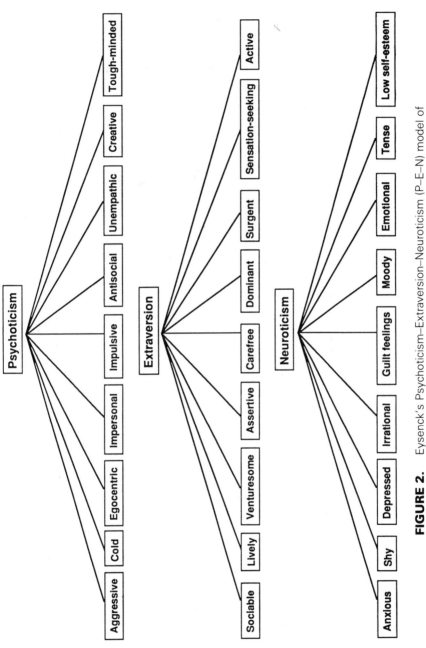

FIGURE 2. Eysenck's Psychoticism–Extraversion–Neuroticism (P–E–N) model of personality traits. From H. J. Eysenck and M. W. Eysenck (1985). Reprinted with permission.

each set are not specified.[2] Figure 3 provides another hierarchical model for personality traits, this one based on the Costa and McCrae (1992) variant of the five-factor structure (R. R. McCrae, personal communication, October 11, 1991); eight items are included in each of the six "facet" scales that are associated with each of the Big Five domains, one of which has been illustrated in complete detail in Figure 3. From this model, it is clear that the facets of fantasy, aesthetics, feelings, actions, ideas, and values fall in the domain of Openness, but the relations among those facets are unspecified.

Horizontal Approaches to Trait Structure

The defining feature of horizontal models is that the relations among the variables are specified by the variables' locations in multidimensional space. When that space is limited to only two dimensions, and the locations of the variables are projected to some uniform distance from the origin, the resulting structures are referred to as "circumplex" representations. The most famous example of such models is the Interpersonal Circle (e.g., Kiesler, 1983; Wiggins, 1979, 1980), which is based on Factors I (Surgency) and II (Agreeableness) in the five-factor model. Other examples of circumplex models include those that incorporate Big Five Factors I, II, and III (Peabody & Goldberg, 1989; Stern, 1970) and Factors I, II, and IV (Saucier, 1992).

A more comprehensive circumplex representation has recently been proposed by Hofstee et al. (1992). Dubbed the "AB5C" model, for Abridged Big Five-Dimensional Circumplex, this representation includes the 10 bivariate planes formed from all pairs of the Big Five factors. In the AB5C model, each trait is assigned to the plane formed by the two factors with which it is most highly associated (e.g., its two highest factor loadings). As evidence for the reasonableness of this limitation to two of the five dimensions, a mere 3% of the varimax-rotated factor loadings from a representative pool of 540 English trait adjectives were .20 or higher on three or more factors; indeed, less than 1% of the factor loadings were

---

[2]The trait of impulsiveness has migrated from Extraversion to Psychoticism in these two versions of Eysenck's theory.

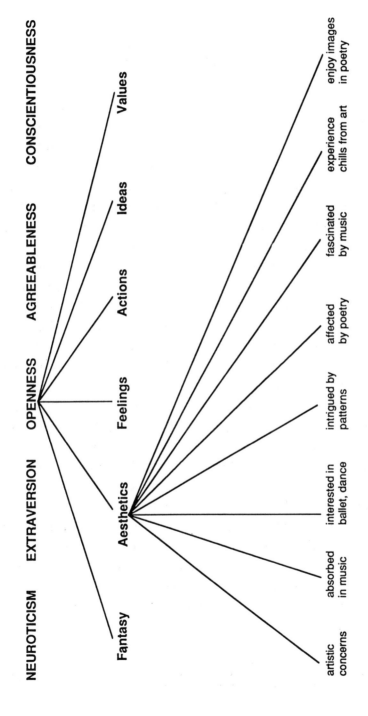

FIGURE 3. Hierarchical structure of the NEO Personality Inventory. From Costa and McCrae (1992). Reprinted with permission.

.25 or higher, and none of the loadings were .30 or higher, on three or more factors.[3]

The article by Hofstee et al. (1992) provided the AB5C locations of these 540 trait adjectives, based on analyses of 636 self- ($n = 320$) and peer ($n = 316$) ratings. The Big Five factor loadings were derived from varimax rotations of the 100 unipolar factor markers from Goldberg (1992), and the resulting five orthogonal factor scores were used to calculate the loadings of the remaining 440 terms. Of the 10 AB5C planes, the most densely populated were those for Factors I and II (the Interpersonal Circle) and for Factors II and IV; the most sparsely populated planes were those associated with Factor V, especially II/V and IV/V. The distributions of terms around the circles varied substantially across the 10 planes. Factors I and II (the Interpersonal Circle) formed a near-perfect circumplex. By contrast, in five planes (II/III, III/V, I/IV, II/IV, and III/IV), there were more terms located in the evaluatively congruent quadrants (e.g., II + /III +) than in the evaluatively incongruent ones (e.g., II + /III −), which resulted in a distinct northeast by southwest orientation of the terms in those planes. Finally, four planes (I/III, I/V, II/V, and IV/V) were relatively devoid of interstitial variables (i.e., factor blends) and thus appeared to be more simple structured.

The three panels in Figures 4a–c provide examples of the 10 bivariate planes: I/II (Figure 4a, a nearly perfect circumplex), I/III (Figure 4b, a configuration relatively close to simple structure), and II/IV (Figure 4c, a configuration that shows the distinct northeast by southwest orientation that results when there are more terms of the same evaluative valence than of different ones). The location of each term in each plane is provided twice, once as defined by its angular position and its distance from the origin within the circle, and again when it is projected onto the circumference of the circle. The triangles in Figures 4a–c indicate the locations of the factor-univocal terms, which by definition have low secondary loadings, in each of the four planes other than the one containing their actual secondary loadings.

---

[3]If it were not for limitations in the ability to display more than two dimensions on a page, one could use the same number of three-dimensional representations as two-dimensional ones. That is, one needs 10 panels to display five dimensions taken either two at a time or three at a time.

Factor I and Factor II

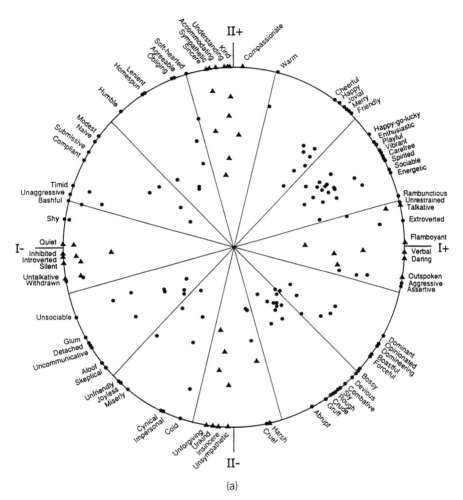

FIGURES 4a–c. Three examples of the ten bivariate planes included in Hofstee et al. (1992). Reprinted with permission.

In Figures 4a–c, solid lines are used to divide each circle into 12 regions, each of 30°, which form the facets of the AB5C model. These facets can be conceptualized as blends of two factors in a matrix in which the columns represent the primary loadings and the rows represent the secondary ones. However, the 10 cells representing combinations of the

Factor I and Factor III

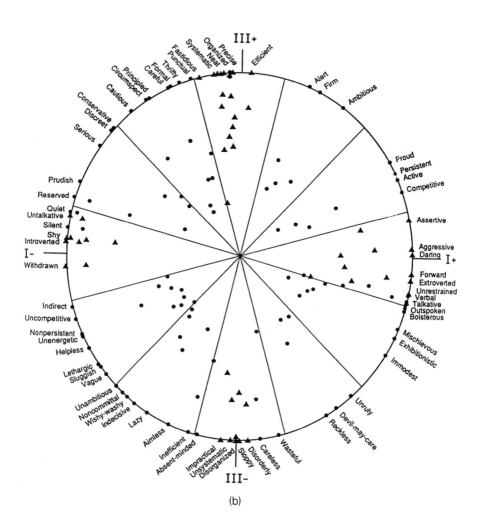

(b)

positive and negative poles of the same factor in this 10 × 10 matrix are necessarily empty. Of the remaining 90 cells, the number of terms per cell varies from 0 for six cells to 24 for the II + /IV + cell. A table providing some of the terms within each of the AB5C facets is given in Hofstee et al. (1992).

As an alternative representation of both the horizontal and the vertical features of these trait terms, one could use a path diagram, such as that presented in Figure 5. Included in this figure are 12 of the trait terms

Factor II and Factor IV

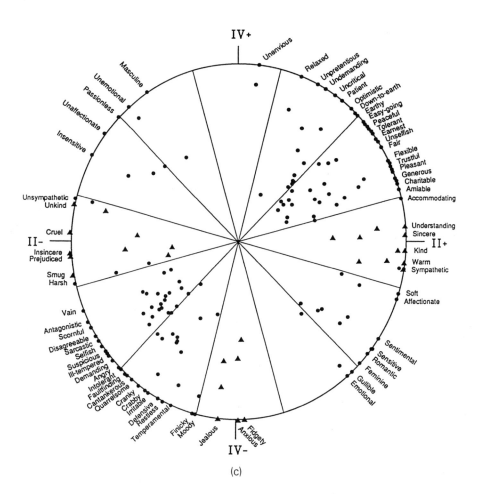

(c)

from Panel A (Factors I and II) of Figure 4. The values in the figure are the factor loadings of each term on each of the two factors. Although such diagrams are now being used with increasing frequency, they normally are used only in studies that include relatively few variables. Indeed, it is not easy to see how one might use path diagrams to display the structure of all 540 of the trait terms used by Hofstee et al. (1992).[4]

[4]On the other hand, one advantage of path models is that they permit the investigation of complex hierarchical structures, in which factors can include variables located at different hierarchical levels.

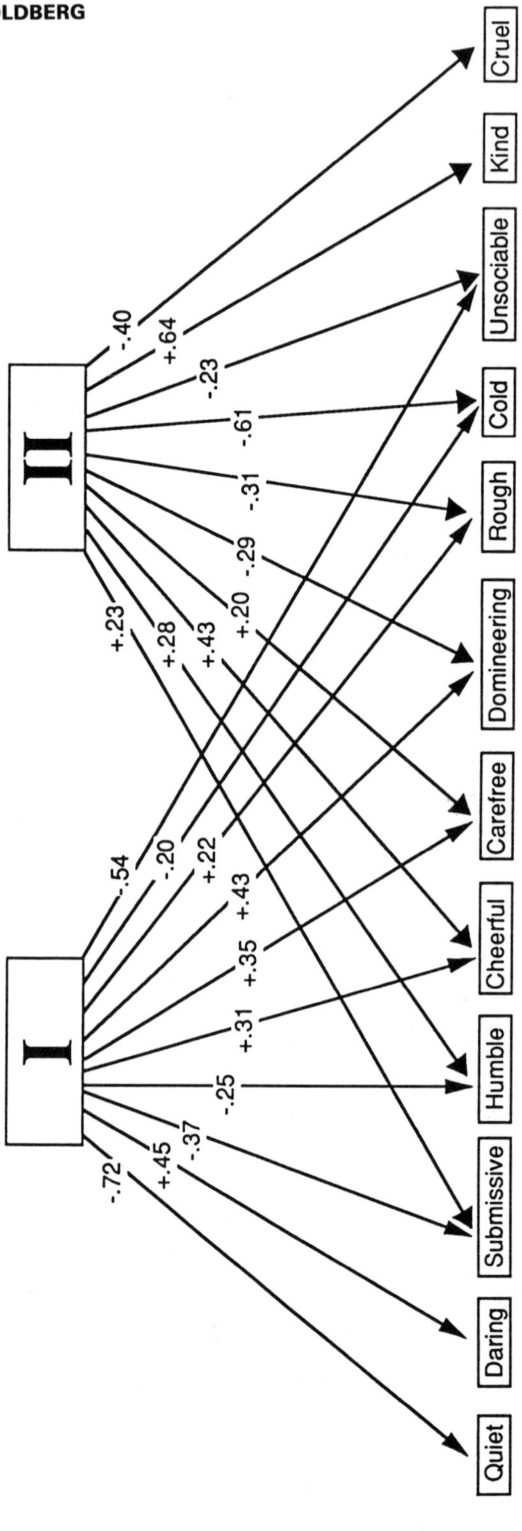

FIGURE 5. An alternative method for displaying some of the trait terms in Panel A of Figure 4. From Hofstee et al. (1992). Reprinted with permission.

Differentiating Vertical From Horizontal Facets

All structural representations based on factor-analytic methodology can be viewed from either vertical or horizontal perspectives. Factor analysis can be used to construct hierarchical models *explicitly* with oblique rotational procedures and *implicitly* even with orthogonal solutions because any factor can be viewed as being located at a level above that of the variables being factored; that is, even orthogonal factors separate the common variance (the factors) from the total (common plus specific) variance of the measures. One could therefore emphasize the vertical aspect by grouping the variables by the factor with which they are most highly associated, thereby disregarding information about factorial blends. Alternatively, one could concentrate on the horizontal features of the representation, as in the AB5C model. What are the advantages associated with each perspective?

McCrae and Costa (1992) have argued that hierarchical structures are to be preferred to the extent to which the variances of the traits are trait specific, as compared with the extent that they are related to the five broad factors. Those investigators demonstrated that, after partialing out the five-factor common variance from both self- and other ratings on the facet scales from the revised NEO Personality Inventory, the residual variance in these scales was still substantial enough to elicit strong correlations among self-ratings, spouse ratings, and peer ratings of the same trait. From this finding, they argued in favor of hierarchical representations, in which relatively small amounts of common variance produce the higher level factors, with ample amounts of specific variance still available for predictive purposes.

This assumption has powerful implications for the role of trait measures when used in multiple regression analyses in applied contexts, such as personnel selection and classification. Because one always loses specific variance as one amalgamates measures, the optimal level of prediction is completely a function of statistical power and thus of sample size. In the population (i.e., samples of unlimited size), optimal prediction by regression analysis will always be at the level of individual items; that is, for huge samples it would be silly even to amalgamate the items into scales because one would inevitably lose some specific variance at the item level that could serve to increase predictive accuracy. Indeed, it is only the problem of capitalization on chance that justifies the use of scales as compared with items, and analogously of factor scores as compared with scale scores, when making predictions by regression analyses in applied contexts.

Failure to understand this psychometric axiom has led to some serious misunderstandings. For example, Mershon and Gorsuch (1988) invoked as a criterion for deciding between different structural representations the "predictability of real-life criteria" (p. 677). Those investigators compared the validity of predictions based on the 16 scales in the Sixteen Personality Factors Questionnaire (16PF) with that based on the six second-order 16PF factors. Not surprisingly, validity tended to be higher when the 16 scales were used in regression analyses than when only the six second-order scales were so used. Had their sample sizes been large enough, they could have similarly "demonstrated" that the use of all of the 16PF items increased predictions over the use of the 16 scales.

Although it is necessary to think hierarchically about the use of trait measures in applied contexts, it is equally necessary to think horizontally about basic taxonomic issues. To compare these two types of representations, I will assume that the total variance of any item i can be decomposed into four parts:

H_i = the variance associated with one or more of the five highest order (H) factors (e.g., the Big Five);

A_i = the variance associated with one or more of any additional (A) factors, orthogonal to the Big Five;

S_i = the reliable variance specific (S) to each item and thus orthogonal to both H and A; and

e_i = measurement error, by definition orthogonal to H, A, and S.

Although McCrae and Costa (1992) have assumed that the amount of specific variance in the measures is the key to differentiating between the two types of representations, this assumption is incorrect. That is, the amount of specific as compared with common trait variance is not relevant to a comparison between the two models because the models differ only in their representation of common variance. Specifically, the common variance is associated with a single factor in the NEO Personality Inventory, whereas it is represented as a blend of two factors in the AB5C model. This may be easiest to see by examining the hypothetical extremes, namely 0% and 100% specific variance. If there were no common variance among the variables, every variable would be completely unrelated to all others, and neither model would be useful in any way; the function of both models is to explain common variance. If 100% of the variance of all variables were included in the five-dimensional representation, it would still be possible to provide a set of factor-univocal marker scales for each of the five factors (e.g., Goldberg, 1992), and it would still be possible to provide the locations of all traits in five-dimensional space (as in the AB5C model). That is, for any particular combination of common and specific variance, one could provide either type of representation of the common variance.

However, the common variance can be decomposed into two parts, that associated with the highest order factors (H-variance) and that associated with all additional factors (A-variance). Researchers now know that at the highest order, there are five broad personality factors and no others with even moderate breadth (e.g., Goldberg, 1990). All additional factors orthogonal to the Big Five are narrow, consisting primarily of small clusters of quasi-synonyms and quasi-antonyms.

Is it possible that the ratio of A:H variances might be relevant to the selection of vertical as compared with horizontal representations? Consider the limiting cases. If 100% of all common variance of the items is associated with the five superfactors and thus there is no A-variance, the items all can be described by their positions in five-dimensional space, plus their specific variances. Such a configuration would imply the existence of a sharp natural break between the sizes of the first five and later factors. However, in the five-dimensional space, there may be sets of items that are located close to each other, thus forming item clusters that can be grouped into scales. These scales, in turn, can be grouped under the factor with which they are most highly associated or they could be represented as a blend of two or more factors; that is, the configuration can be represented by either a vertical or a horizontal model, although it would be hard to argue for the former because it would simply throw away information.

Alternatively, in addition to their specific variances and common variances associated with the Big Five, the items may contain varying amounts of common variance on narrow factors that are unrelated to the Big Five (A-variance). Such a configuration would imply less of a sharp break between the sizes of the first five and later factors. If only five factors are rotated, however, it is only the Big Five common variances that would determine the locations of the items in five-dimensional space. Again, as before, item clusters could be grouped under the factor with which they are most highly associated, or they could be represented as blends of the five factors. Thus, this configuration also can be modeled by either a vertical or a horizontal representation, again with the former providing somewhat less information than the latter. Indeed, if only five factors are extracted and rotated, there is no mix of H- to A- to S-variances that would favor the hierarchical model for taxonomic purposes.[5]

A perfect hierarchical model would consist of L higher order factors, M additional orthogonal common factors, each associated with a particular facet, and then K specific factors, one for each item. Every item would contain some variance associated with one or more of the L higher order factors, some additional variance associated with one of the M lower order factors, plus some specific variance of its own. The eigenvalues of the matrix of correlations among the items should show a break between the sizes of factors L and L + 1, and then again between Factors M and M + 1. All real data sets, however, will doubtless include variables with various combinations of the four types of variance, and thus there will rarely be any huge breaks in the sizes of the eigenvalues. As a consequence, it should be possible to represent any real data set by both vertical and horizontal models.

---

[5]The findings from McCrae amd Costa (1992) do not bear directly on the hierarchical structure of the NEO Personality Inventory because the self–peer correlations from their residual matrices could be a result of A-variance, S-variance, or some combination of both. That is, these analyses merely eliminated the H-variance (by residualization) and the e-variance (by self–peer agreement), leaving the A-variance and the S-variance confounded.

It is for this reason that one must think hierarchically when using multiple regression analyses in applied prediction contexts. With any typical data matrix, as one's sample size increases, one will profit by reaching down lower in the hierarchy to select one's initial predictor variables. For small samples, one must stay with only the H-variances of the highest order factor scores to avoid capitalizing on the chance vagaries of one's derivation sample. For large samples, one should use the M facet scales because each contains some A-variance beyond the highest level factors. For populations (or huge samples), one should use the items because each item contains some S-variance beyond its A-variance and H-variance.

Unidimensional Versus Multidimensional Variables

Investigators of the structure of human abilities often contrast research strategies aimed at the development of unidimensional tests with those that proceed with factorially complex variables. The former strategy is expressly hierarchical, proceeding from the most general to the most specific. By partialing out sources of variance at successively lower levels, the aim is to arrive at unidimensional subsets of items, with each subset being orthogonal to each of the others. In such a model, all sources of common variance have been partialed out of the lowest level factors, and the resulting factor representation is that of perfect simple structure. In this idealized unidimensional model, there is no nonarbitrary basis for ordering the items that load on each lowest level factor.

The attainment of truly unidimensional tests would be a signal achievement for the measurement of psychological attributes: Such tests would satisfy the important additivity assumption of measurement theory, whether viewed from the perspective of classical test theory or of modern item-response theory. Unfortunately, there is increasing evidence that the basic irreducible measurement unit, the item, is in fact more often than not multidimensional in nature. Most items include variance from two or more sources, and thus they measure more than one factor at the same level of generality. Thus, most items—and the resulting tests—tend to be factorially complex rather than factor univocal (i.e., most items and tests tend to have substantial relations with at least two factors rather than with only one).

Personality variables are no exceptions to this general rule, as exemplified by the findings of Hofstee et al. (1992). Trait-descriptive terms are not clustered tightly in five-dimensional space, as would be true if the personality lexicon contained only semantically isolated sets of near-synonyms and near-antonyms; rather, most terms share some features of their meanings with one set of terms while they share other features with another set. Thus, even after rotation of the factors to a criterion of simple structure such as varimax, most variables have substantial secondary loadings and thus must be viewed as blends of two or more factors.

Moreover, it is not always easy to secure agreement on the optimal positions of the factor axes, even among personality theorists who share the same biological orientation toward factor location. For example, Gray (1981) has long argued that Eysenck's (1970) two factors of Extraversion and Neuroticism are located 45° away from the theoretically most useful positions, which Gray labeled Anxiety and Impulsivity. To best understand this theoretical disagreement, one should examine the personality descriptors located in the plane formed by Factors I and IV in the Big Five model, the two factors that conform to Eysenck's dimensions of Extraversion and Neuroticism. One can then locate the variables that define Gray's two dimensions, which are blends of the factors proposed by Eysenck (or, alternatively, one can view the variables that are associated with Extraversion and Neuroticism as being blends of Anxiety and Impulsivity). Because hierarchical models deemphasize these horizontal aspects of trait relations, they provide no information about the nature of such factorial blends. Therefore, for purposes of basic research on the structure of traits, models that emphasize horizontal relations (e.g., Hofstee et al., 1992) will typically be more informative.

References

Cattell, R. B. (1947). Confirmation and clarification of primary personality factors. *Psychometrika, 12,* 197–220.

Costa, P. T., Jr., & McCrae, R. R. (1992). *Revised NEO Personality Inventory (NEO-PI-R) and NEO Five-Factor Inventory (NEO-FFI) professional manual.* Odessa, FL: Psychological Assessment Resources.

Costa, P. T., Jr., McCrae, R. R., & Dye, D. A. (1991). Facet scales for Agreeableness and Conscientiousness: A revision of the NEO Personality Inventory. *Personality and Individual Differences, 12,* 887–898.

Digman, J. M. (1990). Personality structure: Emergence of the five-factor model. *Annual Review of Psychology, 41,* 417–440.

Eysenck, H. J. (1970). *The structure of human personality (3rd ed.).* London: Methuen.

Eysenck, H. J., & Eysenck, M. W. (1985). *Personality and individual differences: A natural science approach.* New York: Plenum Press.

Goldberg, L. R. (1990). An alternative "description of personality": The Big-Five factor structure. *Journal of Personality and Social Psychology, 59,* 1216–1229.

Goldberg, L. R. (1992). The development of markers of the Big-Five factor structure. *Psychological Assessment, 4,* 26–42.

Gray, J. A. (1981). A critique of Eysenck's theory of personality. In H. J. Eysenck (Ed.), *A model for personality* (pp. 246–276). Berlin: Springer-Verlag.

Hampson, S. E., John, O. P., & Goldberg, L. R. (1986). Category breadth and hierarchical structure in personality: Studies of asymmetries in judgments of trait implications. *Journal of Personality and Social Psychology, 51,* 37–54.

Hofstee, W. K. B., de Raad, B., & Goldberg, L. R. (1992). Integration of the Big Five and circumplex taxonomies of traits. *Journal of Personality and Social Psychology, 63,* 146–163.

John, O. P. (1990). The "Big-Five" factor taxonomy: Dimensions of personality in the natural language and in questionnaires. In L. A. Pervin (Ed.), *Handbook of personality theory and research* (pp. 66–100). New York: Guilford Press.

John, O. P., Hampson, S. E., & Goldberg, L. R. (1991). The basic level in personality-trait hierarchies: Studies of trait use and accessibility in different contexts. *Journal of Personality and Social Psychology, 60,* 348–361.

Kiesler, D. J. (1983). The 1982 Interpersonal Circle: A taxonomy for complementarity in human transactions. *Psychological Review, 90,* 185–214.

McCrae, R. R., & Costa, P. T., Jr. (1985). Updating Norman's "adequate taxonomy": Intelligence and personality dimensions in natural language and in questionnaires. *Journal of Personality and Social Psychology, 49,* 710–721.

McCrae, R. R., & Costa, P. T., Jr. (1987). Validation of the five-factor model of personality across instruments and observers. *Journal of Personality and Social Psychology, 52,* 81–90.

McCrae, R. R., & Costa, P. T., Jr. (1992). Discriminant validity of NEO-PIR facet scales. *Educational and Psychological Measurement, 52,* 229–237.

McCrae, R. R., & John, O. P. (1992). An introduction to the five-factor model and its applications. *Journal of Personality, 60,* 175–215.

Mershon, B., & Gorsuch, R. L. (1988). Number of factors in the personality sphere: Does increase in factors increase predictability of real-life criteria? *Journal of Personality and Social Psychology, 55,* 675–680.

Norman, W. T. (1963). Toward an adequate taxonomy of personality attributes: Replicated factor structure in peer nomination personality ratings. *Journal of Abnormal and Social Psychology, 66,* 574–583.

Peabody, D., & Goldberg, L. R. (1989). Some determinants of factor structures from personality-trait descriptors. *Journal of Personality and Social Psychology, 57,* 552–567.

Saucier, G. (1992). Benchmarks: Integrating affective and interpersonal circles with the Big-Five personality factors. *Journal of Personality and Social Psychology, 62,* 1025–1035.

Stern, G. G. (1970). *People in context: Measuring person-environment congruence in education and industry.* New York: Wiley.

Tupes, E. C., & Christal, R. E. (1961). *Recurrent personality factors based on trait ratings* (Tech. Rep. ASD-TR-61-97). Lackland Air Force Base, TX: U.S. Air Force.

Vernon, P. E. (1950). *The structure of human abilities.* London: Methuen.

Wiggins, J. S. (1979). A psychological taxonomy of trait-descriptive terms: The interpersonal domain. *Journal of Personality and Social Psychology, 37,* 395–412.

Wiggins, J. S. (1980). Circumplex models of interpersonal behavior. In L. Wheeler (Eds.), *Review of personality and social psychology* (Vol. 1, pp. 265–294). Newbury Park, CA: Sage.

Wiggins, J. S., & Pincus, A. L. (1992). Personality: Structure and assessment. *Annual Review of Psychology, 43,* 473–504.

Wiggins, J. S., & Trapnell, P. D. (in press). Personality structure: The return of the Big Five. In S. R. Briggs, R. Hogan, & W. H. Jones (Eds.), *Handbook of personality psychology.* San Diego, CA: Academic Press.

CHAPTER 9

Conformity and Conscientiousness: One Factor or Two Stages?

Jane Loevinger

The distinction between conformity and conscientiousness is embedded in Judeo–Christian culture and history. Many modern stage and type theories are built around that or a closely similar distinction. These two syndromes—conformity and conscientiousness—have been delineated empirically by studies with the Sentence Completion Test (SCT). However, mainstream psychology, in particular the five-factor conception of personality, ignores or obscures the distinction. There is a psychometric explanation of why anything so self-evident as that distinction can be hidden from the techniques of modern psychology. That is my argument.

History of the Distinction

The distinction between conformity and conscientiousness is an old one: Paul wrote, "the letter killeth but the spirit giveth life" (II Corinthians, 3:6).[1]

The main message of the Hebrew prophets was a protest against the injustices of the ruling class, hence of conformity to their regime, and a call to conscience and righteousness. Amos preached,

> I hate, I despise your feast days .... Though you offer me burnt offerings and your meat offerings, I will not accept them: Neither will I regard the peace offerings of your fat beasts .... But let judgment run down as waters, and righteousness as a mighty stream. (Amos 5:21–22, 24)

I interpret feast days and burnt offerings to represent conformity and judgment and righteousness to represent conscience.

Shakespeare had many references to the difference between conformity to authority and to conscience. Surely one element in the tragedy of King Lear was that he discerned that difference in his daughters too late. In *Henry VIII* Cardinal Wolsey says, "had I but served my God with half the zeal I served my king, he would not in mine age have left me naked to mine enemies" (Act III, ii).

The most ironic comment on the difference comes from Mark Twain (1884). In the *Adventures of Huckleberry Finn*, Huck's conscience tells him that he ought to let Miss Watson know where her runaway slave, Jim, is, so he wrote her a letter: "I felt good and all washed clean of sin for the first time I had ever felt so in my life." He sat thinking about all the times he and Jim had been together and how good Jim had been to him. Then he saw the unmailed letter.

> It was a close place. I took it up and held it in my hand. I was a-trembling, because I'd got to decide, forever, betwixt two things, and I knowed it. I studied a minute, sort of holding my breath, and then says to myself:
>
> "All right, then, I'll *go* to hell"—and tore it up ... and never thought no more about reforming. I shoved the whole thing out of my head, and said I would take up wickedness again, which was in my line, being brought up to it, and the other warn't. And for a start I would go to work

---

[1]Page references are not given for references to the Bible, Shakespeare, *The Adventures of Huckleberry Finn*, or *On Liberty*. All are widely available in many editions—that is part of my thesis—and the reader is unlikely to have access to the editions I used.

and steal Jim out of slavery again; and if I could think up anything worse, I would do that, too. (Twain, 1884, chapter 31)

The difference between conformity to authority and true conscience has been a major dynamic of Judeo–Christian history from the Hebrew prophets to the early Christian martyrs, through Joan of Arc, both sides of the Reformation—Sir Thomas More and Luther—down to the Nuremberg trials and the Watergate hearings, both of which officially recognized the difference. Nothing could have been clearer than the "Saturday night massacre," when Elliott Richardson and William Ruckelshaus each resigned, successively, as United States attorney general rather than dismiss Archibald Cox as special prosecutor, as President Nixon bade them to do. During the Watergate hearings, Senator Sam Ervin quoted the eloquent words that Shakespeare gave to Cardinal Wolsey.

However different the voice of conscience in those men and women of our history and our literature, all understood the distinction between conscience and conformity. The difference is enshrined in contemporary language in the terms *civil disobedience* and *conscientious objector*.

The Distinction in Stage and Type Theories

Some version of this distinction has turned up in numerous psychological type and stage theories in recent years. My choice of terms, *Conformity* and *Conscientiousness*[2], comes from the conception of ego development that my colleagues and I have been working with. There are many others. For example, Kohlberg's (1969) terms, the best known of them, are *Conventional* and *Postconventional morality*. Peck and Havighurst (1960) used the terms *conformity, irrational conscience,* and *rational conscience*. This chapter is not the place for an extensive list of such distinctions; I have tried to do that elsewhere (Loevinger, 1976). At the heart of all similar stage and type conceptions is the distinction at issue; that is because the vast majority of people are in that range.

---

[2]In this chapter, lower case is used for ordinary human traits or faculties, capitals for corresponding stage names. Conformity does not begin at the Conformist stage nor end at the transition to the Self-aware stage. Similarly, conscience and conscientiousness do not begin or end with the Conscientious stage.

Mainstream Theories

The problem is that psychometric and behavioristic psychologists, the mainstream in the United States today, have adopted a kind of empiricism that ignores and obscures the distinction.

One instance, exemplifying the best application of psychometrics to personality theory, is the five-factor theory of personality (Goldberg, 1990; McCrae & Costa, 1990). Goldberg has assembled an impressive number of studies of personality trait adjectives, with each study culminating in discovering five independent factors in descriptions of adult personality. His historical review begins with a study by Thurstone (1934) and includes a pivotal study by Norman (1963) and then an expanding list of other authors.

Goldberg's (1990) own research includes an exemplary set of studies, using large numbers of cases and different methods for generating the lists of adjectives for factoring and various methods for rotating factors. The results of the several studies, although not identical, are impressively similar.

The five factors are, in Goldberg's (1990) terms, Surgency, Agreeableness, Conscientiousness, Emotional Stability, and Intellect. McCrae and Costa's (1990) factors are Extraversion (for Surgency), Agreeableness, Conscientiousness, Neuroticism (for Emotional Stability), and Openness (for Intellect). The two versions have in common Conscientiousness. (In fairness, McCrae & Costa, 1980, have compared our [my colleagues' and my] conscientious stage to Openness [Intellect] rather than to Conscientiousness in their factors.)

Adjectives describing the positive pole of this factor include predictable, rigid, conventional, prompt, punctual, dependable, and conscientious. The negative pole includes as adjectives rebellious, irreverent, impolite, and informal. This is my selection from the many adjectives Goldberg (1990, p. 1218) listed, based on Norman (1963). Goldberg's Table 3 (p. 1225), showing revised synonym clusters, includes conventional and traditional as definitive of the positive pole of conscientiousness. The negative pole includes nonconforming, rebellious, and unconventional.

Taken as a whole, not concentrating on the particular adjectives I have selected, what is sketched certainly qualifies as a popular conception of conscientiousness, the kind of behavior every mother tries to instill in her children under that heading (e.g., be on time, keep your things in order, and do what your teacher tells you).

That is the set of behaviors that Mischel (1984) called *conscientiousness:* "The behavioral assessment of conscientiousness included such measures as: class attendance, study session attendance, assignment neatness, assignment punctuality, reserve reading punctuality for course sessions, room neatness, and personal appearance neatness" (pp. 286–287).[3] Contrast that conception with the description of conscience Shakespeare gave to one of the murderers in *Richard III:*

> I'll not meddle with it: it is a dangerous thing: it makes a man a coward:
> a man cannot steal, but it accuseth him; he cannot swear, but it checks
> him; he cannot lie with his neighbor's wife, but it detects him: it is a
> blushing shamefast spirit that mutinies in a man's bosom; it fills one full
> of obstacles: it made me once restore a purse of gold, that I found; it
> beggars any man that keeps it: it is turned out of all towns and cities for
> a dangerous thing; and every man that means to live well endeavours to
> trust to himself and to live without it. (Act I, iv)

Conscience: Lost and Found

In modern mainstream psychology the distinction between conformity and conscience has been lost. How could this happen? Is the problem excessive and too-literal behaviorism? That could be one element.

The factor theorists are more deeply involved. The fundamental assumption of factor analysis is linear; test scores are assumed to be weighted sums of the component factor scores. Factorists have to be committed to viewing all elements of personality as polar variables (i.e., as proceeding from little of something-or-other to much of that something). That assumption defines their purview. Any variable that develops in a radically curvilinear or nonmonotonic way generates impossible complexities for a factorial approach.

---

[3]An advertisement for a new test, the Personality Adjective Check List-PACL (21st Century Assessment, 1992, p. 2), listed the following as one of eight traits it measures: "Respectful: Conscientious and conforming; responsible, industrious, rule-abiding; can be moralistic and inflexible."

The stage–type theorists begin with more or less clinical observations of people. Although too little has been revealed about how stage and type theorists get their initial ideas and direction, I think that they begin by observing certain repeated syndromes or types of people (i.e., certain characteristics that often go together and form a pattern in some typical cases).

Having observed several such types, the next step is to postulate that there is a set of types or syndromes that more or less accounts for everyone. Because many type theories were discredited early in the history of differential psychology, today probably everyone concedes that types are rarely pure and that intermediate types are certainly more common.

Many type theorists go one step farther. Noting the age differences in usual exemplars of various types, they then postulate that these are not only types but stages in a developing sequence. Thus, stage theorists differ from the factorists in a second crucial way, for the factorial approach is generally mum about how the various factors develop during the formative years. Many stage theorists further elaborate their stages in terms of the logic of the developmental sequence.

The differences in these two approaches, stage and type theories as opposed to factorial theories, are so great that it is difficult to see how they could ever confront each other on an experimental or statistical ground acceptable to proponents of both. I do not claim to prove that my approach is more "scientific" than that of the factorists, although I certainly do not consider it less scientific. I can only show why I believe it is more powerful and more plausible.

Coming, as I did, from the University of Minnesota, known in my time as the prototypic source of "Midwestern dustbowl empiricism," I began measuring personality with an entirely objective test of mothers' attitudes, composed of two-choice items. In many ways, results with that test did not conform to expectations; my colleagues and I were left with several puzzling results (Loevinger, Sweet, Ossorio, & LaPerriere, 1962). We found no support in our data for the conceptions of personality that seemed most often used in child guidance clinics.

No statistical cluster of items corresponded to the Freudian conceptions of psychosexual stages. "Acceptance of the feminine role," another favorite trait of clinicians at that time, split into two clusters of items: acceptance of women's traditional social role and acceptance of women's biological role. Not only was there no positive correlation between those two traits, but they had a small (but replicable) negative correlation.

Although we found something similar to the then-commonly postulated trait of punitiveness–permissiveness, its outline did not correspond to that description. Some items referring to punishment were not included, and some items having no reference to punishment were excellent measures of this cluster. A more accurate description of what was covered by this cluster, by far the most prominent in our items, was "Authoritarian Family Ideology."

With the help of my clinical colleagues (particularly Kitty LaPerriere and Abel Ossorio), I discovered that what our test displayed as a polar variable—Authoritarian Family Ideology (attitudes)—did not in fact cover the extreme of the continuum that we seemed to be tapping.

There are mothers who cannot be placed on the continuum going from extreme authoritarianism to a liberal-permissive or democratic stance. These are mothers so absorbed in filling their own needs and wants that they do not exercise authority over their children; they simply neglect them. They come not from authoritarian households but from chaotic and disorganized ones. When they arrive at child guidance clinics, often under court order, it is apparent that they are not disciplining their children. In fact, sometimes they do not know where their children are for days at a time. (In one case reported in the newspapers recently, an 11-year-old boy had been chained to a cabinet and not fed for weeks. The child weighed half of his normal weight for his age; his mother was extremely obese.) Such considerations broke the hold of the General Linear Hypothesis on my thinking about personality.

Having abandoned the linear approach to personality measurement (although I did not yet know that was what I was doing), I came on the conception of ego development and its associated variables, proposed under various names by many previous psychologists. In particular, I found the article by C. Sullivan, M. Q. Grant, and J. D. Grant (1957) on "interpersonal integration," as they called it, sketching developmental stages of personality and character and their correspondence with adult types. They traced the origin of their conception to the work of Piaget (1932) and H. S. Sullivan (1953). Thus, their conceptual base was a broad one—Swiss children, delinquent young men, schizophrenic male adolescents. Although their initial focus was on delinquency in men, their conception proved to be well adapted to our study of maternal attitudes in normal women.

As we came to validate our new insights into maternal attitudes, we sought to correlate our test of Authoritarian Family Ideology against a new measure, a sentence completion test, adapted from a similar test used by the group working with the conception of C. Sullivan et al. (1957). However, although they had developed skills at scoring sentence completion tests, they had not codified their method sufficiently for our use. We were consequently forced to construct our own scoring manual for our test, a task that has proved to be rewarding but unending. (Fortunately, a former co-worker of that group, the late Virginia Ives [Word], joined our project when we started using sentence completions.)

In order to construct a scoring manual, we first gave the test as a pilot project to several easily available groups. Analyzing the responses for each stem separately, we sorted the responses for each sample into four stages, corresponding approximately to what we now call the Impulsive, Conformist, Conscientious, and Autonomous stages, using our intuitive understanding of the meaning of those stages. We then sorted total protocols according to the same 4-point scale. The distribution of total protocol scores for subjects whose answers fell in a given category of response provided feedback on our initial guesses. All we had to assume was that we could make a better guess of the person's characteristic level using responses to all 36 stems than from a response to a single stem. That assumption is still the backbone of our manual construction methodology.

From that initial point on, the process was data driven; I do not cede the imprimatur of empiricism to the factorists or behaviorists. Although the methods are difficult to describe briefly (e.g., base rates must be taken into account), they are conceptually simple. The essence is internal consistency. Provided that the initial insights set an appropriate direction, repeated applications of the principle of internal consistency to new, varied samples, followed by repeated reshaping of the conception to accord with results, yields an ever more precise measurement of the initial variable (Loevinger, 1993).

Over the years, by this reshaping, our conception has accrued several additional stages and elaborate descriptions of each stage. A recent revision, incorporating our best insights based on a cumulative total of thousands of cases, is indicated in Table 1 (Lê & Bobbitt, 1992; Loevinger, 1987). We again retained the convention of leaving room for a first stage that is not scored, in order to signal that sentence completions do not give access to the beginning of ego formation.

TABLE 1

Some Characteristics of Levels of Ego Development

Level	Characteristics		
	Impulse control	Interpersonal mode	Conscious preoccupation
Impulsive	Impulsive	Egocentric, dependent	Bodily feelings
Self-protective	Opportunistic	Manipulative, wary	"Trouble," control
Conformist	Respect for rules	Cooperative, loyal	Appearances, behavior
Self-aware	Exceptions allowable	Helpful, self-aware	Feelings, problems, adjustment
Conscientious	Self-evaluated standards, self-critical	Intense, responsible	Motives, traits, achievements
Individualistic	Tolerant	Mutual	Individuality, development, roles
Autonomous	Coping with conflict	Interdependent	Self-fulfillment, psychological causation

Note. Adapted from Loevinger (1976, 1987) and Lê and Bobbitt (1992).

The Distinction in Ego Development

Most psychologists and people in related professions are interested in the lowest and highest stages. The lowest stages are undoubtedly of special importance when they persist beyond the normal childhood period; delinquents and psychopaths, who are overrepresented in the lowest stages, pose serious problems for society. Like it or not, however, most adults in prison are in the normal range of ego development by our measure (Mikel, 1975; Powitzky, 1975).

The highest stages fascinate people because they believe that they themselves are there or rapidly approaching that desideratum; it does exemplify what many people would like to think of themselves as being or in process of becoming. On a few occasions when I tested professional groups and then spoke to them on ego development, many in the group reported that they were at the highest stages. I can say only that the SCT scores of the group (rated mixed in other samples) were not that high.

One of the reasons that I choose to emphasize the Conformist and the Conscientious stages is that that is where the people are. Studies of adolescent and adult populations in various settings usually turn up with subjects either in the Self-aware level and lower levels, in the case of less educated or younger groups, or Self-aware and higher levels, in the case of many college and college-educated groups. The range of Conformist to Conscientious stages includes a large proportion of most populations. (Actually, my colleagues and I have found that many mental health professionals are at the Individualistic level, one step beyond the Conscientious stage.) Moreover, many other writers recognize the Conformist and Conscientious stages, although not always by those names.

I now discuss how the Conformist person and the Conscientious person emerge as distinct types from our studies with the SCT. An early description of the Conformist stage was given by Mill (1859) in his essay *On Liberty*. Most people, he said, are conformists. They do not ask themselves what they prefer, only what is suitable to their circumstances and station in life.

> I do not mean they choose what is customary in preference to what suits their own inclination. It does not occur to them to have any inclination,

except for what is customary .... Peculiarity of taste, eccentricity of conduct, are shunned equally with crimes. (Mill, 1859)

The phenomenon Mill was describing psychometricians now refer to as
"social desirability."

I would disagree with Mill (1859) only by saying that that is no longer
descriptive of "most people." There is no definitive study of what most
people are like, but the preponderance of evidence is that in the United
States, most people are at the Self-aware level, midway between the
Conformist and the Conscientious stages (Holt, 1980).

On the evidence of our studies with the SCT, the Conformist can be
described further. Such a person tends to speak, and presumably to think,
in terms of clichés, often moralistic ones. Interpersonal interaction is seen
primarily in terms of behaviors, often just talking, rather than in terms
of feelings. To the extent that inner life is perceived at all, it is seen in
superficial and banal terms. The vocabulary for feelings tends to be limited
to conventional terms such as happy, sad, glad, fun, mad, and the like.
Appearances and social acceptance are of primary importance. Rules are
obeyed because they are the rules and are socially accepted as such;
exceptions and contingencies are ignored or are seen in terms of broad
categories of people. Sex is a major defining category, as are race or
ethnic group, and, on a smaller scale, family, school, and the local team.

Although conformity commonly coincides with conventionality,
which is its nearest match in Kohlberg's (Colby & Kohlberg, 1987) conception of moral development, they are not the same thing. A hippie who
rigidly conforms to his or her life-style is a conformist but not conventional. A person can adhere to a conventional way of life out of conviction
rather than conformity; outward conformity can mask or make easier a
fiercely independent intellectual life.

The transitional level between the Conformist and the Conscientious
levels is what we call Self-aware. One way that the transformation that
leads out of the Conformist stage may occur is for the person to become
aware that he or she does not always conform exactly to the socially
prescribed role. That discovery goes along with some self-consciousness,
whether as cause or effect. The person at this level begins to perceive

some qualifications to general rules, some circumstances that might alter the way things are or ought to be.

That characteristic of the level has been best described by Perry (1970) as "multiplicity." The person becomes aware of many alternatives for circumstances that previously seemed to have a single appropriate kind or way of behaving. Instead of just one right answer to a question, for example, for an issue raised in a college course, the person becomes aware of many alternative answers. A weakness of the level, Perry noted, is that the student cannot see why any answer is preferable to any other. The professor or teacher is just "giving his own opinion," so on what basis can the papers of students who have different opinions be graded? (At the next "position," as Perry called it, the student learns that better answers are founded on better reasoning or supported by more facts.)

The Conscientious stage has also been recognized by many authors. It is characterized, not necessarily by nonconformity but by self-evaluation of rules in terms of their position in the person's system of beliefs. Where the Conformist feels guilty for breaking rules, the Conscientious person feels guilty about the consequences of his or her actions. Achievements are cherished as an important part of life, not merely in terms of recognition by others, which is important to Conformists and cannot be irrelevant to anyone, but achievements are evaluated in terms of the Conscientious person's own standards. Long-term goals and ideals are much more prominent at this level than at the Conformist level.

People at this stage have a rich vocabulary for describing differentiated facets of inner life; cognitive shading allows for a far wider range of emotions. Similarly, they are aware not merely of group differences but also of a wide array of individual differences in traits. Interpersonal relations are highly valued, and they are framed in terms of feelings rather than merely behaviors. Behavior is not merely "emitted"; it has psychological causes.

The classical psychometric criticism of ego development and similar stage conceptions is to say that because there is usually a correlation with intelligence, what is being measured is nothing but intelligence, or social class, or even fluency. One answer is that psychologists have studied intelligence since about 1905, but no one has captured these syndromes from that study. The people who described similar syndromes were not at all the same ones studying intelligence. Moreover, there are some conspicuous examples of highly intelligent people at the Conformist or (rarely) even lower ego levels. We confirmed this by scoring the protocols for a study of middle-aged men who had been selected during their career as Harvard University students for their high potential. There were indeed more examples of people at a very high level and fewer examples of people at low levels in this than in other groups, but there were also some who tested at the Conformist level or Self-aware level (Vaillant & McCullough, 1987). Studies of reliability and validity have been reported elsewhere (Hauser, 1976; Loevinger, 1979).

A Psychometric Explanation

Suppose that the continuum described as ego development, or something like it, does indeed exist or at least make sense. The hypothetical model of development assumed to account for its manifestations is illustrated in Figure 1. Each behavioral or attitudinal manifestation of ego level has its own response curve (i.e., it starts at some point on the ego scale, becomes increasingly prominent with increasing ego level, and then decreases in frequency). Abilities, such as learning to walk, once gained are in general maintained. However, preferences and attitudes tend to be age related; they rise with age and then fall off, although not necessarily to zero.

Figure 1 depicts some hypothetical examples (Loevinger, 1984). In this model, Sign A depicts the item-response curve for a sign that peaks at Stage L; Sign B peaks at Stage M. A sample drawn from individuals in the range L–M will show a highly negative correlation between lines A and B, even though both are manifestations of the same underlying continuum.

Thus, the correlation between two manifestations of a single underlying variable can be anything whatsoever, depending on the particular manifestations chosen and the range of ego levels of the people being measured. There can even be a high negative correlation between two manifestations of ego level within some range, as in Figure 1.

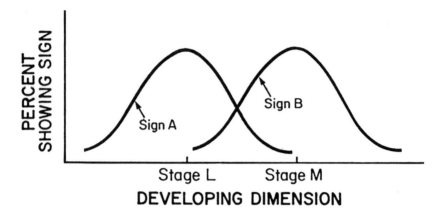

FIGURE 1. General model for signs of a developing personality dimension. From Loevinger (1984). Reprinted with permission.

That fact is one way of seeing the incompatibility between the developmental (milestone) approach and the behavioristic–psychometric (linear) approach to personality measurement. Because those approaches differ so radically, there is no easy way to document the differences or to bring evidence from one research tradition to show its greater validity. That incommensurability is one reason I have broken the taboo against appeals to common sense and cultural history to make my case.

Confusion of the two approaches, that of polar variables and milestone sequences (Loevinger, 1966), has also plagued the expositions of some developmentalists (see Kohlberg, 1969, Figures 2 and 3).

A number of psychologists, hearing my argument, have countered that the developmental approach and the factorial approach are complementary rather than opposed. Stages of ego development have from the beginning (Loevinger, 1966) been presented as partial approaches, not covering all aspects of development or of personality. Ego development has some claim to being the master trait but none to being the only trait. Some advocates of the factorial approach seem to be claiming, on the contrary, that they were not simply presenting five more personality factors, or traits, but the essential five, the "Big Five" (Goldberg, 1990).

The problem is that factor analysis as it was originally presented in many expositions was supposed to make obsolete and replace the kind of thinking represented at the beginning of this chapter. Common sense and the wisdom of the ages were no longer needed; a purely technological fix, factor analysis, would take their place.

The topic of this chapter is only one small corner of a large canvas, the psychology of personality. Seen from the perspective of ego-development theory, the five-factor theory belongs to a different universe of discourse and is not the centerpiece of personality, as proponents seem to claim. How theory of ego development is viewed from the five-factor perspective I cannot say; the suggestion that they are complementary perspectives does not seem consistent with the hegemony that had been claimed for the five factors. From the perspective of personality theory as a whole, McAdams (1992) has shown that the five-factor theory has an established place in personality psychology, but not the place its proponents claim for it. I believe the instant example, the conflation of conformity and conscience in the factorial (and in other psychometric) approaches, illustrates McAdams's thesis.

Conformity and conscientiousness are by no means diametrically opposed in all contexts. There are, however, some limited contexts, such as the Nuremberg trials and the Watergate hearings and "conscientious objector" status, where their opposition is clear. My argument is that factorial methods, or other methods based on the General Linear Hypothesis, have not succeeded so far and cannot be counted on to reveal the difference between the Conformist and Conscientious stages in the development of people. But we all know the difference exists, in our lives, in our history, and in our culture.

References

Colby, A., & Kohlberg, L. (1987). *The measurement of moral judgment.* Cambridge, England: Cambridge University Press.

Goldberg, L. R. (1990). An alternative "description of personality": The Big-Five factor structure. *Journal of Personality and Social Psychology, 59,* 1216–1229.

Hauser, S. T. (1976). Loevinger's model and measure of ego development: A critical review. *Psychological Bulletin, 83,* 928–955.

Holt, R. R. (1980). Loevinger's measure of ego development: Reliability and national norms for male and female short forms. *Journal of Personality and Social Psychology, 39,* 909–920.

Kohlberg, L. (1969). Stage and sequence: The cognitive-developmental approach to socialization. In D. A. Goslin (Ed.), *Handbook of socialization theory and research* (pp. 347–480). Chicago: Rand-McNally.

Lê, H. X., & Bobbitt, K. H. (1992). *Ego development theory and methods: A review of developmental levels, test forms, and scoring rules.* Manuscript submitted for publication.

Loevinger, J. (1966). The meaning and measurement of ego development. *American Psychologist, 21*, 195–206.

Loevinger, J. (1976). *Ego development: Conceptions and theories.* San Francisco: Jossey-Bass.

Loevinger, J. (1979). Construct validity of the Sentence Completion Test for ego development. *Applied Psychological Measurement, 3*, 281–311.

Loevinger, J. (1984). On the self and predicting behavior. In R. A. Zucker, J. Aronoff, & A. I. Rabin (Eds.), *Personality and the prediction of behavior* (pp. 43–68). San Diego, CA: Academic Press.

Loevinger, J. (1987). *Paradigms of personality.* San Francisco: Freeman.

Loevinger, J. (1993). Measurement of personality: True or false. *Psychological Inquiry, 4*, 1–160.

Loevinger, J., Sweet, B., Ossorio, A., & LaPerriere, K. (1962). Measuring personality patterns of women. *Genetic Psychology Monographs, 65*, 53–136.

McAdams, D. P. (1992). The five-factor model in personality: A critical appraisal. *Journal of Personality, 60*, 329–361.

McCrae, R. R., & Costa, P. T., Jr. (1980). Openness to experience and ego level in Loevinger's Sentence Completion Test: Dispositional contributions to developmental models of personality. *Journal of Personality and Social Psychology, 39*, 1179–1190.

McCrae, R. R., & Costa, P. T., Jr. (1990). *Personality in adulthood.* New York: Guilford Press.

Mikel, E. (1975). *Preliminary research studies of character development among imprisoned offenders.* Unpublished manuscript, Department of Psychology, Washington University, St. Louis.

Mill, J. S. (1859). *On liberty.*

Mischel, W. (1984). On the predictability of behavior and the structure of personality. In R. A. Zucker, J. Aronoff, & A. I. Rabin (Eds.), *Personality and the prediction of behavior* (pp. 269–305). San Diego, CA: Academic Press.

Norman, W. T. (1963). Toward an adequate taxonomy of personality attributes: Replicated factor structure in peer nomination personality ratings. *Journal of Abnormal and Social Psychology, 66*, 574–583.

Peck, R. F., & Havighurst, R. J. (1960). *The psychology of character development.* New York: Wiley.

Perry, W. G., Jr. (1970). *Forms of intellectual and ethical development in the college years.* New York: Holt, Rinehart & Winston.

Piaget, J. (1932). *The moral judgment of the child.* New York: Free Press of Glencoe.

Powitzky, R. J. (1975). *Ego levels and types of federal offenses.* Unpublished doctoral dissertation, University of Texas Health Science Center at Dallas.

Sullivan, C., Grant, M. Q., & Grant, J. D. (1957). The development of interpersonal maturity: Applications to delinquency. *Psychiatry, 20,* 373–385.

Sullivan, H. S. (1953). *The interpersonal theory of psychiatry.* New York: Norton.

Thurstone, L. L. (1934). The vectors of mind. *Psychological Review, 41,* 1–32.

Twain, M. (1884). *The adventures of Huckleberry Finn.*

21st Century Assessment. (1992). Advertisement for Personality Adjective Check List (PACL). Pasadena, CA: Author.

Vaillant, G. E., & McCullough, L. (1987). The Washington University Sentence Completion Test compared with other measures of adult ego development. *American Journal of Psychiatry, 144,* 1189–1194.

CHAPTER 10

Methodological Implications of a Peephole Perspective on Personality

David Magnusson, Tommy Andersson, and Bertil Törestad

One characteristic of empirical research in the areas of personality, developmental psychology, and developmental psychopathology is the emphasis on variables; the focus of interest is on a single variable or a combination of variables, their interrelations, and their relations to a specific criterion. The problems are *formulated* in terms of variables and the results are also *interpreted* in such terms. This is the case in studies on the interrelationships among variables as a basis for factor analysis, in studies on the stability of single variables across time, in studies of the links between environmental factors and individual functioning in various respects, in studies on the developmental background of adult functioning, and so on. A good example is research focusing on the relation between various aspects of individual functioning and environmental upbringing conditions, on the one hand, and the development of alcohol abuse and criminal behavior, on the other. Frequently, this research is concerned with aspects of individual functioning that are defined in terms of hypothetical variables, regarded and treated as nomothetical variables, equally valid for all human beings.

One characteristic of variable-oriented research, pertinent to the issue dealt with here, is the frequent application of linear regression methods to the treatment of data. In variable-oriented studies in the areas of personality, individual development, and developmental psychopathology, the interest is normally focused on the extent to which a specific variable or a set of variables, regarded as the independent variables, contribute to the statistical prediction of a specific criterion, regarded and treated as the independent variable. The extent to which a variable or a combination of variables contributes to the prediction of the criterion is usually estimated by the application of linear regression methods for data treatment and the result expressed in coefficients of correlations or regression.

The real contribution of this kind of study to scientific progress depends on the character and quality of the data, the initial treatment of the data, the relevance of the statistical method used, and how the transition from statistical figures to psychologically meaningful conclusions are handled by the researcher. An illustrative example of the role of some of these conditions was presented by Olweus (1983). The introduction of certain antecedent factors such as demographic and familial conditions changed the picture as to the earlier obtained relationships between aggressive behavior and school grades. The outcome and interpretation of the results changed conspicuously when new statistical analyses were introduced. This type of finding draws attention to the importance of the appropriate application of statistical methods and the correct interpretation of results from statistical analyses.

The first basic requirement for the correct use of statistics in personality research is that the method applied in a specific study matches the characteristics of the phenomena under investigation and the character of the data. Because this issue has been discussed in detail in Magnusson, Bergman, Rudinger, and Törestad (1991), we do not focus on it here.

A second requirement is that the results of statistical analyses are correctly interpreted in psychological terms. Statistical significance is not always directly interpretable as psychological significance. Although this statement may seem self-evident, empirical research is too often characterized by lack of attention to this important element in the research work (Ford & Carr, 1990; Harford & Spiegler, 1982; Robins & Ratcliff, 1979; Temple & Fillmore, 1986). The purpose of this chapter is to illustrate how such neglect has consequences with respect to the conclusions that can be drawn from the statistical analyses. We do this by applying frequently used traditional linear regression methods for data treatment to data that are common in research in the areas of personality, development, and developmental psychopathology. The data pertain to the relationships among indicators of individual functioning at age 13 and their links to alcohol abuse in young adulthood. More often than not, independent variables of this type are intercorrelated. This is also the case in our study. The issue of multicollinearity is taken as a point of departure for a discussion of the supremacy of psychological meaningfulness over statistical significance in research on individual functioning (Magnusson, 1992).

Data

The data considered here were derived from the longitudinal research program, Individual Development and Adjustment (IDA; Magnusson, 1988; Magnusson, Dunér, & Zetterblom, 1975). The group studied consisted of all boys who attended Grade 6 in the school system in one community in Sweden in 1968 (N = 540). The only boys not included in the study were those who were severely retarded or in mental hospitals (about 1% of the cohort). The subjects were representative of boys of the same age in Sweden.

Antecedents of Adult Alcohol Problems

As antecedents of later alcohol problems among 13-year-olds, we chose seven variables: *aggressiveness, motor restlessness, concentration difficulties, lack of school motivation, disharmony, peer rejections,* and *school achievement.* The data were collected when the majority of the subjects were 13 years old. The basis for the selection of these variables was that each of them has been reported in the literature to be early indicators of later antisocial problems (see, e.g., Andersson, Bergman, &

Magnusson, 1989; Cloninger, Sigvardsson, & Bohman, 1988; Donovan, Jessor, & Jessor, 1983; Hesselbrook et al., 1984; Jones, 1968; McCord & McCord, 1960; Robins, Bates, & O'Neal, 1962).

The first five variables were obtained by teachers' ratings. When the ratings were obtained, each teacher had known his or her students for about 3 years. The ratings were performed on 7-point scales. The instruction to the teachers aimed at a normal distribution of ratings, and the total distribution of ratings did not deviate from normality for any of the variables. Data for rejection by peers were obtained by sociometric ratings of the extent to which the boys were rejected by their peers. Data for school achievement were obtained by summing the grades, which were given on 5-point scales, in Swedish and mathematics. Data for all seven variables were obtained for all boys attending the school system during the school year.

Data for Adult Alcohol Problems

We studied alcohol problems in adulthood via official records. Data were collected from the police, the social authorities, and open and closed psychiatric care facilities (Andersson, 1988). The data were complete for all subjects aged 18–24 years. Specifically, we obtained information on arrests for public drunkenness, convictions for drunken driving, measures taken in accordance with the temperence law, and a *Diagnostic and Statistical Manual of Mental Disorders* (3rd ed., rev.) diagnosis of alcohol abuse and alcohol dependence (American Psychiatric Association, 1987). In total, 80 of the subjects were registered for alcohol abuse during this period.

The statistical criterion on adult alcohol problems was dichotomized, yielding two groups of young men: those with and those without alcohol records. This implies that the distribution of criterion values was skewed. Thus, for some purposes it was not the optimal criterion. However, for the specific purpose of this study, it did not bias the results.

Calculations and Results

In Table 1, the coefficients for the correlations among the independent variables are presented. As can be seen in Table 1, there was a certain

TABLE 1

Intercorrelations Among the Independent Variables

Variable	AB	MR	CD	LSM	DIS	SA	PR
AB	—	.668	.538	.571	.614	−.278	.242
MR		—	.674	.611	.512	−.385	.193
CD			—	.797	.587	−.639	.309
LSM				—	.646	−.591	.278
DIS					—	−.361	.335
SA						—	−.193
PR							—

Note. AB = aggressive behavior, MR = motor restlessness, CD = concentration difficulties, DIS = disharmony, LSM = lack of school motivation, SA = school achievement, and PR = peer rejection.

degree of collinearity, especially among the teacher-based variables. Multicollinearity implies that the shared variances among the variables are substantial. The largest common variance (64%) was that between concentration difficulties and lack of school motivation.

Single Early Indicators of Later Problems

Table 2 shows the correlation coefficients for the relationship between each of the independent variables and the dependent variable, which were obtained as point-biserial coefficients. The semipartial correlations are

TABLE 2

Point-Biserial Correlations and Semipartial Correlations Between the Independent Variables and the Dependent Variables (Registered Alcohol Abusers Aged 18–24)

Independent variable	Correlation	
	Point biserial	Semipartial
AB	.221	.025
MR	.236	.036
CD	.262	.048
LSM	.259	.030
DIS	.248	.079
SA	−.180	−.018
PR	.055	−.049

Note. AB = aggressive behavior, MR = motor restlessness, CD = concentration difficulties, LSM = lack of school motivation, DIS = disharmony, SA = school achievement, and PR = peer rejection.

also presented. Each semipartial coefficient reflects the unique relation between the variable under consideration and the criterion when the role of the other independent variables was partialed out.

Each of the independent variables had a significant linear relationship with the dependent variable, except one: poor peer relations. So far, the significant coefficients for the correlation between single early indicators of problem behaviors and adult alcohol problems were consistent with results from a large number of earlier studies using the same methodology.

The existence of multicollinearity is reflected in the semipartial correlations (also called part correlations) in Table 2. None of them was more than .10, which meant that data for each of the independent variables shared less than 1% with the total variance for registered alcohol abuse at ages 18–24, when the variance, common with all of the other variables, was removed. Thus, the specific contribution of each single variable per se to the prediction of alcohol problems at adulthood was limited.

Comments

Most often, the role of various aspects of individual functioning at an early age in the developmental process, assumed to lead to adult problems, is studied in terms of the predictive value of each of a number of relevant variables, (i.e., in terms of the type of correlation coefficients shown in Table 2). Frequently, each specific study on the developmental background of adult antisocial behavior is concerned with only one or a limited number of the variables studied here. As illustrated by the semipartial coefficients also shown in Table 2, the specific role of each of the single variables will be conspicuously overestimated when they are studied in isolation from other related aspects.

The intercorrelations presented in Table 1 indicate that the measures of each of the studied variables to some extent reflect an overall judgment of the ratees. That this is the case is often concealed in all the cases in which each of the variables is studied on a separate group of subjects.

The size of the semipartial coefficients, demonstrating the unique contribution of each of the variables to the relation between the independent variables and adult alcohol problems, can be interpreted from both a statistical and a substantive perspective. Statistically, the size of the semipartial coefficients is a consequence only of the collinearity among the independent variables. Substantively, the size of the semipartial coefficients is understandable in the light of a holistic view on individual functioning as a dynamic, multidetermined, and complex process. The independent variables used in the analysis were all hypothetical variables. Each of them was fuzzy without clear boundaries and reflected one aspect of the same total dynamic process. This implies that many particular elements are operating jointly and simultaneously in forming individuals' functioning and malfunctioning. The important conclusion for empirical research is that the specific contribution of single variables to the understanding and explanation of individual ways of dealing with reality, in a current and developmental perspective, will be overestimated and, consequently, overinterpreted when coefficients are presented in isolation from coefficients for other related variables.

Combination of Early Indicators of Later Problems

To study the predictive value of the combination of early problem indicators, we used the SPSSX (1990) program for multiple regression in its stepwise, backward elimination variant.

In the first step in this program, all independent variables are entered. Next, the variables with the least explanatory power are removed one by one until an optimal solution, according to specified criteria, is obtained. In Table 3, the deletion process is depicted and the end result presented.

The optimal linear prediction of alcohol problems in adulthood from a combination of the independent variables was reflected in a multiple correlation of .300. The deletion procedure ended with a solution in which the combination of disharmony and concentration difficulties predicted the criterion at a level of .287. (Note that the semipartial correlations in Table 2, if squared, are estimations of the unique contribution to the dependent variable in percentage of each of the two variables: .117 and .144, respectively.) The solution—with the program's default level for statistical significance applied—implied that aggressiveness, lack of

TABLE 3

Multiple Regression Analysis and Stepwise Backward Deletion With Registered Alcohol Abusers as the Dependent Variable and PR, AB, SA, CD, LSM, MR, and DIS as Independent Variables

Step	R	β	Semipartial
1. All variables	.300		
2. SA removed	.300		
3. AB removed	.299		
4. LSM removed	.297		
5. PR removed	.293		
6. MR removed	.287		
Variables in the final equation with $R = .287$			
DIS		.144	.117
CD		.178	.144

Note. SA = school achievement, AB = aggressive behavior, LSM = lack of school motivation, PR = peer rejection, MR = motor restlessness, DIS = disharmony, and CD = concentration difficulties. *R*s are presented for each removal step and standardized beta weights for the final solution.

school motivation, peer rejection, school achievement, and motor restlessness did not significantly contribute to the multiple correlation with adult alcohol problems.

The psychometrically sophisticated researcher should be careful not to interpret the results of the statistical analysis with respect to the relative importance of each of the single variables in the developmental background of alcohol problems in adulthood. However, not infrequently, these types of results of a statistical analysis would be looked on as indicating that the most important antecedent factors in the developmental background of adult alcohol problems would be disharmony and concentration difficulties, whereas agressiveness, lack of school motivation, peer rejection, school achievement, and motor restlessness would be less important.

The Significance of Insignificant Variables

In order to illustrate the danger of the second kind of conclusion, we performed a supplementary analysis. In this analysis, the five independent variables that did not contribute significantly to the multiple correlation with alcohol problems in adulthood—aggressiveness, lack of school motivation, peer rejection, school achievement, and motor restlessness—

were introduced as independent variables, with the dichotomized distribution of data for alcohol problems as the criterion. The result is presented in Table 4.

As can be seen in Table 4, the optimal solution with the five variables as predictors resulted in a multiple correlation of .284. After elimination of peer rejection, school achievement, and aggressiveness, the remaining two variables—motor restlessness and lack of school motivation— yielded a multiple correlation of the same size, indicating that data for the first three variables did not contribute any unique variance to the multiple correlation in this analysis.

The coefficient of .284, obtained with aggressiveness, lack of school motivation, peer rejection, school achievement, and motor restlessness as independent variables in the supplementary analysis, should be compared with the coefficient of .287, which was obtained in the original statistical analysis in which data for disharmony and concentration difficulty were enough to yield an optimal multiple correlation with data for adult alcohol problems. The first of these multiple coefficients accounted for 8.1% of the variance in the distribution of alcohol records, whereas the second coefficient, obtained in the original analysis, accounted for 8.2%.

TABLE 4
Multiple Regression Analysis and Stepwise Backward Deletion With Registered Alcohol Abusers as the Dependent Variable and AB, MR, LSM, SA, and PR as Independent Variables

Step	R	β	Semipartial
1. All five variables	.284		
2. PR removed	.283		
3. SA removed	.281		
4. AB removed	.277		
Variables in the final equation with $R = .277$			
MR		.123	.098
LSM		.184	.146

Note. AB = aggressive behavior, MR = motor restlessness, LSM = lack of school motivation, SA = school achievement, and PR = peer rejection. The five dependent variables in this table were removed in the original solution, presented in Table 3. *R*s are presented for each removal step and standardized beta weights for the final solution.

Thus, the variables that were eliminated from the prediction equation in the first multivariate analysis, because they did not contribute significantly to the prediction of the criterion, had, in fact, a predictive value of the same magnitude as those that were accepted as the important ones in the supplementary analysis.

As emphasized earlier, there was nothing peculiar or unexpected in the results from a purely statistical viewpoint. They followed logically from the existence of collinearity among the variables (see Darlington, 1968, Gordon, 1968, and Kerlinger & Pedhazur, 1973, for elaborations on the issue of multicollinearity).

As long as the purpose of the calculations of multiple correlations was restricted to estimate the optimal linear relationship of a set of independent variables to a criterion, the multiple coefficient gave a correct answer, which was also easy to interpret. However, as demonstrated earlier, the statistical analysis did not contribute to a psychologically meaningful knowledge about the relative role of each of the single variables with respect to its differential impact on the independent variables.

Discussion

Individual functioning can be described as a dynamic, multidetermined, stochastic process when analyzed from both current and developmental perspectives. The characterization of individual functioning as a multi-determined, stochastic process implies that many factors are involved—psychological and biological factors in the individual and physical and social factors in the environment—and that these factors are continuously and functionally interacting. This understanding of individual functioning is fundamental for the understanding and explanation of the phenomena with which psychologists are concerned in personality and developmental research.

The theoretical methodological and research strategical consequences of dynamic systems in general have recently been discussed and formulated in what has been called "chaos theory," which was originally developed on the basis of careful analysis and simulation of the weather (see Gleick, 1987). (The term *chaos* is misleading in this context. Chaos theory actually deals with lawful but unpredictable processes.) One aspect of dynamic processes, which is emphasized in chaos theory and has direct relevance for the study of individual functioning, is their holistic character.

Under special conditions, the study of single aspects—for example, intelligence, attachment, and aggressiveness—may be helpful (e.g., in the identification of possible operating factors; Magnusson, in press). However, a consequence of the dynamic, holistic character of individual functioning is that only under special conditions does the study of single aspects of the total process, taken out of context, contribute to the understanding and the explanation of the total process. The problems connected with the study of single aspects of the dynamic processes of individual functioning grow still more complicated if they are regarded and treated as nomothetic variables in statistical analyses of data across individuals, as is frequently done in the application of linear regression models for the treatment of data in personality and development research.

These conclusions, which refer to the view of individual functioning as a dynamic, multidetermined, stochastic process, lead, among other things, to the conviction that researchers have to complement the variable approach with a person-oriented approach for further progress in research in the areas of personality, development, and developmental psychopathology. In a person approach, individuals are studied in terms of their individual patterning of values for (or configurations across) variables relevant for the study under consideration, as advocated theoretically and illustrated empirically by Block (1971) in his classic book, *Lives Through Time* (see also Magnusson, 1988; Magnusson, Stattin, & Dunér, 1983). A crucial problem in pattern analysis is the appropriate choice of variables to be used in each specific case. The theoretical basis for that choice has been discusssed in Magnusson (in press). A person approach of this kind does not mean that each single analysis has to cover all aspects of the total functioning of the individual. The implications are twofold. First, the starting point for the formulation of the problem should be an analysis of the specific level of the phenomena under investigation with reference to the functioning of the individual as a totality. Second, this analysis implies the identification of the subsystem involved (e.g., the cognitive system, the immune system, the coronary system, the behavioral system, and the social system) and of the operating factors, within the system, that best serve as the basis for the pattern analysis.

The development of appropriate and effective methodologies that can be applied to the study of individual functioning as a dynamic process is full of conceptual and methodological problems and pitfalls (see Bergman, in press; Bergman & Magnusson, 1984a, 1984b; Magnusson & Bergman, 1987). At the same time, this dynamic process constitutes one of the most important and challenging tasks for future research in the areas of personality, developmental psychology, and developmental psychopathology. The development of methods for data treatment that match the character of the phenomena and problems researchers are interested in is necessary if they want to handle them in a truly scientific manner. Researchers must not be satisfied with producing empirical results that may be statistically significant but psychologically meaningless.

References

American Psychiatric Association. (1987). *Diagnostic and statistical manual of mental disorders* (3rd ed., rev.). Washington, DC: Author.

Andersson, T. (1988). *Alkoholvanor i ett utvecklingsperspektiv* [Drinking habits in a developmental perspective]. Unpublished doctoral dissertation, Department of Psychology, University of Stockholm, Stockholm, Sweden.

Andersson, T., Bergman, L. R., & Magnusson, D. (1989). Patterns of adjustment problems and alcohol abuse in early adulthood: A prospective longitudinal study. *Journal of Development and Psychopathology, 1,* 119–131.

Bergman, L. R. (in press). Some methodological issues in longitudinal research: A forward look. In D. Magnusson & P. Casaer (Eds.), *Longitudinal research on individual development: Present status and future perspectives.* Cambridge, England: Cambridge University Press.

Bergman, L. R., & Magnusson, D. (1984a). *Patterns of adjustment problems at age 10: An empirical and methodological study* (Tech. Rep. No. 615). Department of Psychology, Stockholm University, Stockholm, Sweden.

Bergman, L. R., & Magnusson, D. (1984b). *Patterns of adjustment problems at age 13: An empirical and methodological study* (Tech. Rep. No. 620). Department of Psychology, Stockholm University, Stockholm, Sweden.

Bergman, L. R., & Magnusson, D. (1987). A person approach to the study of the development of adjustment problems: An empirical example and some research strategy considerations. In D. Magnusson & A. Öhman (Eds.), *Psychopathology: An interactional perspective* (pp. 383–401). San Diego, CA: Academic Press.

Block, J. (1971). *Lives through time.* Berkeley, CA: Bancroft Books.

Cloninger, C. R., Sigvardsson, S., & Bohman, M. (1988). *Childhood personality predicts alcohol abuse in young adults.* Unpublished manuscript, Department of Child and Youth Psychiatry, University of Umeå, Umeå, Sweden.

Darlington, R. B. (1968). Multiple regression. *Psychological Bulletin, 69,* 161–182.

Donovan, J., Jessor, R., & Jessor, L. (1983). Problem drinking in adolescence and young adulthood. A follow-up study. *Journal of Studies on Alcohol, 44,* 109–138.

Ford, D. S., & Carr, P. G. (1990). Psychosocial correlates of alcohol consumption among black college students. *Journal of Alcohol and Drug Education, 36,* 45–51.

Gleick, J. (1987). *Chaos: Making a new science.* New York: Penguin Books.

Gordon, R. A. (1968). Issues in multiple regression. *American Journal of Sociology, 73,* 592–616.

Harford, T., & Spiegler, D. (1982). Environmental influences in adolescent drinking. *Alcohol and Health Monograph* (Whole No. 4).

Hesselbrook, M. N., & Hesselbrook, V. M., Babor, T. F., Stabenau, J. R., Meyer, R. E., & Weidenman, M. (1984). Antisocial behavior, psychopathology and problem drinking in the natural history of alcoholism. In D. W. Goodwin, K. T. van Dusen, & A. Mednick (Eds.), *Longitudinal research in alcoholism* (pp. 197–214). Norwell, MA: Kluwer Academic.

Jones, M. G. (1968). Personality correlates and antecedents of drinking patterns in adult males. *Journal of Consulting and Clinical Psychology, 32,* 2–12.

Kerlinger, F. N., & Pedhazur, E. J. (1973). *Multiple regression in behavioral research.* New York: Holt, Rinehart & Winston.

Magnusson, D. (1988). *Individual development from an interactional perspective.* Hillsdale, NJ: Erlbaum.

Magnusson, D. (in press). Human ontogeny: A longitudinal perspective. In D. Magnusson & P. Casaer (Eds.), *Longitudinal research on individual development: Present status and future perspectives.* Cambridge, England: Cambridge University Press.

Magnusson, D., Bergman, L. R., Rudinger, G., & Törestad, B. (Eds.). (1991). *Problems and methods in longitudinal research: Stability and change.* Cambridge, England: Cambridge University Press.

Magnusson, D., Dunér, A., & Zetterblom, G. (1975). *Adjustment: A longitudinal study.* New York: Wiley.

Magnusson, D., Stattin, H., & Dunér, A. (1983). Aggression and criminality in a longitudinal perspective. In K. T. van Dusen & S. A. Mednick (Eds.), *Prospective studies of crime and delinquency* (pp. 277–301). Boston: Kluwer-Nijhoff.

McCord, W., & McCord, J. (1960). *Origins of alcoholism.* Stanford, CA: Stanford University Press.

Olweus, P. (1983). Low school achievement and aggressive behavior in adolescent boys. In D. Magnusson & V. L. Allen (Eds.), *Human development: An interactional perspective* (pp. 353–365). San Diego, CA: Academic Press.

Robins, L. N., Bates, W. M., & O'Neal, P. (1962). *Adult drinking patterns of former problem drinking children. Society, culture and drinking patterns.* New York: Wiley.

Robins, L. N., & Ratcliff, K. S. (1979). Risk factors in the continuation of childhood antisocial behavior into adulthood. *International Journal of Mental Health, 7,* 76–116.

SPSS, *Statistical Data Analysis* (1990). Chicago, Illinois: SPSS, Inc.

Temple, M. T., & Fillmore, K. M. (1986). The variability of drinking patterns and problems among young men, age 16–31: A longitudinal study. *International Study of Addiction, 20,* 1595–1620.

PART TWO

Weighing
the Evidence

CHAPTER 11

Interpersonal Memories as Maps for Personality Consistency

Avril Thorne and Eva Klohnen

$\textbf{A}$fter several decades of concern about whether personality is consistent across time, interest has begun to shift toward understanding the *psychological processes* that underlie personality consistency and change. For example, how do some people consistently manage to push other people's limits, whereas other people manage to avoid all sorts of conflict and connection? The processes by which personality consistency is maintained are far from being understood.

The study of personality processes has required new measures to augment the language of adjectives and single-word person descriptors

This research was supported by National Institute of Mental Health Grant MH 16080 to Jack Block and Jeanne H. Block and by faculty research funds from the University of California, Santa Cruz, and Wellesley College.

We would like to thank David Funder, Per Gjerde, Dan McAdams, David Pillemer, Nancy Cantor, and an anonymous reviewer for their valuable feedback.

that is basic to personality research. The new measures are often more explicitly motivational as well as more contextualized within the person's own experience than is the vocabulary of traits. As such, the interest in personality processes has revived the concerns of such forebearers as Henry Murray, Karen Horney, and Erik Erikson. This group shares the conviction that personality and behavior cannot be understood without knowing what the person is trying to do (although knowing the person's conscious intent may not be enough); that people are basically trying to satisfy particular needs; and that past experiences provide contexts for current concerns. Recent work on self-narratives (McAdams, 1989) and on life tasks (Cantor & Kihlstrom, 1987), for example, calls to mind Erik Erikson's (1959) work on psychosocial crises. Studies of self-discrepancies (Higgins, 1987; Strauman & Higgins, 1987) and of feared and hoped-for possible selves (Markus & Nurius, 1986) are reminiscent of Horney's (1945) distinction between real and ideal selves. The almost-ancient concept of transference (Freud, 1912/1976) has inspired work on nuclear scripts (Carlson, 1981; Tomkins, 1979) and conditional patterns (Thorne, 1989), whereas Murray's (1962) revisionist work on needs–aims seems to foreshadow studies of personal strivings (Emmons, 1989) and personal projects (Little, 1989).

Although old and new dynamic approaches share certain fundamental assumptions about personality, the earlier work was not often concerned with connecting motivations and behavior. Current research, by contrast, is centrally concerned with understanding how motivations get transformed into behavior and vice versa. Of particular interest to current dynamic approaches are the kinds of assumptions or strategies that people use, implicitly or explicitly, to get what they want in specified circumstances (see the review by Cantor & Zirkel, 1990). These strategies are presumed to derive at least in part from previous emotionally significant experiences, which in some way or another help to organize and direct current behavior.

A practical problem with these new approaches is that they tend to require different kinds of information than is customarily collected in personality research. Most longitudinal personality archives do not contain much information about how people go about trying to satisfy particular needs. Such archives are not unique in overlooking personal scenarios or strategies, for it has not been customary in personality psychology to ask people how they go about getting what they want under certain conditions (Thorne, 1993).

Confronted with the yawning abyss of new questions, the tendency of new researchers has been to cast broad and flexible nets through the use of narratives: People are asked more or less directly to describe how they stay the same, how they change, and how they get what they want or fail to get it. McAdams (1989), for example, collected autobiographies as people related them in lengthy interviews, listening to the accounts with the ear of a biographer. Norem (1989) and Cantor and Kihlstrom (1987) translated current life tasks into the language of specific goals and behavioral strategies, or scripts. Emmons (1989) asked people to list the types of goals they typically pursued in daily life and related these personal strivings to more familiar measures of motives such as the Thematic Apperception Test (TAT). Thorne (1987) asked subjects to watch videotapes of themselves interacting and to provide play-by-play accounts of what they were doing and why.

In this chapter we examine personality processes through the lens of interpersonal memories. Relative to other current approaches, the study of autobiographical memories is unusually centered on the past. However, because past episodes can contour current expectations, personal memories would seem to be a potentially valuable source of information about current functioning. In the course of reviewing recent work on the psychological function of personal memories, we identify one particular kind of memory—memories in which people fail to get what they want from others—as being potentially pivotal for maintaining personality consistency across time. We then describe our ongoing research with a longitudinal sample. Because the work has only recently gotten underway, we cannot provide firm findings. This chapter is a prelude, not a coda, but we hope it is sufficiently tantalizing to encourage others to include autobiographical memories in longitudinal research.

Negative Memories as the Unfinished Business of Current Functioning: Clinical Leads

The founders of psychoanalysis (Breuer & Freud, 1893–1895/1957) were the first psychologists to suggest the possibility that memories of moments can have consequences for a lifetime. The essence of Freud's clinical theory is that the recovery and working through of traumatic memories is the key to personality change. Although a century of psychoanalytic hours have proceeded on the assumption that alterations in awareness of memories of negative or traumatic episodes is pivotal for personality change, only recently has this assumption been systematically studied in empirical research.

Transference is the psychoanalytic term for the dynamic mechanism through which memories of traumatic episodes come to influence current functioning. Transference, according to Freud, does not just happen in the therapy hour but occurs whenever a core, perpetually unmet need is aroused, such as the need for attention or for security. At such times, a well-rehearsed personal script ensues in which old expectations are projected onto new people in such a way that one comes to elicit the very frustrations that one wished to avoid. According to Freud, such repetition compulsions are not restricted to psychotics but are prevalent to a greater or lesser extent in everyone because each individual has some basic needs that were not adequately gratified. Lack of early need gratification results in repeated and often unsuccessful attempts to meet the needs elsewhere. Such repetitions are a rough and broad translation of what Freud meant by "transference patterns."

Basic to the notion of transference, then, is the assumption that individuals tend to have idiosyncratic kinds of unfinished business and that people come to develop routines or scripts for negotiating this perpetually unfinished business. Particular scripts, in turn, are associated with particular effects on others. Such effects, in turn, may result in perceptions on the part of observers about the existence of certain dispositions (e.g., Kiesler, 1979; Murray, 1938; Patterson, 1988).

The notion that personality dispositions stem from perpetually unmet needs has been carried forward by a number of psychodynamic personality theorists. The power of early frustrations is well elaborated in Adler's (1927) work, which focused on the significance of early memories of family relationships for understanding a person's unique modes of adjustment. In an eloquent passage, McAdams (1990) described Adler's view that

> [the earliest memory is] something like a personal creation myth or scene that implicitly foreshadows and symbolizes the overall tone of the person's subsequent life story .... Adler describes the case of a man whose first memory was that of being held in his mother's arms, only to be summarily deposited on the ground so that she could pick up his younger brother. His adult life involved persistent fears that others would be preferred to him, including extreme mistrust of his fiancee. (p. 411)

Roughly similar claims that traumatic episodes can have enduring effects on personality can be found in Murray's (1938) concept of unity thema, Sullivan's (1953) concept of parataxic distortion, Horney's (1945) notion of inner conflicts, and Tomkins's (1979; Carlson, 1981) work on nuclear scripts.

Although a number of empirical measures of transference have been developed in recent years, only a few methods have been systematically applied in empirical research. Luborsky's (1990a) core conflictual relationship theme (CCRT) method has been the most systematically developed and thoroughly studied. The Luborsky method uses narratives of relationship episodes as its basic unit. Such episodes are often the stuff of stories, anecdotes, and other recollections that occur during psychotherapy sessions as well as during many everyday conversations. Each episode is characterized in terms of what the subject wants from the other person (the wish) and the primary responses of other and of self in regard to the wish. For example, the wish in the Adlerian memory might be coded as wanting to feel securely loved by mother; the mother's response is rejection, and the boy's response is mistrust. Episodes such as this in which wishes are not gratified are referred to as negative, and episodes in which wishes are gratified are referred to as positive.

Applications of the CCRT method to transcripts of psychotherapy sessions have supported several basic hypotheses about transference (Crits-Christoph & Luborsky, 1990; Luborsky, Barber, & Crits-Christoph, 1990; Malan, 1976; Marziali, 1984). First, patients tend to have one core conflictual relationship theme, such as the need for love being perpetually frustrated. Second, these themes pervade anecdotes about encounters within therapy as well as outside of therapy. Third, the therapist's focusing on such themes in the course of psychotherapy is the key to positive psychotherapeutic change. Outcome studies have also shown that the content of the most pervasive wish is less likely to change over the course of successful therapy than is the outcome of the wish. For example, as a result of successful therapy, the man in the Adlerian memory would still wish that others would love him as much as they do his competitors, but he would be less likely to feel that this wish is not being gratified.

The fact that core conflictual relationship themes are pivotal to psychotherapeutic change suggests that such themes are also pivotal in maintaining the status quo. Evidence from a variety of sources indicates that negative memories are particularly difficult to change (e.g., Aronoff & Wilson, 1985; Duhl & Duhl, 1981; Emmons & King, 1988; Freud, 1912/1976; Horney, 1945; Markus & Nurius, 1986; Murray, 1938; Sternberg & Dobson, 1987; Sternberg & Soriano, 1984; Sullivan, 1953; Zeigarnik, 1927). Some of this work has been systematic and empirical, whereas other evidence comes from clinical case studies. Markus and Nurius (1986) found that people expected their negative or conflictual past selves to endure into the future more than their positive past selves. Only the negative past selves showed a substantial correlation with the selves imagined as possible ($r = .55$). Emmons and King (1988) reported that the content of conflictual strivings, such as trying to keep one's jealousy under control, was stable over a 1-year follow-up.

Might core conflictual relationship themes be implicated in processes of personality consistency and change in nonclinical samples? Until now, Luborsky's (1990a) method of identifying core conflictual relationship themes has not been systematically explored in nonclinical samples, nor have the themes identified by Luborsky's method been examined in terms of their relation to personality dispositions at one point in time or across time.

The purpose of our ongoing study was to explore the feasibility of identifying core conflictual relationship themes in the memories of a nonclinical sample; the possible association between such themes and personality characteristics as measured by self-reports and by impacts on others; and, most important, the possible association between such themes and personality consistency across time. Before describing this research, we consider leads that emerge from nonclinical studies of personality and personal memory.

Links Between Personality and Features of Personal Memory

To date, personality researchers have primarily focused on whether self-report measures of personality are correlated with particular features of autobiographical memories. In studies that seem to be benchmarks in the revival of interest in personality and autobiographical memory, Carlson (1981), Kihlstrom and Harackiewicz (1982), and McAdams (1982) examined a number of features of personal memories, such as age at the time of the event, clarity, imagery, and affect. Some of those features were significantly associated with personality, as measured by self-report inventories and projective tests.

In the past decade, personality researchers have reported numerous significant correlations between features of memory and personality tests scores, TAT themes, and other measures of self-concept or self-schemata. The consensus of this research is that people have a repertoire of memories that vary in affect, age, and salience (e.g., Kihlstrom & Harackiewicz, 1982); that personally salient memories are particularly likely to reflect social motives and self-concepts (McAdams, 1982); and that attributes associated with social or emotional difficulties, such as neuroticism and depression, are particularly likely to be associated with the retrieval of negative memories (Acklin, Sauer, Alexander, & Dugoni, 1989; Bower, 1981; Ireland & Kernan-Schloss, 1983; Mayo, 1983, 1989).

The focus of much of this research has been on the emotional component originally highlighted by Freud—affect or trauma— with relatively little elaboration of the content of the trauma. The neglect of memory content serves to obscure differences between "negative" personality traits such as depression and introversion, which are both associated with negative affect in memories. The neglect of memory content also obscures the particular kinds of scenarios or expectations that are associated with particular attributes.

In addition to examining the interpersonal scenarios that pervade personal memories, there is also a need for longitudinal studies of personality and personal memory. Because subjects in most studies of personality and memory are only examined at one point in time, researchers do not know whether links between personality and memory represent enduring or fleeting patterns. A common assumption in recent research is that current concerns guide the retrieval of memories, that current concerns vary with mood and situational factors, and that recollections of the same event vary remarkably from one time to the next (see the review by Ross, 1991). The durability of recollections—in core themes if not in specific details—is, of course, pivotal to establishing a generative relationship between personal memories and personality consistency. To date, researchers do not know the extent to which core conflictual relationship themes are durable features of memories because longitudinal studies of memory themes outside of psychotherapy contexts are rare.[1]

The Durability of Personal Memories: The View From Cognitive–Developmental Psychology

The cognitive structures through which memorable experiences are organized and empowered are often referred to as schemata, or unified sets of coordinated generalized actions (Piaget, 1951). *Scheme* and *schema* are global terms for various kinds of knowledge, such as memories, expectations, and propositions (Markus & Wurf, 1987). Schemata are thought to originate from interactions with the environment and to be subsequently invoked and applied to analogous occurrences. Some schemata, for example, develop early on to coordinate actions with caretakers (e.g., Main, Kaplan, & Cassidy, 1985).

---

[1]An exception to the neglect of longitudinal studies of personality and memory is a study by Kihlstrom and Harackiewicz (1982). About 60% of their subjects identified the same earliest memory as the memory they had identified 3 months earlier.

Can schemata change? According to Piaget (1951) and many personality theorists (e.g., Allport, 1937; Murray, 1938), personality is the result of an organized set of structures, or schemata, that prescribe more or less permanent modes of behavior but are also capable of accommodation or change. Schemata are not set in stone; they do not just assimilate experience. Assimilation provides continuity through the persistent use of existing schemata, whereas accommodation yields new or modified schemata to integrate discrepant experiences. However, assimilation is probably more pressing than accommodation because it requires less work. "Assimilate if you can, accommodate if you must!" is a compelling statement of this adaptive imperative for personality functioning (J. Block, 1982, p. 286).

Just as schemata can change, memories (which are specific instances of schemata) can also change. Changes in memories are not necessarily in the direction of being less accurate. Piaget demonstrated that memories can increase in accuracy over a period of months or years in accord with a child's cognitive development (Ross, 1991). The concept of reconstructive memory has been used both to signify changes toward greater as well as lesser veridicality to the actual event. Reconstructions in the direction of greater veridicality lie at the heart of some assumptions about the psychoanalytic process (e.g., Fine, Joseph, & Waldhorn, 1971). However, changes toward less accuracy are more frequently reported, and Spence's (1982) view seems to be more widely held: "Memory is more fallible than we realize, and it is vulnerable to a wide range of interfering stimuli . . . . In fact, one might ask whether any kind of veridical memory exists" (p. 91). The assumption that retrospective reports are bound to be inaccurate has been recently challenged by Brewin, Andrews, and Gotlib (in press). Their review of autobiographical memory research focused on studies of the personal memories of depressed subjects; they concluded that claims about the unreliability and invalidity of autobiographical memory reports, particularly of early childhood experiences, have been exaggerated.

Although a definitive conclusion cannot be reached about the veridicality of recollections, the truth probably lies somewhere between absolute veridicality and absolute confabulation. Perhaps more important for our purposes than the issue of veridicality is the issue of the personal function of memories. After reviewing studies of changes in personal memory, Ross (1991) concluded that personal memory exists to help people interact with the environment moreso than to accurately record events. In line with that conclusion, research on natural memory has begun to show a more social–developmental than brute factual cast.

Why Remember This? The Psychological Function of Personal Memories

Inspired by the richness of Freud's clinical observations about memory and his lack of empirical data, cognitive psychologists have begun to make impressive strides in understanding the personal function of autobiographical memories. A core feature of personal memory is that in the telling, the teller approximates a reliving of his or her subjective experience during the earlier episode. This reliving, in fact, can be so vivid that it has a profound emotional impact on the rememberer (e.g., Brewer, 1988; Pillemer, 1992; Spence, 1982). A memory is not just a retelling of the past; in the retelling, the memory becomes the present.

Why do some events become vivid memories and other events fade? Stein and Levine (1987) found that specific events are likely to be remembered that are unusual or surprising, such as unanticipated disaster or good fortune. A number of cognitive psychologists view personal memories as functioning to guide current actions and to anticipate future events (e.g., Neisser, 1988; Schank, 1982; Stein & Levine, 1987). The vividness of personal memories seems to enhance their imperativeness, sending an urgent message about the probable consequences of a particular course of action. The content of the memory, then, conveys the conditions under which analogous consequences are likely to occur.

Psychologists tend to posit different psychological functions for positive and negative memories. Because people seem to be primarily oriented by the pleasure principle, explaining memory for positive events seems less problematic than explaining memory for negative events. Why, as Bruner (1987) asked, does the tongue seem to continually seek the sore tooth? Stein and Levine (1987) suggested that negative memories can serve as reminders about what can go wrong and can thus help people to know what to avoid in the future. In a similar vein, Schank (1982) proposed that people remember failures so that when they next encounter a similar situation, they will not fail that way again. Stein posited a similar, if proactive rather than prohibitive, function for positive memories: Positive memories can be reassuring by reminding people that things can go right, thereby providing a positive signpost. Thus, memories of past successes and failures can very much inform current functioning. The metaphor of a highway comes to mind, in which the vehicle (the self) is channeled by green lights (positive memories) and red lights (negative memories).

It is easy to think of a number of examples of new experiences being influenced by old memories. To revive the Adlerian example, the man whose mother replaced him with a sibling is now on the alert for reoccurrences of replacement, and his sensitivity to such events seems to render him more likely to remember and perhaps to help create instances in which similar kinds of events occur. And so we return once again to the hypothesis with which we began: The matching of new events with potent old memories may contribute to consistency in personality across time. Failure-based memories may be particularly likely to become part of the personality structure of the individual and begin to guide future interpretations of experience and behavior (Cantor, 1990; Markus & Nurius, 1986).

We now summarize what still needs to be known in order to understand how personal memories might be involved in maintaining personality consistency. Do interpersonal memories show repetitious wish-response themes in nonclinical samples? Are such themes associated with particular personality characteristics, as measured by self-reports and observer ratings of personality? Are negative memories mostly related in a monolithic fashion to attributes such as depression and impulsivity, or can dispositions be usefully differentiated in terms of the *kinds* of disappointments that are remembered? Finally, the most generative question of all: Are negative memories more strongly associated with enduring personality impacts than are positive memories?

Infusing Memories Midstream Into a Longitudinal Study, or Boarding the Agile Elephant

In pursuit of a longitudinal data set that included systematic collection of interpersonal memories, we searched longitudinal archives on the East and West coasts, to no avail.[2] We could find no longitudinal personality study that had systematically collected autobiographical memories. This meant that we had to shelve our interest in studying the relation between memory consistency and personality consistency for the time being. However, we still hoped to be able to begin to collect memories from a longitudinal sample. Fortunately, our search coincided with Jack Block's interest in devising an interview protocol for the age 23 assessment of his longitudinal study of personality development. Jack and Jeanne Block's longitudinal archive is legendary for the quality, quantity, and versatility of its assessment data (J. H. Block & Block, 1980). It was a great privilege to be able to hop aboard what David Harrington has aptly described as "the agile elephant."

Developmentally, age 23 seemed an auspicious time to collect relationship memories because young adulthood in American society is typically a time when an individual begins to develop a life story, when reconciling past and present selves and achieving an identity becomes an important developmental task (cf. Cohler, 1982; Erikson, 1959; McAdams, 1989). Although the consolidation of a personal narrative becomes more important in later years, motivations for developing a self-narrative begin in young adulthood. An interest, if not a sense of urgency, is brought to bear on constructing a self-narrative that is sensibly coherent across time.

The subjects in our study were 48 men and 47 women who had participated in J. H. Block and Block's (1980) longitudinal study for the past 20 years, beginning in preschool at age 3. About two thirds of the sample were White, with about one quarter Black and a small percentage of Asians, Hispanics, and Native Americans. Excellent rapport had been maintained with the subjects and their families across the years, shown

---

[2]Our pursuits were bicoastal because of our bicoastal residences during the last few years; we did not intentionally discriminate against the Midwest.

by the fact that sample attrition had been low (see J. H. Block & Block, 1980, for a more extensive description of the sample).

In the course of their involvement with the longitudinal study, the subjects had answered many kinds of questions about themselves and their lives. Our assessment, however, was the first time that they had been asked to focus entirely on memories of themselves in specific encounters with other people. The interview protocol was derived from the Relationship Anecdotes Paradigm interview devised by Luborsky (1990b). Each subject was asked to describe approximately 10 specific memories of *personally important or problematic encounters* between himself or herself and another person. The memories could be about anyone (self with a parent, sibling, teacher, peer, lover, etc.) and could have taken place at any time. We emphasized the importance of describing memories of specific encounters rather than memories of events that happened frequently. For each memory, the subject was asked to describe what happened and when, whom he or she was with, and how each person felt or reacted. After at least 10 memories had been described, the subject was probed for particular kinds of memories: earliest memory, next earliest memory, earliest memory of mother, earliest memory of father, a memory of feeling guilty or ashamed, a high point, and a low point. The latter questions were derived from a procedure suggested by Mayman (1968).[3] Each interview lasted about 90 minutes and was videotaped. The interviewer was a White woman with more than 10 years of clinical experience. Probing was kept to a minimum to enhance free-flowing narratives.

This task was experienced in diverse ways. Some subjects seemed to feel at home, whereas others seemed nearly baffled at first and wanted to know exactly what kinds of memories to recount. Once they got started, some subjects were able to remember many events; others seemed to struggle. To what extent did the form we demanded—narratives of specific interpersonal interactions—influence the kind of memories we obtained? This is one of many unanswered questions. However, the interview resulted in an average of 16 codable memories for each subject, a good-sized sampling totaling almost 1,600 memories.

---

[3]In this report we combine memories from both parts of the interview.

TABLE 1

Primary Components for Coding Memories of Specific Encounters

Component	Definition
Age	Subject's age at time of memory
Other person	Identity of the other person with whom the subject is primarily interacting
Wish	What the subject wishes, needs, or intends in relation to the other person
Response of other	How does the other person respond, feel, or react? Does the other person gratify the wish?
Response of self	How does self respond, feel, or react? Does self feel gratified?
Outcome	Positive (positive response of other and of self) Mixed (negative response of other or of self, but not both) Negative (negative response of other and of self)

Coding of Memories

Our coding system owed much of its existence to several decades of work by Lester Luborsky and his colleagues (Luborsky & Crits-Christoph, 1990). Our version of the Luborsky system was designed for use by student coders instead of psychiatrists, and various criteria for identifying codable units were refined so as to require less inference (Thorne & Hogan, 1992).[4] Each memory was coded for age of the subject at the time of the memory; wish content; outcome (positive, mixed, or negative); and identity of the primary other (e.g., mother, boss, best friend). These components are summarized in Table 1, and an example of a coded episode from a subject we will call Edith Fay is shown in Table 2.

The idiographic content of each wish was placed into one of seven standard wish categories. Each wish category was explicitly relational in that it referred to what the subject wanted from the other person: to be approved of or validated, to be helped, to play with, to be securely loved, to assert self or control the other, to help other, and avoid conflict with other. Descriptions of each category, along with interjudge reliabilities and agreed-on frequencies in the reliability sample, are shown in Table

[4]Kimberley Hogan, Ari Blum, Melissa Brand, and Pilar Gonzalez-Doupe of Wellesley College assisted in refining the coding scheme.

TABLE 2

Example of a Coded Episode

Subject:	Edith Fay
Memory number:	10
Age:	3
Other:	Parents

One night my bear had fallen from the crib. I was yelling that the bear fell so I could get them to come. Dad said the bear had to lie on the ground until tomorrow. I thought, "If I get out of the crib and get hurt it will be their fault." I was really mad at them, that they wouldn't come to help me. Crying wouldn't help.

Wish:	To be helped	
Response of other:	Wouldn't help.	(negative)
Response of self:	Really mad.	(negative)
Outcome:	Negative	

TABLE 3

Content, Reliability, and Distribution of Wish Categories in Memories

Wish content and example	Reliability[a]	Distribution[b]
1. To have approval, validation from other; recognition; esteem		
Example: I wanted my parents to have confidence in me.	.79	.18
2. To be helped, taught, nurtured by other		
Example: I wanted him to teach me to read.	.83	.17
3. To play with, have adventures with, fun with		
Example: I wanted him to explore the park with me.	.77	.09
4. To love and be securely loved by		
Example: I wanted us to be a family again.	.74	.18
5. To assert self against other, control, dominate		
Example: I wanted to win the argument.	.67	.12
6. To help other, be concerned about other's welfare		
Example: I wanted mom to be healthy again.	.75	.06
7. To avoid conflict, pain; move away from		
Example: I wanted him to quit yelling and to leave me alone.	.79	.19

[a]Percentage agreement between coders.

[b]Average ipsative percentage of memories in each wish category.

3. It can be seen that the wish to control the other was the least reliable wish, with an agreement percentage of .67. The other wish categories showed better agreement, ranging from .74 to .83. Wishes to play and to help others, although judged reliably, were relatively infrequent. We focus on wish categories that showed interjudge reliabilities of at least .70 and on wishes that showed reasonably high base rates: wishes for approval, help, love, and avoiding conflict.

Some Preliminary Findings

Because analyses were still underway as of this writing, we cannot present firm findings but instead touch on several interesting trends to date; more extensive reports of the findings will appear shortly. The trends we briefly describe here concern age-graded changes in memories, relations between negative memories and self-report measures of depression, and relations between particular kinds of negative memories and personality consistency across time.

Age-Graded Changes in Memories

Recall that the primary task was not to recall memories of a particular age but to recall specific interactions that had happened at any time as long as the encounters were personally important or problematic. If the subjects did not state their age at the time of the episode, we probed for age afterward. Although subjects were not asked to characterize their life histories in terms of their significant others and primary wishes that characterized each age period, we were able to construct a normative relationship history by aggregating across specific memories. Some of these age-graded changes are graphed in Figure 1, which shows the frequency of each of the four most frequent wish categories arrayed across 5-year age periods.

The figure shows that the wish to be helped predominated at ages 1–5 and decreased dramatically thereafter. The wish to avoid conflict with others peaked at ages 6–10 and declined gradually thereafter. The wish for approval increased gradually over time but was eclipsed by the wish to be loved at ages 16–20. The wish to play, not shown in Figure 1, showed

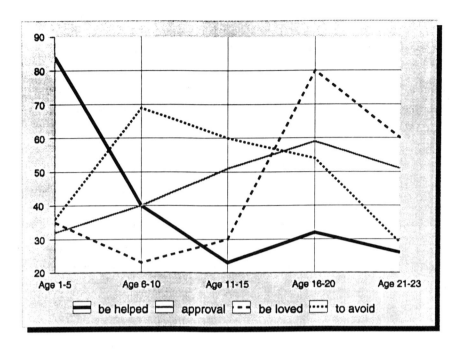

FIGURE 1. Total frequencies of wishes in memories as a function of age at time of memory.

a pattern much like that of the wish to be helped but at a much lower elevation. The wish to help others, also not shown in Figure 1, showed a pattern similar to that of wishes for approval but at a much lower elevation.

A second developmental trend concerned the identities of memorable significant others. Not surprisingly, parents (particularly the mother) were the most prevalent other people in memories up to age 5. By late adolescence (ages 16–20), best friends and lovers outnumbered parents in memories of important or problematic encounters. Memories of teachers, siblings, and peers were relatively infrequent across the five age periods.

A third developmental trend concerned the affect of memories. Negative memories were the most prevalent at ages 6–10, the grade school years. Memories about siblings and about nonprimary peers tended to be more negative than were memories about best friends, lovers, and parents.

Thus, parents and friends appeared to be safe havens compared with siblings and acquaintances, who were more hazardous.

These findings, taken together with some additional analyses of sex differences, yielded the following developmental portrait: At ages 1–5, subjects wanted to be helped by parents. At ages 6–10, subjects wanted to avoid conflict with parents and same-sex peers and were typically unable to do so. At ages 11–15, subjects continued to want to avoid conflict with same-sex peers and were getting more successful at it (boys), or they wanted to get approval from teachers and same-sex peers (girls). By age 16, subjects wanted a secure, reciprocal love, a wish that continued up to their present age of 23.

What is the significance of these age-graded changes? The changes seem developmentally reasonable and, because of that, surprising. If memory is reconstructed (and hardly anyone argues otherwise), what maintains the developmental verisimilitude of what is wanted, from whom it is wanted, and when it is wanted? One possibility is that the apparent developmental trends reflect subjects' knowledge of narrative conventions about how to tell stories about certain periods of the life cycle. Such an interpretation can account for nomothetic trends, but not for deviations from the trends such as adolescent memories of wanting help. There may also be a kernel of truth in these memories that goes beyond conventions about storytelling. A recent review by Brewin et al. (in press) supports the existence of such truths. However, to select between the truth and the invention interpretation requires corroboration that we do not presently have.

Negative Memories and Depression: Not Always

Interjudge agreements were high for ratings of wish gratification, exceeding percentages of .90. Negative wish outcomes showed the highest base rates (45%), followed by positive outcomes (37%) and mixed outcomes (18%) or memories in which either the response of self or other did not gratify the wish. Once it was apparent that relatively few episodes showed mixed outcomes, we hoped to be able to combine mixed episodes with negative episodes. Our rationale in so doing was that neither type of episode would yield complete gratification of the wish. However, as we report shortly, we could find little empirical justification for combining negative and mixed outcomes and more reason for retaining the distinction.

Prior research on personality and memory has often shown that the tendency to recall negative memories is associated with depression. Although our measure of wish outcome was not precisely the same as a measure of affect, it seemed reasonable to expect that relatively high frequencies of ungratified wishes would also be associated with depression because one of the hallmarks of depression is rumination about past disappointments and injuries. Subjects at age 23 were administered an extensive personality inventory that contained items from the General Behavior Inventory's Depression scale (Depue, Krauss, Spoont, & Arbisi, 1989), the Beck Depression Inventory (BDI; Beck, Ward, Mendelson, Mock, & Erbaugh, 1961), and the Center for Epidemiological Studies Depression Scale (Radloff, 1978). These scales showed moderately high intercorrelations for both men and women, averaging about .50. Each scale was correlated with frequencies of negative, mixed, and positive memories.[5] Correlations were computed separately for men ($n = 48$) and for women ($n = 47$), yielding a total of 18 correlation coefficients (3 depression measures × 3 memory outcomes × 2 sexes).

The findings did not confirm expectations. The largest correlation between depression and negative memories was a coefficient of .20 ($p < .20$) with the Beck Depression Inventory for females. In addition, no statistically significant correlations were found between depression and frequencies of positive memories. The only statistically significant correlations with the depression scales were found for mixed memories. The General Behavior Inventory's Depression scale correlated $-.32$ ($p < .05$) with mixed outcomes for males, and the BDI correlated $-.35$ ($p < .05$) with mixed outcomes for females. Mixed memories—memories in which the response of self and of other diverged in gratifying one's wish—

---

[5]Because distributions of memory frequencies were often skewed, we calculated Spearman correlation coefficients instead of Pearson coefficients whenever memory frequencies were analyzed. Analyses of memory data using percentages yielded approximately the same findings as did frequencies, reflecting the fact that individual differences in total number of codable memories showed few significant correlations with any personality variables.

appeared to be a kind of unfinished business with positive or at least nonnegative ramifications for emotional functioning.

The results did not support prior findings of positive correlations between depression and frequencies of negative memories. However, prior research has usually focused on relatively few memories and often only one kind of memory, such as the earliest memory, instead of patterns across an average of 16 specific interpersonal memories. As we report shortly, certain kinds of negative memories in our study were significantly and positively associated with depression. In future research we will examine relationships between depression and wish gratification in specific kinds of memories, including earliest memories and memories with mother and father.

Unfinished Business and Personality Consistency

We now examine our hypothesis that ungratified wishes in memories would be associated with personality characteristics that are relatively enduring across time. This idea, it may be recalled, was derived from theories that perpetually frustrated wishes are especially likely to emerge as insistent social motives. The unfinished business of negative memories, we reasoned, may result in particularly enduring kinds of impacts on others.

Our measure of consistent personality impacts was the California Q-Sort (J. Block, 1961/1978). This instrument was used to encode impressions about each subject at ages 3–4, 7, 11, 14, 18, and 23. Because our analyses of consistency have just gotten underway, we must limit our discussion to examining consistency across the past 5 years. At age 18 and again at age 23, each subject was described on the California Adult Q-Set (CAQ) by independent observers. A different set of observers was used at each age period. Interrater reliabilities averaged .72, allowing Q-sorts to be averaged to form a composite Q-sort description of each subject at age 18 and again at age 23.

The CAQ consists of 100 carefully assembled items that comprehensively sample the domain of personality and ego development. The items are sorted into a quasi-normal distribution so that descriptors judged most and least characteristic of a person form the tails of a bell-shaped distribution. Particular personality constructs can be measured by computing a Q correlation between a person's actual Q-sort composite and an a priori Q-sort prototype that is specially constructed to measure the construct (see, e.g., J. Block, 1961/1978). Although any number of such prototypes are possible, we limit ourselves to two constructs chosen for their relevance to this particular longitudinal study: ego overcontrol and adolescent depression. Each prototype was constructed by asking separate panels of personality psychologists to independently describe a prototypical ego-overcontrolling person and a prototypical depressed adolescent. Interrater reliabilities for these prototypical judgments exceeded .90, allowing a composited prototype to be formed for each construct. The overcontrol and depression prototypes correlated .38, indicating adequate differentiation between constructs.

The CAQ adolescent depression prototype highlights qualities such as feeling an acute lack of personal meaning in life, ruminating excessively, and noticeably lacking in cheerfulness and humor. The CAQ overcontrol prototype emphasizes fastidiousness, unnecessary delay of gratification, and lack of rebelliousness and open expression of hostility. Each subject's level of depression and overcontrol was assessed by computing the similarity between the actual Q description and each prototypical description. High correlations indicate similarity to the prototype. As an indication of convergent validity, similarity to the depression prototype correlated in the .40s to .50s with the depression scales described earlier. Similarity to the overcontrol prototype correlated about $-.45$ with Block's Ego-Control Scale (J. Block, personal communication, October 31, 1991), on which high scores indicate undercontrol. Most of these self-report measures were used only at age 23.

Cross-time consistencies on the CAQ measures of depression and overcontrol, computed separately by sex, ranged from .54 to .70, with an average Pearson correlation of .63. This represents a substantial degree of consistency, meaning that the same people who ranked high on overcontrol at age 18, for example, also tended to rank high on overcontrol at age 23. However, we were actually interested in a more specific kind of consistency. We wanted to know whether specific kinds of ungratified wishes could postdict who had scored consistently high on particular personality measures for the past 5 years. This kind of consistency is more complicated than is usually implied by the notion of consistency because it requires consistent relations between two different variables: patterns in personal memory and personality impacts. *Coherence* seems to be a more appropriate term for this kind of consistency because consistent relationships are required across different domains.[6]

To investigate this question, we correlated memory patterns with personality impacts at ages 18 and 23. We reasoned that a similar relation between personality and memory at each age could indicate a generative psychological link. The memory patterns explored were frequencies of negative, mixed, and positive memories in each of the four most frequent and reliable wish categories: approval, help, love, and avoidance. We expected that consistently significant personality and memory correlations would be more likely to be found for negative than for positive memories. We henceforth refer to parallel and statistically significant personality–memory correlations at ages 18 and 23 as a "coherence pattern." Analyses were conducted separately for each sex.

Although sex differences were plentiful, the structure of both the male and the female correlation matrices confirmed the hypothesis that ungratified wishes in memories (i.e., negative or mixed outcomes) would be more strongly associated with perpetual personality impacts than would gratified wishes. However, the wishes that showed coherence for women were different from the wishes that were coherent for men. Wishes for approval and love showed coherence for men, whereas wishes for help and to avoid conflict showed coherence for women. Table 4 displays the specifics of these male and female coherence patterns.

Consistent undercontrol in women was associated with memories in which there was a repeated scenario of wanting help and not getting it. This memory pattern correlated significantly ($-.35$) with overcontrol at age 18 and at age 23 ($-.30$). Because the pattern is correlational, we do not know whether the perception of a repeatedly obstructive environment was the cause or consequence (or both) of tendencies toward rebellion, impulsivity, and other aspects of undercontrol. A similar am-

[6]We would like to thank Dan McAdams for sensitizing us to this issue.

TABLE 4

Correlations Between California Adult Q-Set (CAQ) Measures at Ages 18 and 23 and Frequencies of Memories Showing Particular Kinds of Wish Gratification

CAQ measure and age	Wishes for help			Wishes to avoid other		
	Negative	Mixed	Positive	Negative	Mixed	Positive
		Women				
Depression						
18	−.10	.20	−.12	.25*	.16	.13
23	−.03	.24*	−.18	.35**	.04	.07
Overcontrol						
18	−.35**	.29*	−.10	.11	−.11	.11
23	−.30*	.08	−.07	.16	−.02	.13
		Men				
Depression						
18	.04	.00	.29*	.27*	.17	−.19
23	−.19	.07	.10	.24*	.40**	−.09
Overcontrol						
18	−.24*	−.04	.19	.05	.18	−.09
23	−.39**	−.11	−.10	−.07	.28*	.00

Note. Coherent patterns are underlined.

*$p < .05.$ **$p < .01,$ one-tailed.

biguity surrounds findings for consistencies in male undercontrol, which was associated with repeated memories of disapproval from others.

Consistent depression[7] in women was associated with memories of failing to avoid conflict. This pattern is reminiscent of the proposed link between depression and learned helplessness in women (Radloff & Rae, 1979). Consistent depression in men, on the other hand, was associated with memories of failed bids for intimacy. As can be seen in Table 4, wishes for love that had negative outcomes correlated .27 with depression at age 18 and .24 with depression at age 23. The association of male depression with ungratified love relationships is difficult to evaluate in terms of prior research because depression has mostly been conceptualized in the context of women's experience. In future research we will identify the significant others who are primarily involved in the negative

[7]It is important to note that we are referring to subclinical depression. This was not a clinical sample and average scores on the depression scales were not in the clinical range.

patterns and the developmental periods in which the episodes are most likely to be reported. We are also expanding our analyses to cover longer periods of time and a more diverse array of personality constructs and of memory patterns.

Summary and Conclusions

A skeptical view of the relation between memory and personality is that autobiographical memories reflect current needs and provide a psychological sense of continuity for the person but do not reflect publically observable consistencies in personality across time. So far we have found little evidence for such skepticism. Results thus far support hypotheses derived from clinical and cognitive research that negative outcomes can become part of the personality structure of the individual and come to guide perceptions and social behavior. Memories of negative encounters were more likely to be associated with consistent personality impacts than were memories of positive encounters.

It is important to note that by the term *consistency*, we mean the maintenance of relatively high rank orderings at ages 18 and 23 on two particular characteristics: depression and undercontrol. Also, it is important to note that although we predicted the relationship between negative outcomes in memories and personality consistency, we did not predict specific linkages. The association between personality consistency and negative memories interacted with subject's sex and with the type of wish that was frustrated. For example, depression was not related to all negative memories but only to some kinds of memories, and the kind of memory depended on the subject's sex. The specificity of the interactions suggested that the psychological scenarios associated with personality consistency are highly differentiated, certainly moreso than the authors' crude understandings of personality could anticipate. The highly specific nature of these linkages may eventually contribute to the refinement of our understandings of personality. For example, our findings suggest that depression is not rumination about all past disappointments and injuries but about specific kinds of disappointments that, in turn, differ by sex.

Because of the exploratory nature of our research, we did not feel confident hypothesizing about which dispositions would be enduringly related to wishes for love, which characteristics would be related to wishes for approval, and so forth. To do so seemed too far a reach. It was particularly difficult to hypothesize about features of personality that seem more intrapersonal than interpersonal, such as impulsivity or undercontrol. In addition, predictions for depression were difficult because depression has usually not been construed in the context of men's experience. The obtained link between male depression and failures at love, although seemingly reasonable, has less precedent in prior research than does the obtained link between depression in women and failures at avoiding conflict (Radloff & Rae, 1979).

As we expand our exploration of links between memory outcomes and kinds of personality impacts, we may find that positive memories also relate to patterns of personality, especially impacts construed in terms of positive coping, such as generosity or generativity. If clinical theory is correct, however, such patterns may not be as enduring as are patterns associated with memories of negative outcomes.

Exploratory research such as this requires cross-validation. We recently finished interviewing a second sample that roughly paralleled the age and demographics of the longitudinal sample and on which, unlike the longitudinal sample, memories were collected at two periods of time. Whatever this second study confirms will be better understood through case studies of subjects who typify particular patterns. As an example, we have begun to examine individual cases in an effort to understand the connection between undercontrol in women and repeated scenarios of wanting help and not getting it. The young woman whom we referred to earlier as Edith Fay (see Table 2) consistently impressed the research staff as being undercontrolled. Edith Fay reported a number of memories in which she failed to receive the help she wanted and thus showed the core pattern that typified women who consistently impressed others as being prone toward impulsivity, pushing limits, and expressing hostility directly. A summary of Edith Fay's repertoire of memories about failing to get help is shown in Table 5. The content of this repertoire helps to elaborate the nature of Edith Fay's unfinished business on the help front.

In reading through these and other memories, Edith Fay's parents and other authorities appear as ineffectual figures. At ages 2–3, neither

TABLE 5
Edith Fay's Memories About not Being Helped

Age 2 or 3 with older sister. Everyone is rushing around getting ready for something. My sister is pinning my diaper and yelling at someone and I was feeling scared and in all the hubbub she stuck me with a pin and it hurt like anything.

Age 3 with parents. Won't get my bear until morning and I'm very mad (see Table 3).

Age 6 with dad. When I was about 6, I casually mentioned to my dad that I wanted to learn how to whistle. So every day at 5 p.m. I had to meet him at his rocking chair and learn how to whistle for half an hour. I regretted having mentioned it. He was just such a tyrant—"you're gonna learn this." I felt dumb for having mentioned I wanted to whistle. I was bored doing this thing I didn't want to do.

Age 7 with older brother. My brother was my buddy, my playmate while I was growing up even though he was so much older than me. My oldest sister S. is very protective of me, very much a parental figure, moreso than my mother—"No, you can't do that, you'll get hurt," etc. Me and my brother used to roughhouse and I'd run a lot and I broke open my head on a table and my brother was useless and hysterical. He told S. "I killed her." I thought "he's so dumb, it not so bad," but then I saw the blood . . . . I wanted him to calm down and not be hysterical. He was acting the way my mother would act if she had been there.

Age 15 with high school principal. I wanted the principal to get the boys who assaulted me in the office and tell them off. I overheard them being interviewed and they acted like I was crazy and said I asked for it, at one point I yelled as loud as I could "bullshit" and they only suspended a few guys for a few days and I told the principal he was useless. I got back at him later for being such a dork—I knew they wouldn't do enough.

parent responds to Edith Fay's pleas for help. At age 6, dad spoils her curiosity. At age 7, older brother and mother are described as being useless and hysterical in a crisis. By age 15, it is clear that Edith Fay has come to expect little help from authorities in a crisis. These five memories were all negative in outcome and were the most pervasive scenario across Edith Fay's recollections. A second, less pervasive scenario was also about help, but in this case about helping others. Edith Fay's attempts to help her older siblings were rebuffed in early memories, but a recent memory had a different outcome: She describes an episode in which she did all she could to help her mother and then walked away to start her own life.

She was basically helping herself. Other aspects of Edith Fay's memories also suggest that with her move away from home she may finish her business on the help front, or at least that her expectations for help will no longer be so urgent. If we were to interview Edith Fay again in, say, 5 years and her memory patterns change so that help is no longer thematic, we will expect her personality impacts to have also changed.

Finally, the finding that age-graded changes in memories showed developmentally reasonable patterns suggests that there may be some truth to the stories that people tell about their encounters. Edith Fay, the youngest child in a large family, seemed to frequently fall between the cracks and to have good reason to wish that others would help her. Perhaps she really did get stuck with diaper pins and perhaps her brother and her mother were hysterical and did not have the sense to call the doctor when she was hurt. Was Edith Fay actually the product of an early and prolonged environment that was unusually neglectful or incompetent? If there is some kernel of truth to autobiographical memories, then longitudinal study of personality and memory cannot only serve to uncover the psychological scenarios that become part of the personality structure but also to reveal the social conditions that foster personality development and change.

References

Acklin, M. W., Sauer, A., Alexander, G., & Dugoni, B. (1989). Predicting depression using earliest childhood memories. *Journal of Personality Assessment, 53*, 51–59.

Adler, A. (1927). The significance of early recollections. *International Journal of Individual Psychology, 3*, 283–287.

Allport, G. (1937). *Pattern and growth in personality.* New York: Holt, Rinehart & Winston.

Aronoff, J., & Wilson, J. P. (1985). *Personality in the social process.* Hillsdale, NJ: Erlbaum.

Beck, A. T., Ward, C. H., Mendelson, M., Mock, J., & Erbaugh, J. (1961). An inventory for measuring depression. *Archives of General Psychiatry, 4*, 561–571.

Block, J. (1978). *The Q-sort method in personality assessment and psychiatric research.* Palo Alto, CA: Consulting Psychologists Press. (Original work published 1961)

Block, J. (1982). Assimilation, accommodation, and the dynamics of personality development. *Child Development, 53*, 281–295.

Block, J. H., & Block, J. (1980). The role of ego-control and ego-resiliency in the organization of behavior. In W. A. Collins (Ed.), *Minnesota Symposia on Child Psychology* (Vol. 13, pp. 39–101). Hillsdale, NJ: Erlbaum.

Bower, G. H. (1981). Mood and memory. *American Psychologist, 36,* 129–148.

Breuer, J., & Freud, S. (1957). *Studies on hysteria.* (J. Strachey Ed. and Trans.). New York: Basic Books. (Original work published 1893–1895)

Brewer, W. F. (1988). Memory for randomly sampled autobiographic events. In U. Neisser & E. Winograd (Eds.), *Remembering reconsidered: Ecological and traditional approaches to the study of memory* (pp. 21–90). Cambridge, England: Cambridge University Press.

Brewin, C. R., Andrews, B., & Gotlib, I. H. (in press). Psychopathology and early experience: A reappraisal of retrospective reports. *Psychological Bulletin.*

Bruner, J. S. (1987). Life as narrative. *Social Research, 54,* 11–32.

Cantor, N. (1990). From thought to behavior: "Having" and "doing" in the study of personality and cognition. *American Psychologist, 45,* 735–750.

Cantor, N., & Kihlstrom, J. F. (1987). *Personality and social intelligence.* Englewood Cliffs, NJ: Prentice-Hall.

Cantor, N., & Zirkel, S. (1990). Personality, cognition, and purposive behavior. In L. A. Pervin (Ed.), *Handbook of personality: Theory and research* (pp. 135–164). New York: Guilford Press.

Carlson, R. (1981). Studies in script theory: Adult analogs of a childhood nuclear scene. *Journal of Personality and Social Psychology, 40,* 501–510.

Cohler, B. J. (1982). Personal narrative and the life course. *Life-Span Development and Behavior, 4,* 205–241.

Crits-Christoph, P. & Luborsky, L. (1990). Changes in CCRT pervasiveness during psychotherapy. In L. Luborsky & P. Crits-Christoph (Eds.), *Understanding transference— The CCRT method* (pp. 133–146). New York: Basic Books.

Depue, R. A., Krauss, S., Spoont, M., & Arbisi, P. (1989). General Behavior Inventory identification of unipolar and bipolar affective conditions in a nonclinical university population. *Journal of Abnormal Psychology, 98,* 117–126.

Duhl, B. S., & Duhl, F. J. (1981). Integrative family therapy. In A. S. Gurman & D. P. Kniskern (Eds.), *Handbook of family therapy* (pp. 483–513). New York: Brunner/Mazel.

Emmons, R. A. (1989). Exploring the relations between motives and traits: The case of narcissism. In D. M. Buss & N. Cantor (Eds.), *Personality psychology: Recent trends and emerging directions* (pp. 22–44). New York: Springer-Verlag.

Emmons, R. A., & King, L. A. (1988). Conflict among personal strivings: Immediate and long-term implications for psychological and physical well-being. *Journal of Personality and Social Psychology, 54,* 1040–1048.

Erikson, E. H. (1959). Identity and the life cycle: Selected papers. *Psychological Issues, 1,* 5–165.

Fine, B. D., Joseph, E. D., & Waldhorn, H. F. (Eds.). (1971). *Recollection and reconstruction. Reconstruction in psychoanalysis* (Monograph No. 4 of the Kris Study Group of the New York Psychoanalytic Institute). New York: International Universities Press.

Freud, S. (1976). *Therapy and technique.* New York: MacMillan. (Original work published 1912)

Higgins, E. T. (1987). Self-discrepancy: A theory relating self and affect. *Psychological Review, 94,* 319–340.

Horney, K. (1945). *Our inner conflicts: A constructive theory of neurosis.* New York: Norton.

Ireland, M. S., & Kernan-Schloss, L. (1983). Pattern analysis of recorded daydreams, memories, and personality type. *Perceptual and Motor Skills, 56,* 119–125.

Kiesler, D. J. (1979). An interpersonal communication analysis of relationship in psychotherapy. *Psychiatry, 42,* 299–311.

Kihlstrom, J. F., & Harackiewicz, J. M. (1982). The earliest recollection: A new survey. *Journal of Personality, 50,* 134–148.

Little, B. R. (1989). Personal projects analysis: Trivial pursuits, magnificent obsessions, and the search for coherence. In D. M. Buss & N. Cantor (Eds.), *Personality psychology: Recent trends and emerging directions* (pp. 15–31). New York: Springer-Verlag.

Luborsky, L. (1990a). A guide to the CCRT method. In L. Luborsky & P. Crits-Christoph (Eds.), *Understanding transference—The CCRT method* (pp. 15–36). New York: Basic Books.

Luborsky, L. (1990b). The Relationship Anecdotes Paradigm (RAP) interview as a versatile source of narratives. In L. Luborsky & P. Crits-Christoph (Eds.), *Understanding transference—The CCRT method* (pp. 102–116). New York: Basic Books.

Luborsky, L., Barber, J., & Crits-Christoph, P. (1990). Theory-based research for understanding the process of psychotherapy. *Journal of Consulting and Clinical Psychology, 58,* 281–287.

Luborsky, L., & Crits-Christoph, P. (1990). *Understanding transference—The CCRT method.* New York: Basic Books.

Main, M., Kaplan, N., & Cassidy, J. (1985). Security in infancy, childhood, and adulthood: A move to the level of representation. *Monographs of the Society for Research in Child Development* (50, Serial No. 209).

Malan, D. M. (1976). *Toward the validation of dynamic psychotherapy.* New York: Plenum Press.

Markus, H., & Nurius, P. (1986). Possible selves. *American Psychologist, 41,* 954–969.

Markus, H., & Wurf, E. (1987). The dynamic self-concept: A social psychological perspective. *Annual Review of Psychology, 38,* 299–337.

Marziali, E. (1984). Prediction of outcome of brief psychotherapy from therapist interpretive interventions. *Archives of General Psychiatry, 41,* 301–304.

Mayman, M. (1968). Early memories and character structure. *Journal of Projective Techniques, 32,* 303–316.

Mayo, P. R. (1983). Personality traits and the retrieval of positive and negative memories. *Personality and Individual Differences, 4,* 465–471.

Mayo, P. R. (1989). A further study of the personality-congruent recall effect. *Personality and Individual Differences, 10,* 247–252.

McAdams, D. P. (1982). Experiences of intimacy and power: Relationships between social motives and autobiographical memory. *Journal of Personality and Social Psychology, 42,* 292–302.

McAdams, D. P. (1989). The development of a narrative identity. In D. M. Buss & N. Cantor (Eds.), *Personality psychology: Recent trends and emerging directions* (pp. 160–174). New York: Springer-Verlag.

McAdams, D. P. (1990). *The person: An introduction to personality psychology.* San Diego, CA: Harcourt Brace Jovanovich.

Murray, H. A. (1938). *Explorations in personality.* New York: Oxford University Press.

Murray, H. A. (1962). Toward a classification of interaction. In T. Parsons & E. A. Shils (Eds.), *Toward a general theory of action* (pp. 434–464). New York: Harper & Row. (Original work published in 1951)

Neisser, U. (1988). Time present and time past. In M. M. Gruneberg, P. E. Morris, & R. N. Sykes (Eds.), *Practical aspects of memory: Current research and issues: Vol. 2. Clinical and educational implications* (pp. 545–560). New York: Wiley.

Norem, J. (1989). Cognitive strategies as personality: Effectiveness, specificity, flexibility, and change. In D. M. Buss & N. Cantor (Eds.), Personality psychology: Recent trends and emerging directions (pp. 45–55). New York: Springer-Verlag.

Patterson, G. R. (1988). Family process: Loops, levels, and linkages. In N. Bolger, A. Caspi, G. Downey, & M. Moorehouse (Eds.), *Persons in context* (pp. 114–151). Cambridge, England: Cambridge University Press.

Piaget, J. (1951). *Play, dreams and imitation in childhood.* New York: Norton.

Pillemer, D. B. (1992). Remembering personal circumstances: A functional analysis. In E. Winograd & U. Neisser (Eds.), *Affect and accuracy in recall: The problem of "flashbulb" memories* (pp. 236–264). New York: Cambridge University Press.

Radloff, L. S. (1978). The CES-D Scale: A self-report depression scale for research in the general population. *Applied Psychological Measurement, 1,* 385–401.

Radloff, L. S., & Rae, D. S. (1979). Susceptibility and precipitation factors in depression: Sex differences and similarities. *Journal of Abnormal Psychology, 88,* 174–181.

Ross, B. M. (1991). *Remembering the personal past: Descriptions of autobiographical memory.* New York: Oxford University Press.

Schank, R. (1982). *Dynamic memory.* Cambridge, England: Cambridge University Press.

Spence, D. P. (1982). *Narrative truth and historical truth: Meaning and interpretation in psychoanalysis.* New York: Norton.

Stein, N. L., & Levine, L. J. (1987). Thinking about feelings: The development and organization of emotional knowledge. In R. E. Snow & M. Farr (Eds.), *Aptitude, learning, and instruction: Cognition, conation, and affect* (Vol. 3, pp. 165–197). Hillsdale, NJ: Erlbaum.

Sternberg, R. J., & Dobson, D. M. (1987). Resolving interpersonal conflicts: An analysis of stylistic consistency. *Journal of Personality and Social Psychology, 52,* 794–812.

Sternberg, R. J., & Soriano, L. J. (1984). Styles of conflict resolution. *Journal of Personality and Social Psychology, 47,* 115–126.

Strauman, T. J., & Higgins, E. T. (1987). Automatic activation of self-discrepancies and emotional syndromes: When cognitive structures influence affect. *Journal of Personality and Social Psychology, 53,* 1004–1014.

Sullivan, H. S. (1953). *The interpersonal theory of psychiatry.* New York: Norton.

Thorne, A. (1987). The press of personality: A study of conversations between introverts and extraverts. *Journal of Personality and Social Psychology, 53,* 718–726.

Thorne, A. (1989). Conditional patterns, transference, and the coherence of personality across time. In D. M. Buss & N. Cantor (Eds.), *Personality psychology: Recent trends and emerging directions* (pp. 150–159). New York: Springer-Verlag.

Thorne, A. (1993). On contextualizing Loevinger's stages of ego development. *Psychological Inquiry, 4,* 53–55.

Thorne, A., & Hogan, K. B. (1992). *Coding wish-response patterns in interpersonal memories.* Unpublished manuscript, University of California, Santa Cruz.

Tomkins, S. S. (1979). Script theory: Differential magnification of affects. In H. E. Howe, Jr. & R. A. Dienstbier (Eds.), *Nebraska Symposium on Motivation* (Vol. 26, pp. 741–746). Lincoln: University of Nebraska Press.

Zeigarnik, B. (1927). Über das Behalten von erledigten und unerledigten Handlungen. *Psychologische Forschungen, 9,* 1–85.

CHAPTER 12

Depressive Symptoms in Young Adults: A Developmental Perspective on Gender Differences

Per F. Gjerde

D evelopmental psychopathologists aim to understand the origins and course of psychological disorders at different age levels and to clarify the developmental pathways whereby early patterns of maladaptation evolve into later patterns of maladaptation (Bowlby, 1988; Rutter & Garmezy, 1983; Sroufe & Rutter, 1984). It is now widely recognized that longitudinal research strategies are central to achieving the aims of developmental psychopathologists (e.g., Rutter, 1988), and longitudinal prospective studies have detailed pathways from childhood to adulthood in both clinical and nonclinical samples (J. Block, 1971; Robins & Rutter, 1990).

The study was supported by National Institute of Mental Health Grant MH 16080 to Jack Block. I gratefully acknowledge additional support from the Social Sciences Division, University of California, Santa Cruz.

I want to thank Jack Block for having made available the data on which these analyses are based. Jeanne H. Block, who died a decade ago, played an indispensable role in designing and developing the longitudinal study that made this research possible.

The purpose of this chapter is to demonstrate the unique contribution that longitudinal analyses can make to the understanding of the development of depressive symptoms by examining both the concurrent and the preadolescent personality antecedents of dysphoria in young adults.[1] Longitudinal analyses of depression are particularly called for because the manifestations and prevalence of depression change with age, and the complex link between childhood and adult depression is not well understood (e.g., Bemporad & Wilson, 1978; Rutter, 1986). A central issue concerns the relation between childhood attributes and circumstances and depressive symptoms during the transition to young adulthood. Is it possible to discern adaptational failures, or risk factors, in childhood (e.g., poor peer relations, inadequate impulse control, social isolation, antisocial tendencies, unstable or conflict-ridden relationships to parents, insufficient intellectual competence, etc.) that increase the probability of subsequent depressive experiences? Moreover, are there gender differences in the vulnerability (or risk) factors that influence the probability of depressive symptoms in young adults? Understanding the greater proneness toward depression in women as compared with men (Nolen-Hoeksema, 1987) is a major challenge, and longitudinal research may play a pivotal role in clarifying why, after puberty, women experience depressive feelings more frequently than do men.

Early Personality Attributes as Risk Factors for Depression

The importance of identifying long-term personality antecedents of subsequent depressive disorders has long been recognized (e.g., Chodoff,

---

[1]The focus of this chapter is on depressive symptoms rather than on clinical depression per se. Hence, I use the terms *depressive symptoms*, *dysphoric mood*, and *dysphoria* interchangeably to acknowledge that depression symptoms in a nonclinical sample may or may not generalize to clinical depression as defined in psychiatry. That is, the despair and extreme sadness of "depressed" or dysphoric subjects may not constitute a clinically recognizable major depressive disorder. As Rutter (1986) noted, there is no clear way in which to determine which types of depression constitute distinct disease entities and therefore represent qualitative deviations from normality. Moreover, depressive tendencies in children and adolescents warrant study in their own right, of course, but also a considerable proportion of individuals manifesting subclinical depression early in life subsequently appear to develop clinical depression (e.g., Kovacs et al., 1984). Considerable psychiatric research on depression has also relied on self-report depression inventory scales.

1970, 1972; Salzman, 1975), and cross-sectional studies have established links between attributes such as dependency, self-criticism, introversion, and low self-esteem and susceptibility to depressive mood (e.g., Akiskal, Hirschfeld, & Yerevanian, 1983; Arieti & Bemporad, 1980; Blatt, 1974; Hirschfeld, Klerman, Chodoff, Korchin, & Barrett, 1976). However, the personality factors identified by these studies as possible antecedents of depression may merely be concomitants, or symptoms, of depression that emerge with the onset of a depressive episode and vanish with its remission. Because these factors may or may not precede the onset of the depressive disorder itself, their causal significance remains equivocal (e.g., Barnett & Gotlib, 1988).

Most studies in this area have relied on self-report data. The effort to tease out causal factors from concurrent symptomatic manifestations is therefore further complicated because depressive states appear to influence concurrent self-perceptions of personality (e.g., Hirschfeld et al., 1983). Moreover, although the character structure of depressed and nondepressed individuals has been found to differ, it is unclear whether these observed differences precede the depressive disorder itself or whether they merely reflect personality changes induced by the experience of depression (Akiskal et al., 1983). In conclusion, it is exceedingly difficult to distinguish empirically between variables occurring contemporaneously with depressive symptoms and those that serve either as antecedents or as consequences of this disorder.

For all of these reasons, then, a longitudinal methodology offers a unique promise of a clearer understanding of the role of personality in the origin and developmental course of depressive disorders. Do depressive symptoms emerge in response to age-specific stress and therefore have few and relatively weak early characterological antecedents? Or can researchers trace backward, developmentally, the personality antecedents of depressive symptoms that emerge in young adults? That is, using a longitudinal prospective methodology, can one discern a relatively enduring personality structure, can this vulnerability be identified early in life, and does its nature differ for boys and girls?

Depression and Personality: Gender Differences in Origin and Developmental Course

Several years ago, I undertook in collaboration with Jack Block a program of research aimed at understanding the personality context surrounding depressed affect in late adolescence and factors related to its origin. Special emphasis was placed on understanding gender differences in the psychological dynamics of depression. Adolescence is not only an emergent time for depression, it is also the period when depressive disorders become notably more common among girls than among boys (Rutter, 1986). Attempts to account for this finding have considered factors such as reproduction-related events, personality, role and status, victimization and poverty, and diagnostic bias (McGrath, Keita, Strickland, & Russo, 1990). Moreover, women and men may not only be differentially exposed to various risk factors, but they may also react in significantly different ways to the experience of depression itself.

In our initial studies (J. Block, Gjerde, & Block, 1991; Gjerde & Block, 1991; Gjerde, Block, & Block, 1988), we suggested that gender differences in the psychological dynamics of depression evolve from more general considerations of gender-differentiated socialization patterns. J. H. Block (1973, 1976, 1979, 1983), in particular, outlined the different orientations toward self and the world that emerge as a consequence of differential socialization—orientations, we conjectured, that are likely to have implications for the nature and developmental course of depressive mood. J. H. Block proposed that traditional sex role socialization extends the range of available experiences for boys but is relatively restrictive for girls. Because boys are permitted relatively greater freedom to explore and tend to receive greater reinforcement for curiosity, independence, competition, and achievement-related behaviors, they are inclined to "develop a premise system about the self that presumes or anticipates having consequences, instrumental competence, and mastery" (J. H. Block, 1983, p. 1345). Boys are also more likely than girls to rely on assertive, even aggressive behaviors to achieve important life goals (Eron, 1980). By contrast, at least partly because socialization pressures on girls tend to circumscribe or delineate their spheres of experience and to reduce their exposure to situations that encourage awareness of "the evocative role they themselves play in eliciting effects from the environment" (J. H. Block, 1983, p. 1345), girls are less likely to develop a sense of personal resourcefulness on which later competence builds. The self-perceptions of girls, relative to those of boys, are therefore less likely to include attributes such as agency, initiative, and a sense of personal mastery. Expressed in slightly different terms, socialization patterns may increase the tendency in girls to view events as being outside of their control (i.e., to experience helplessness). Supportive evidence for the view that girls are more likely to perceive the world as noncontingent comes from studies reporting that girls are more likely than boys to attribute their failures to stable internal personal causes (e.g., lack of ability) and their successes to unstable external causes (e.g., luck), whereas boys, by contrast, are more likely to perceive their failures as fortuitous and coincidental and their successes as personally based (Dweck, Davidson, Nelson, & Enna, 1978).

Applying these conceptual recognitions to the domain of depression, we anticipated that when depressive symptoms occur, their dynamics and manifestations—in particular, the directionality (inner vs. outer) of symptom expression—are likely to differ significantly for boys and girls. We expected that dysphoric boys would manifest an outer- or action-oriented mode of symptom expression and express their internal unhappiness directly, visibly, and without hesitation by acting on the world. In particular, we expected anger and hostility, feelings that frequently co-occur with sadness, to be readily expressed by dysphoric boys in social interactions. Hence, depressive symptoms in boys were anticipated to be embedded within a context of aggression and interpersonal antagonism. A different pattern was expected for dysphoric girls. On the basis of their socialization history, girls were expected to display a more inner- or thought-oriented mode of symptom expression and be more strongly characterized by self-focus, introspection, and a mostly hidden preoccupation with self. In particular, an open expression of hostile feelings was deemed less likely in dysphoric girls than in dysphoric boys (see also Nolen-Hoeksema, 1987, for a related conceptual view). As McCraine (1971) noted, when feelings of helplessness (or hopelessness) dominate, the consequent tendency may be to submit to depression without the overt expression of anger because instrumental responses to feelings of despair are considered unlikely to succeed. Due at least partly to gender differences in socialization experiences, we expected this situation to be more likely to occur for girls than for boys. Despair resulting in openly expressed anger is likely to be predicated on a personal sense of autonomy and independence (Stein & Levine, 1987), requiring perhaps a sense of personal agency that the female depressive has not yet acquired. Open expression of anger means to "satisfy one's impulses without considering the effect on others .... It requires a sense of self that the depressive has not developed" (Bemporad, 1980, p. 170).

Other theories and findings also suggest that relative to dysphoric boys, dysphoric girls are more likely to be self-focused and to keep their unhappiness within themselves (Blumberg & Izard, 1985; Ingram, Cruet, Johnson, & Wisnicki, 1988; Stapley & Haviland, 1989) and to respond to dysphoric mood in a more thought-oriented, self-focusing, and behaviorally (but perhaps not cognitively) less active manner than boys (Nolen-Hoeksema, 1987; Panter & Tanaka, 1987). Sroufe and Rutter (1984) also noted that boys, through socialization pressure, are more likely to be shaped toward an externalizing symptomatology and that depression, at least in young boys, is nested within a context of conduct disorders—a conjecture now supported by other research (Edelbrock & Achenbach, 1980; Ostrov, Offer, & Howard, 1989; Puig-Antich, 1982).

These conjectures about gender differences in the directionality of impulse expression were initially tested when our longitudinally followed subjects had reached late adolescence (Gjerde et al., 1988). Obtained results were generally consistent with the hypotheses insofar as dysphoric 18-year-old boys displayed a more outer-directed mode of impulse expression: They were judged, concurrently, by others as being openly angry, antagonistic, behaviorally unrestrained, discontented, and unconventional (i.e., the social stimulus value of dysphoric adolescent boys was consistent with their privately held feelings of aggression and alienation from others). Dysphoric 18-year-old girls, by contrast, displayed a more inner-directed mode of impulse expression, and relatively few observable behavioral qualities distinguished them from their nondysphoric female peers. Although these dysphoric young women were not judged by others as being visibly aggressive or as having problems in the interpersonal domain, they nevertheless described themselves as being relatively aggressive, unrestrained, and alienated from others. This discrepancy between privately held feelings and observable behaviors suggested the possibility that dysphoric adolescent girls withhold or avoid the behavioral expression of self-perceived characteristics that might be aversive to others. This discrepancy between observer and self-report data is consistent with our hypothesis that an inner-directed mode of impulse expression would characterize dysphoric girls at this age.

To identify long-term personality antecedents of subsequent depressive disorders, we evaluated longitudinally the antecedents of depressive tendencies at age 18 using data from nursery school through high school (J. Block et al., 1991). As early as age 7, boys who subsequently acknowledged depressive mood in late adolescence appeared to be more active, aggressive, self-aggrandizing, and undercontrolled (an outer-directed pattern of impulse expression), whereas at age 7, girls who later acknowledged depressive leanings tended to be more passive, intropunitive, oversocialized, and overcontrolling (an inner-directed pattern of impulse expression). Similar gender differences in personality antecedents were observed in pre- and early adolescence. Moreover, preschool intelligence correlated positively with depressive mood in 18-year-old girls and negatively with depressive mood in 18-year-old boys, a finding suggesting that the role of intelligence in the genesis of depression differs markedly for the sexes. In another prospective study (Gjerde & Block, 1991), prepubertal play patterns were found to be moderately related to subsequent depressive tendencies in late adolescence. Particularly noteworthy was the finding that in prepubertal girls, play patterns expressive of concern with moral issues (indicative of a strong superego) foretold subsequent depressive tendencies in girls, perhaps reflecting the greater emphasis placed on conscientiousness and fostering an interpersonal orientation in the socialization of girls (J. H. Block, 1983). In sum, the consistency of these prospective findings suggested that there is a gender-differentiated personality structure vulnerable to depression and that this vulnerability can be identified early in life. Both prospectively and concurrently, depressive mood in boys, as a group, tended to be associated with an outer-directed behavioral mode, whereas depressive mood in girls, as a group, tended to be associated with an inner-directed behavioral mode.

Personality and Depressive Mood in Young Adults

Are our previous findings specific to adolescence or do they reflect more enduring personality patterns of depression-prone individuals? In addressing this question, two issues are of particular interest. First, depressive symptoms in adolescence may constitute ephemeral or transient phenomena that emerge in response to age-specific experiences, such as increasing—yet perhaps transitional—stresses, lack of experience, limited time perspective, and inadequate knowledge with which to mitigate affective reactions. The dynamics of depressive mood during adolescence may therefore bear only moderate resemblance to the dynamics of depressive mood during young adulthood, when depressive symptoms may be more strongly related to a continuing and enduring character structure and therefore manifest stronger developmental antecedents.

Second, we cannot exclude that our findings of gender differences in the directionality of symptom expression merely illustrate an adolescence-specific intensification of gender role differentiation. As children pass through adolescence, gender role differentiation may increase (J. H. Block, 1976; Hill & Lynch, 1986). Adolescent girls appear to be more self-conscious and more motivated than adolescent boys to avoid behaviors that might alienate others. It is therefore of interest to observe whether the gender-differentiated patterns of symptom expression persist into young adulthood. Eighteen-year-old dysphoric girls did not express in behavior their subjectively experienced anger and alienation. Do these self-experienced, yet withheld, emotions "burst through" and manifest themselves in actual behavior by young adulthood?

Perhaps because the transition to young adulthood is less demarcated by dramatic biological and cognitive changes than the transition to adolescence, psychopathology research has neglected the immediate postadolescent years. Historically, adolescence has been viewed as a stage most likely to be characterized by psychological maladjustment. Young adulthood, by contrast, has been seen as "the time to stop sowing one's wild oats and to settle down to sober, conforming, and productive adult life" (Hallowell, Bemporad, & Ratey, 1989, p. 177). Not surprisingly, however, young adulthood is also associated with intensifying stress, psychological maladjustment, and suicide (cf. Bemporad, Ratey, & Hallowell, 1986; Fredrichs, Aneshansel, & Clark, 1981; Looney, 1989). This phenomenon has been attributed to sociocultural factors that increasingly emphasize individual achievement and excessive reliance on self at the expense of family ties (Bemporad et al., 1986; Hallowell et al., 1989). Empirical research, however, is just beginning to struggle with these issues.

To summarize, this study examined whether (a) the personality context surrounding depressive symptoms in young adults would be differentiated according to gender in a manner consistent with our findings obtained for adolescents and (b) depressive symptoms in young adults would have early, prepubertal personality antecedents and whether these antecedents would differ by gender.

Method

Subjects

Subjects were 98 young adults (51 women and 47 men), participating in an ongoing study of ego and cognitive development initiated by Jack Block and Jeanne H. Block in 1968 at the University of California, Berkeley (J. H. Block & Block, 1980). Number of subjects varied somewhat at each stage of analysis. Subjects lived primarily in urban settings and were heterogeneous with respect to social class and parents' educational backgrounds. About two thirds of the subjects were European American, one quarter were African American, and one twentieth were Asian American.

Subjects were initially recruited into the study at age 3 while attending a university-run nursery school or a parent-run cooperative nursery school. The children, now young adults, were assessed by means of wide-ranging batteries of personality, cognitive, and interpersonal measures at ages 3, 4, 5, 7, 11, 14, 18, and 23.

Measuring Depressive Symptoms: The General Behavior Inventory (GBI) Depression Subscale

The age 23 assessment consisted of six separate sessions, each of which lasted 2–3 hours. As part of the age 23 assessment, the subjects responded to an extensive pool of personality items measuring various aspects of personality functioning and family relations.

Among the scales administered was the GBI (revised 1987 version), a comprehensive self-report inventory designed to identify both unipolar and bipolar affective conditions in clinical and nonclinical samples (Depue & Klein, 1988; Depue, Krauss, Spoont, & Arbisi, 1989). The GBI consists of 73 items—45 depression items, 21 hypomania items, and 7 biphasic items—each responded to on a 4-point scale. The GBI scoring system yields two scores: a depression score (based on the 45 depression items) and a hypomania and biphasic score (based on the sum of all the remaining items). In this study, only results for the Depression subscale are reported. Because our intent was to estimate depressionlike tendencies as a continuous dimension in a nonclinical population, rather than to derive a diagnostic estimate based on actual cutoff points separating clinical from nonclinical cases, we scored the GBI Depression subscale according to a 4-point (0–3) Likert format as recommended in the GBI manual (Depue, 1987). This approach yields a continuous score of depressive symptoms, with possible scores ranging from 0 to 135 (higher scores indicate higher depressive mood).

The GBI Depression subscale was administered during two separate sessions that were several days, often a week or more, apart. Even-numbered items were administered during the first session and odd-numbered items during the second session. The mean GBI Depression subscale scores for women ($M = 34.12$, $SD = 17.52$; $n = 51$) were marginally higher than the mean GBI Depression subscale scores for men ($M = 27.77$, $SD = 20.46$; $n = 47$), $t(96) = 1.65$, $p = .10$. In this study, the internal consistency reliability of the full GBI depression scale was .93.

The GBI scale correlated .34 ($p < .05$) for women and .38 ($p < .05$) for men with the Center for Epidemiological Studies Depression Scale (CES-D; Radloff, 1977) administered to this sample 5 years earlier, when the subjects were 18 years old. Hence, moderate longitudinal (rank order) consistency characterized depressive symptoms over the 5-year period. Concurrently at age 23, the GBI and the CES-D Depression subscales correlated .29 ($p < .05$) for women and .64 ($p < .0001$) for men. This difference was statistically significant ($z = 2.19, p < .05$).[2]

Measuring Personality: Encoding Observer Evaluations by Means of the California Adult and Child Q-Sets

At each stage of the longitudinal study, the personality characteristics of the subjects were described using the California Child Q-Set (CCQ; J. Block & Block, 1980; J. H. Block & Block, 1980) or the California Adult Q-Set (CAQ; J. Block, 1978). The CCQ is an age-appropriate modification of the CAQ. Each Q-set consists of 100 widely ranging statements about the personality, cognitive, and social characteristics of the person being described.

At age 3, each child was described using the CCQ by three nursery school teachers who had observed the child for a minimum of 6 months before offering their descriptions. Previously, teachers had received training and calibration regarding the use of the Q-sort method in this context. At age 4, when attending a later nursery school, each child was again described by means of the CCQ procedure but by an entirely different set of three trained nursery school teachers. At age 7, each child was

[2]As can be expected on the basis of this gender difference, the personality correlates of the two depression inventories differed substantially for young women but not for young men. For example, the age 23 congruence correlation resulting from comparing the vector of 100 California Adult Q-Sort (CAQ) correlations of the Center for Epidemiological Studies Depression Scale (CES-D) with the vector of 100 CAQ correlations of the General Behavior Inventory (GBI) Depression subscale was only .51 for young women compared with .94 for young men. At age 23, GBI Depression scores were also associated with many more concurrent significant CAQ correlates than was the CES-D scale. The different personality correlations associated in young women with GBI-measured dysthymia at age 23 and CES-D-measured dysthymia at age 18 should therefore not immediately be attributed to the effect of age. The GBI Depression scale may simply differentiate better between the behavioral qualities of dysthymic and nondysthymic young adult women than the CES-D scale, the scale used by Gjerde, Block, and Block (1988) with 18-year-olds. Further analyses are underway to clarify why the GBI Depression scale yielded stronger personality correlates than the CES-D Depression scale in the female sample.

described on the CCQ by one elementary school homeroom teacher and by two psychologist examiners. At the age 3 assessment, CCQ descriptions were completed by a total of 11 nursery school teachers; at the age 4 assessment, CCQ descriptions were completed by an entirely different set of 9 nursery school teachers; and at the age 7 assessment, the CCQ descriptions were completed by 67 elementary school teachers. At the age 11 assessment, a total of 4 psychologist examiners who observed and administered a variety of experimental procedures tapping different aspects of personality and cognitive functioning provided CCQ descriptions using only 63 of the 100 CCQ items. At the age 23 assessment, a different set of 5 psychologist examiners described each subject on the CAQ. Three of these assessors based their evaluation on extensive, in-depth interviews with the subjects, whereas the remaining 2 assessors observed the subject during experimental sessions.

Judges described each subject by arranging the Q-set items in a forced nine-step distribution according to the evaluated salience of each item with respect to the subject. The judges worked independently of each other. At the age 3 and age 4 assessments, the three independent Q-sort formulations of the child were averaged to form a composite Q-sort description. These two composite Q descriptions were, in turn, composited to form an overall composite for each child during the preschool years. This last overall composite was used in the analyses reported here. At each of the later assessments, the several Q descriptions available for each subject were also composited. Because no judge contributed Q descriptions more than once for a given subject, the personality assessments at each time period were strictly independent of each other.

Results

Concurrent Personality Correlates of Depressive Symptoms in Young Adults

To identify the concurrent personality characteristics of young adults who privately acknowledged depressive symptoms, GBI Depression subscale scores were correlated with age 23 observer CAQ evaluations for each sex separately.

The Sample of Men

Table 1 contains the statistically significant ($p < .05$, two-tailed test) CAQ correlates of depressive symptoms for men. For the sake of comparisons,

TABLE 1

Concurrent Personality Correlates of Subsequent Depressive Symptoms (GBI Scores) at Age 23: Young Men

CAQ items	Young men (n = 47)	Young women (n = 51)
Positive correlates		
78. Feels cheated, victimized by life	.66***	.37**
22. Feels a lack of personal meaning in life	.52***	.47**
38. Has hostility toward others	.49***	.35*
49. Basically distrustful of people	.48***	.31*
55. Is self-defeating	.46**	.54***
45. Has brittle ego-defense system	.45**	.41**
30. Withdraws in face of adversity	.44**	.32*
36. Is subtly negativistic	.43**	.29*
82. Has fluctuating moods	.43**	.41**
23. Is extrapunitive, transfers blame	.42**	.25
53. Unable to delay gratification	.42**	.09
37. Guileful, deceitful, manipulative	.39**	.23
34. Overreacts to minor frustrations	.38**	.21
79. Tends to ruminate	.37**	.42**
39. Unconventional thought processes	.35*	.24
42. Tends to delay or avoids action	.35*	.39**
67. Is self-indulgent	.35*	−.11
76. Projects own feeling onto others	.34*	−.21
46. Has personal fantasy, daydreams	.33*	.29*
50. Is unpredictable in behavior, attitudes	.33*	.29*
62. Tends to be rebellious, nonconforming	.33*	.38**
65. Tries to stretch limits	.33*	.21
13. Is sensitive to criticism	.32*	.17
Negative correlates		
84. Is cheerful	−.52***	−.47***
2. Dependable, responsible person	−.50***	−.30*
77. Appears straightforward, candid	−.48***	−.23
26. Productive, gets things done	−.43**	−.32*
74. Is subjectively unaware of self-concern	−.42**	−.58***
17. Sympathetic, considerate	−.38**	−.19

(continued)

TABLE 1
(continued)

CAQ items	Young men (n = 47)	Young women (n = 51)
20. Has a rapid personal tempo	−.38*	−.18
75. Has clearcut, consistent personality	−.38**	−.40**
70. Behaves in ethically consistent manner	−.37**	−.15
92. Has social poise and presence	−.36*	−.37**
29. Is turned to for advice	−.35*	−.43**
8. Has high degree of intellectual capacity	−.34*	.05
35. Warm, capacity for close relations	−.34*	−.23
24. Prides self on being objective, rational	−.33*	−.14
31. Regards self as physically attractive	−.33*	−.28
81. Is physically attractive	−.33*	.18
3. Has a wide range of interests	−.30*	.12
54. Emphasizes being with others, gregarious	−.30*	−.51***
28. Liked, accepted by people	−.28*	−.15

Note. GBI = General Behavior Inventory and CAQ = California Adult Q-Sort.
*p < .05. **p < .01. ***p < .001.

I also report the corresponding results for the equivalent CAQ items—significant or not—for the sample of women.

The social stimulus value of young depressed men was striking and unambiguous: They were evaluated as ego-brittle, undercontrolled, interpersonally antagonistic, discontented, and unconventional. By contrast, young men with low GBI scores were judged by others to be cheerful, subjectively unaware of self-concern, sympathetic, socially poised, and intelligent, as well as enjoying positive social relations. The psychological portrait summarized by these CAQ attributes was generally consistent with the psychological portrait concurrently associated with depressive symptoms 5 years earlier—at age 18. At ages 23 and 18, dysphoric men channelled their impulses outward into overt, easily recognizable behaviors often indicative of undercontrol of impulse, interpersonal antagonism, and visible discontent with self. Previously, this behavioral orientation was described as "externalizing" (Gjerde et al., 1988) or "outer oriented" (J. Block et al., 1991). For young men, therefore, there appeared to be longitudinal continuity in the personality organization concurrently associated with depressive symptoms from late adolescence to young adulthood.

The Sample of Young Women

Table 2 contains the equivalent age 23 CAQ correlations for the sample of young women and, for the sake of comparisons, the results for the same CAQ items for young men. A coherent, recognizable constellation of personality characteristics also characterized dysphoric young adult women. Twenty-three-year-old women with depressive tendencies were seen as concerned with adequacy of self; vulnerable, brittle, anxious; and experiencing difficulties in relations with others. Interpersonal antagonism, although present, appeared to be less characteristic of dysphoric women than of dysphoric men. By contrast, young nondysphoric women tended to be seen as unaware of self-concern, cheerful, socially outgoing, and interpersonally engaged.

The number of statistically significant concurrent CAQ correlates of depressive symptoms was much higher for this sample at age 23 than it was at age 18 (cf. Gjerde et al., 1988; 38 correlates at age 23 vs. 6 at age 18). As noted earlier, although dysphoric 18-year-old young women perceived themselves as being vulnerable, interpersonally alienated, and aggressive, these self-perceptions were not expressed behaviorally and therefore were not discernible by observers; hence, there were few behavioral correlates. By contrast, at age 23, observers interacting with dysphoric women were readily able to discern self-concern, vulnerability, and interpersonal distance, even antagonism. It appears that relative to 18-year-old dysphoric young women, 23-year-old dysphoric women showed a greater tendency to channel impulses into overt, recognizable behaviors. Thus, on this behavioral level, there appeared to be noticeable longitudinal discontinuity in the personality organization concurrently associated with depressive symptoms in late adolescence and in young adulthood. The self-experienced—yet hidden and withheld—vulnerability, concern about the adequacy of self, and (to a lesser extent) inter-

TABLE 2

Concurrent Personality Correlates of Subsequent Depressive Symptoms (GBI Scores) at Age 23: Young Women

CAQ items	Young women (n = 51)	Young men (n = 47)
Positive correlates		
55. Is self-defeating	.51***	.41**
22. Feels a lack of personal meaning in life	.48***	.52***
78. Feels cheated, victimized by life	.43**	.54***
72. Concerned with own adequacy as person	.42**	.25
79. Tends to ruminate	.42**	.37*
45. Has a brittle ego-defense system	.41**	.45**
82. Has fluctuating moods	.41**	.43**
42. Tends to delay or avoid action	.39*	.34*
62. Tends to be rebellious, nonconforming	.38**	.33*
40. Vulnerable to threat	.37**	.28
85. Communicates through action	.36**	.18
38. Has hostility toward others	.35*	.49***
21. Arouses nurturant feelings in others	.34*	−.12
48. Keeps people at a distance	.34*	.33*
30. Withdraws in face of adversity	.32*	−.44**
49. Basically distrustful of people	.31*	.48***
68. Is basically anxious	.31**	.13
36. Is subtly negativistic	.29*	.43**
46. Has personal fantasy, daydreams	.29*	.33*
50. Is unpredictable in behavior, attitudes	.29*	.33*
10. Anxiety outlet in body symptoms	.28*	.04
Negative correlates		
74. Is subjectively unaware of self-concern	−.58***	−.42**
95. Tends to proffer advice	−.49***	−.11
84. Is cheerful	−.47***	−.52***
54. Emphasizes being with others, gregarious	−.45***	−.30*
29. Is turned to for advice	−.43**	−.35*
4. Is talkative individual	−.40**	−.12
75. Has clearcut consistent personality	−.40**	−.38**
92. Has social poise and presence	−.37**	−.36*
11. Is protective	−.36**	−.18
7. Favors conservative values	−.35*	−.19
52. Is assertive	−.35*	−.07
91. Is power oriented	−.32*	.16
26. Productive, gets things done	−.31*	−.43**
63. Judges self, others in conventional terms	−.29*	−.22
64. Perceptive of interpersonal cues	−.29*	.03
2. Dependable, responsible person	−.28*	−.50***
31. Regards self as physically attractive	−.28*	−.33*

Note. GBI = General Behavior Inventory and CAQ = California Adult Q-Sort.
*p < .05.   **p < .01.   ***p < .001.

personal antagonism observed at age 18 seemed to have found a more direct and unmitigated behavioral expression in young adulthood.[3]

Prepuberty Personality Antecedents of Depressive Symptoms in Young Adults

To identify the personality antecedents during preadolescence, childhood, and preschool of subjects who later at age 23 privately acknowledged depressive symptoms, we correlated, for each sex separately, the CCQ item data based on assessments at ages 11, 7, and 3–4 with later obtained GBI scores.

The Sample of Young Men

Table 3 shows the significant prospective correlations between early CCQ evaluations and the subsequently administered GBI Depression subscale scores for the sample of young men.

Depressive symptoms in young men were found to have many and psychologically coherent early CCQ personality correlates. Young men who reported depressive symptoms at age 23 tended to be described 12 years earlier, at age 11, as restless, manipulative, unable to delay gratification, emotionally labile, limit stretching, deviant from peers, attention seeking, immature under stress, and aggressive. By contrast, young men scoring low on the GBI Depression subscale at age 23 tended to be described in preadolescence as able to concentrate, planful, reflective, intelligent, responsive to reason, ambitious, verbally fluent, neat, persist-

---

[3]As was noted in Footnote 2, however, one cannot exclude the possibility that the different personality correlates associated with dysthymia in our sample of young women at ages 18 and 23, respectively, partly resulted from the use of different self-report depression inventories at the two ages. As I noted earlier, the General Behavior Inventory Depression scale appears to differentiate better between the behavioral qualities of dysthymic and nondysthymic female young adults than does the Center for Epidemiological Studies Depression Scale (CES-D). An alternative interpretation of this age difference in the personality correlates of dysthymia in the female sample would emphasize that the personality characteristics (e.g., hostility and interpersonal antagonism) withheld from overt expression at age 18 now have "burst through" and found open manifestation in behavior at age 23, perhaps because of a reduction in the intensity of gender role expectations in young adulthood. However, given the finding that the CES-D scale, when used both at ages 18 and 23, generates few personality correlates among young women, it appears premature to conclude that the results reported by Gjerde, Block, and Block (1988) for 18-year-olds merely illustrate an adolescence-specific intensification of gender role differentiation that leads to a withholding of behavioral qualities that might be aversive to others.

PER F. GJERDE

TABLE 3

Preschool, Childhood, and Preadolescence Personality Antecedents of Subsequent Depressive Symptoms (GBI) at Age 23: Young Men

CCQ items	Boys	Girls
Age 11		
Positive correlates		
34. Is restless and fidgety	.56***	−.15
22. Manipulate by ingratiation	.53***	−.20
65. Is unable to delay gratification	.50***	−.07
54. Emotionally labile	.48***	−.01
13. Generally stretches limits	.43**	−.06
27. Is visibly deviant from peers	.39**	−.05
21. Tries to be center of attention	.37**	−.13
12. Immature behavior under stress	.36*	−.06
85. Aggressive (physically or verbally)	.31*	.08
Negative correlates		
66. Attentive and able to concentrate	−.57***	.10
67. Is planful, thinks ahead	−.55***	.19
99. Is reflective	−.54***	.18
68. High intellectual capacity	−.53***	.18
25. Uses and responds to reason	−.51***	.14
47. Performance standards for self high	−.49***	.03
69. Is verbally fluent	−.42**	.14
59. Neat and orderly in dress	−.39**	.17
41. Persistent, does not give up	−.38**	−.03
30. Tends to arouse liking in adults	−.36*	−.03
89. Is competent, skillful	−.36*	.08
43. Recoups after stressful experiences	−.33*	−.04
92. Physically attractive, good looking	−.30*	.07
Age 7		
Positive correlates		
91. Is inappropriate in emotive behavior	.52**	−.01
65. Is unable to delay gratification	.50***	−.17
33. Cries easily	.46**	−.05
7. Seeks physical contact with others	.44**	−.29
49. Shows specific mannerisms	.43**	.01
48. Others sought to affirm self-worth	.41**	−.07
97. Has an active fantasy life	.40*	−.11
13. Generally stretches limits	.39*	−.11
21. Tries to be center of attention	.36*	−.20
38. Has unusual thought processes	.36*	−.17
12. Immature behavior under stress	.35*	.09
90. Is stubborn	.35*	.02
54. Emotionally labile	.33*	−.16
34. Is restless and fidgety	.32*	−.12

TABLE 3

CCQ items	Boys	Girls
Negative correlates		
25. Uses and responds to reason	−.55***	−.01
47. Performance standards for self high	−.46**	.11
68. High intellectual capacity	−.45**	.21
76. Can be trusted, is dependable	−.43**	−.06
61. Tends to be judgmental of others	−.42*	−.03
66. Attentive and able to concentrate	−.42**	.16
89. Is competent, skillful	−.42**	.04
37. Competitive	−.39*	−.28
41. Persistent, does not give up	−.37*	−.04
67. Is planful, thinks ahead	−.36*	.23
88. Is self-reliant, confident	−.35*	−.02
6. Helpful and cooperative	−.33*	.06

Ages 3–4

	Boys	Girls
Positive correlates		
56. Is jealous and envious of others	.53***	−.29
34. Is restless and fidgety	.43**	−.17
10. Has transient interpersonal relationships	.42*	−.11
21. Tries to be center of attention	.37*	−.21
94. Tends to be sulky or whiny	.37*	−.11
39. Immobilized under stress	.35*	−.17
85. Aggressive (physically or verbally)	.34*	−.17
55. Is afraid of being deprived	.32*	−.22
Negative correlates		
68. High intellectual capacity	−.49***	.28*
69. Is verbally fluent	−.37*	.32*
47. Performance standards for self high	−.36*	.15
96. Is creative	−.36*	.25
83. Seeks to be independent	−.35*	−.03
6. Helpful and cooperative	−.33*	.15
31. Recognizes feelings of others	−.33*	.03
73. Responds to humor	−.33*	.06
75. Is cheerful	−.33*	.06
66. Attentive and able to concentrate	−.31*	.33*
92. Physically attractive, good-looking	−.30*	.11
15. Shows concern for moral issues	−.29*	.06
30. Tends to arouse liking in adults	−.29*	.00
76. Can be trusted, is dependable	−.29*	.26

Note. GBI = General Behavior Inventory and CCQ = California Child Q-Sort. At age 11, there were 48 boys and 50 girls. At age 7, there were 35–40 boys and 39–46 girls. At ages 3–4, there were 47 boys and 52 girls.
*$p < .05$. **$p < .01$. ***$p < .001$.

ent, likable, competent, able to recoup from stress, and physically attractive.

Turning to the 7 year assessment of young men, the distinguishing CCQ items characterizing later depressive symptoms also portrayed an undercontrolled, vulnerable, and emotionally labile boy. Young men who reported many depressive symptoms at age 23 tended to be described 16 years earlier, at age 7, as being inappropriate in emotive behavior, unable to delay gratification, crying, contact seeking, manneristic, seeking others to affirm self-worth, fantasy oriented, limit stretching, attention seeking, as having unusual thought processes, immature under stress, stubborn, emotionally labile, and restless. By contrast, young men scoring low on the GBI Depression subscale at age 23 tended to be described at age 7 as being responsive to reason, ambitious, intelligent, dependable, judgmental, attentive, competent, persistent, planful, self-reliant, and helpful.

Extending these analyses back to nursery school (ages 3–4), we found that boys who acknowledged depressive symptoms at age 23 tended to be seen by their nursery school teachers as jealous of others, restless, transient in their relationships, attention seeking, sulky and whiny, immobilized under stress, aggressive, and afraid of being deprived. By contrast, young men scoring low on the GBI scale at age 23 tended to be described in nursery school as being intelligent, verbally fluent, ambitious, creative, independence seeking, helpful, empathic, humorous, cheerful, attentive, physically attractive, concerned with moral issues, likable, and dependable.

In sum, from nursery school and through preadolescence, a coherent pattern of personality attributes prospectively characterized the boys who many years later as young adults acknowledged depressive experiences. From ages 3–4 through age 11, subsequently dysphoric boys evinced an outer-directed behavior pattern that strongly resembled the behavior pattern concurrently associated with depressive symptoms at age 23: At all age levels, young men were seen to channel their impulses into easily recognizable, overt behaviors indicative of insufficient modulation of impulse, interpersonal antagonism, and low intellectual competence.

The Sample of Young Women

Table 4 shows the significant prospective correlations between early CCQ evaluations and the subsequently administered GBI Depression scores for the sample of young women.

Notice, first of all, that the number of prepuberty personality antecedents of depressive symptoms at age 23 was far smaller for young women than for young men. For example, in preadolescence there were

TABLE 4

Preschool, Childhood, and Preadolescence Personality Antecedents of Subsequent Depressive Symptoms (GBI Scores) at Age 23: Young Women

CCQ items	Girls	Boys
Age 7		
Positive correlates		
86. Likes to be by himself or herself	.55***	.02
79. Suspicious of others	.42**	.20
1. Prefers nonverbal communication	.37*	.30
98. Is shy and reserved	.37*	.00
99. Is reflective	.32*	−.19
8. Keeps thoughts, feelings to self	.31*	.02
Negative correlates		
58. Is emotionally expressive	−.40**	.14
40. Is curious and exploring	−.39**	−.10
16. Proud of accomplishments	−.34*	.00
85. Aggressive (physically or verbally)	−.33*	.15
28. Is vital, energetic, lively	−.32*	−.14
Ages 3–4		
Positive correlates		
45. Withdraws under stress	.34*	.06
66. Attentive and able to concentrate	.33*	−.31*
69. Is verbally fluent	.32*	−.37*
68. High intellectual capacity	.28*	−.49***
Negative correlates		
13. Generally stretches limits	−.35*	.26
95. Overreacts to minor frustrations	−.32*	.20
56. Is jealous and envious of others	−.29*	.52***

Note. There were no significant correlates at age 11. GBI = General Behavior Inventory and CCQ = California Child Q-Sort. At age 11, there were 48 boys and 50 girls. At age 7, there were 35–40 boys and 39–46 girls. At ages 3–4, there were 47 boys and 52 girls.
*$p < .05$.   **$p < .01$.   ***$p < .001$.

no statistically significant CCQ precursors of high GBI Depression scores for young women at age 23 as compared with 22 precursors in the male sample. At age 7, the distinguishing CCQ items anticipating subsequent depressive symptoms portrayed a young girl who preferred solitude, was suspicious of others, preferred nonverbal communication, was reflective, and kept her thoughts and feelings to herself. By contrast, young women who received low GBI Depression scores at age 23 were described by their elementary school teachers as being emotionally expressive, curious, proud of their accomplishments, aggressive, vital, energetic, and lively. These age 7 CCQ antecedents of age 23 depressive symptoms in young women, indicative of an inner-directed mode of impulse expression, were much different from the age 7 CCQ antecedents of age 23 depressive symptoms in young men. This inner-directed, socially avoidant behavior pattern at age 7 also contrasted sharply with the relatively more outer-directed behavior pattern concurrently associated in young women with depressive symptoms at age 23. Few CCQ items at ages 3–4 anticipated subsequent depressive symptoms in the female sample. Hence, the longitudinal continuity between preadolescent antecedents and concurrent, young adulthood manifestations of depressive symptoms so clearly visible in the sample of young men was essentially absent in the sample of young women.

Evaluating the Congruence of Personality Correlations of Depressive Symptoms

In order to evaluate the congruence of findings across age and gender, we correlated sets of Q correlates of the GBI Depression scale. For example, within the male sample, a vector of 100 age 23 CAQ correlates of depressive symptoms in young men may be correlated with a vector of 100 age 23 CAQ correlates of depressive symptoms in young women. The resulting correlation summarizes the congruence, or degree of pattern similarity, that characterized the personality correlates of depressive symptoms in young men and women at age 23. In the following analysis, I use this procedure to summarize patterns of Q correlates of GBI Depression scores.

Congruence of Correlation Patterns Within Gender Across Age

To summarize the degree of across-age similarity in the personality correlates of depressive symptoms from preschool through young adulthood, we correlated vectors of Q-item correlates (one for each assessment period). In order to evaluate the congruence of correlation patterns from preschool all the way through young adulthood, we limited these analyses to the 55 Q items that had approximately analogous items in the CCQ and the CAQ. The ensuing matrix of congruence correlations is presented in Table 5, separately by sex.

The congruence correlations for young men were all highly positive, ranging from .53 to .80 (mean $r = .65$), indicating that the personality correlates of depressive symptoms at age 23 were highly similar across the 20-year period encompassed by this study. For example, when the vector of 55 CAQ-item correlations obtained at age 23 was correlated with the vector of the 55 analogous CCQ-item correlations obtained at ages 3–4, the ensuing congruence correlation equaled .70.

By contrast, within the sample of young women, the pattern of congruence correlations showed much greater variability, with correlations ranging from −.18 to .52 ($M = .17$). For example, when the vector of 55 CAQ-item correlations obtained at age 23 was correlated with the vector of the 55 analogous CCQ-item correlations obtained at ages 3–4, the ensuing congruence equaled .18, considerably lower than the equivalent correlation of .70 obtained for young men.

TABLE 5

Congruence of Correlation Patterns of Age 23 Depressive Symptoms Across Age From Preschool to Young Adulthood Within Each Sex

Age	Age of assessment			
	23	11	7	3–4
23	—	.59	.62	.70
11	−.12	—	.80	.53
7	.52	.16	—	.56
3–4	−.18	.38	.11	—

Note. Correlations for boys are above the diagonal; correlations for girls are below the diagonal.

Congruence of Correlation Patterns Across Gender

To examine, at each age level, the degree of between-sex similarity characterizing the personality correlates of age 23 depressive symptoms, vectors of 100 Q correlates of depressive symptoms obtained for young men
were correlated with vectors of 100 Q correlates of depressive symptoms
obtained for young women. Note that concurrently at age 23, the personality correlates of depressive symptoms were remarkably similar for the
sexes ($r = .77$). By contrast, the prospective congruence correlations
indicated that prior to puberty, the personality antecedents of depressive
symptoms in young adults differed markedly by sex, with the congruence
correlations being $-.58$ at age 11, $-.07$ at age 7, and $-.70$ at ages 3–4.[4]

Gender Differences in Preschool CCQ Antecedents of Depressive Symptoms at Age 23

The congruence of correlation patterns across gender indicated that the
preschool personality precursors of depressive symptoms were markedly
different in 23-year-old young men and women. To examine more closely
the extent and nature of these differences, we evaluated directly the
gender differences in the nursery school CCQ antecedents of later-ob-
served depressive symptoms in young adulthood, using McNemar's (1969)
test for evaluating differences between independent correlations. Table
6 shows, in descending order of magnitude, the 32 CAQ items associated
with reliably different correlates for preschool boys and girls.

As shown in Table 6, preschool boys who later acknowledged depressive symptoms as young adults, when compared with preschool girls
who later acknowledged depressive symptoms as young adults, were more
likely to be seen by observers as being jealous, restless, limit stretching,
transient in their interpersonal relationships, attention seeking, afraid of
being deprived, overreactive to minor frustrations, immobilized under

---

[4]Additional analyses showed that after puberty, the personality antecedents of age 23 depressive
symptoms became more similar for young men and women, with the between-sex congruence correlations being .37 at age 14 and .30 at age 18. When compared with the low or negative between-sex
congruence correlations obtained prior to puberty, these findings provide additional evidence for the
view that noticeable changes appear to occur in the antecedents of adulthood dysthymia as girls pass
through puberty. Between ages 11 and 14, the personality antecedents of subsequent dysthymia in girls
become markedly more similar to the personality antecedents of subsequent dysthymia in boys.

TABLE 6

Preschool Sex Differences in Personality Antecedents of Depressive Symptoms (GBI Scores) at Age 23

CCQ item	Young men $(n = 47)$	Young women $(n = 52)$	z
Male r > female r			
56. Is jealous and envious of others	.53	−.29	4.30***
34. Is restless and fidgety	.37	−.24	3.07***
13. Generally stretches limits	.26	−.35	3.04***
10. Has transient interpersonal relationships	.42	−.11	2.73**
21. Tries to be center of attention	.34	−.21	2.71**
55. Is afraid of being deprived	.32	−.22	2.70**
95. Overreacts to minor frustrations	.20	−.32	2.61**
39. Immobilized under stress	.35	−.17	2.58**
85. Aggressive (physically or verbally)	.34	−.17	2.53**
94. Tends to be sulky and whiny	.37	−.11	2.37*
100. Is easily victimized by other children	.28	−.20	2.35*
12. Immature behavior under stress	.21	−.25	2.24*
65. Is unable to delay gratification	.21	−.24	2.19*
57. Tends to exaggerate mishaps	.28	−.16	2.18*
20. Tries to take advantage of others	.28	−.15	2.10*
46. Tends to go to pieces under stress	.27	−.15	2.07*
80. Teases other children	.25	−.16	2.05*
33. Cries easily	.30	−.10	2.00*
Male r < female r			
68. High intellectual capacity	−.49	.28	3.97***
69. Is verbally fluent	−.37	.32	3.42***
66. Attentive and able to concentrate	−.31	.33	3.20***
96. Is creative	−.36	.25	3.03***
76. Can be trusted, is dependable	−.29	.26	2.70**
47. Performance standards for self are high	−.36	.15	2.53**
67. Is planful, thinks ahead	−.28	.23	2.51**
6. Helpful and cooperative	−.34	.15	2.43*
89. Is competent, skillful	−.22	.27	2.41*
25. Uses and responds to reason	−.28	.18	2.27*
2. Is considerate of other children	−.28	.15	2.13*
99. Is reflective	−.17	.26	2.11*
92. Physically attractive, good-looking	−.30	.11	2.02*
75. Is cheerful	−.33	.07	1.96*

Note. GBI = General Behavior Inventory and CCQ = California Child Q-Sort.
*p < .05. **p < .01. ***p < .001.

stress, aggressive, sulky, easily victimized, immature under stress, unable to delay gratification, likely to exaggerate mishaps and take advantage of others, likely to go to pieces under stress, teasing, and likely to cry. By contrast, relative to depression-prone young men, depression-prone young women were seen in preschool as being more intelligent, verbally fluent, attentive, creative, dependable, ambitious, planful, helpful, competent, responsive to reason, considerate, reflective, physically attractive, and cheerful. In nursery school, the girls who later acknowledged depressive symptoms appeared to be more mature and intellectually competent than depression-prone boys.

Discussion

Although young adults of both sexes appeared to experience and reflect depression in relatively similar ways, individual differences in personality prior to puberty were prospectively related to subsequent depressive mood at age 23 in a manner that differed substantially according to sex. For young men, there were multiple early personality precursors of adult depressive symptoms stretching back all the way to nursery school, and the nature of these personality antecedents was, when their age-appropriateness was taken into account, remarkably similar to the concurrent personality correlates of depressive symptoms at age 23. For young men, therefore, a coherent pattern of personality characteristics was related to adulthood depressive symptoms both prospectively and concurrently. For young women, the number of early antecedents of subsequent depressive symptoms was far smaller, and the nature of such antecedents differed markedly from the early antecedents obtained for same-aged young men *as well as* from the concurrent personality manifestations of depressive symptoms observed many years later for young women at age 23. In sum, although the concurrent personality manifestations of depressive symptoms at age 23 showed only minor gender differences, the early personality structure that anticipates subsequent adult depressive symptoms differed considerably by sex. Only for boys were the prepuberty personality antecedents of adult depressive symptoms self-evidently and directly congruent with the concurrent personality manifestations of adult depressive symptoms.

Developmental psychopathologists describe psychopathology in terms of deviant pathways of development (Bowlby, 1988). One important pathway pattern is the *final common pathway:* where different paths eventually lead to an identical outcome (e.g., Masten & Braswell, 1990). Despite a relative congruence in the nature of depressive symptom expression in young adulthood, the gender-differentiated prepuberty personality antecedents suggested that the developmental trajectories that eventually result in depressive symptoms in young adults differ sharply for young men and women. In the sample of young men, the antecedents of depressed affect demonstrated impressive longitudinal consistency: An outer-directed, allocentric constellation of personality attributes indicative of undersocialized undercontrol, lack of intellectual resourcefulness, and troubled social relations predicted subsequent depressed mood from preschool through preadolescence. In the sample of young women, on the other hand, the personality antecedents of depressed affect were weaker, less consistent over time, and significantly different from the concurrent personality correlates observed at age 23. The lack of straightforward, linear longitudinality in the antecedents of depression in young women suggested that the course that eventually results in dysphoric mood in young adulthood is developmentally more complex in young women than in young men. It was only following puberty (at ages 14 and 18) that the antecedents of adulthood depressive symptoms in girls began to resemble the concurrent personality constellation surrounding depressive symptoms at age 23 (Gjerde, 1993). In sum, young women exhibited comparatively fewer prepuberty personality antecedents of depressive symptoms than did young men and, in contrast to young men, the prepuberty antecedents of depressive symptoms in young women were noticeably different from the postpuberty antecedents of depressive symptoms.

These gender-differentiated results indicating that correlations between childhood behaviors and postadolescence outcomes are less consistent for girls than for boys are consistent with data from the Berkeley

Growth Study (Hunt & Eichorn, 1972) and suggest that the transition to adolescence has particularly important implications for adjustment in girls. Better predictability for boys than for girls has also been reported by others (e.g., Lewis, Feiring, McGuffog, & Jaskir, 1984). Although consistent with the findings of others, our findings do not shed light on the specific mechanisms that underlie this phenomenon, nor is it known how extensive this gender difference in predictability is. Better predictability for boys than for girls certainly does not extend to all behavioral domains, but the occurrence of such differences in independent studies suggests that our results may be an illustration of a more general sex difference in psychodynamic organization. The reorganization of psychological structures is frequently associated with critical transitions in the life course. Puberty is a cardinal transitional event in the lives of girls (e.g., Caspi & Moffitt, 1991) and the transition to adolescence may represent a greater developmental challenge for girls than for boys. With specific reference to depression, Petersen, Sarigiani, and Kennedy (1991) suggested that girls are at greater risk than boys for developing depressive symptoms in early adolescence because they experience more challenges during this period. Further studies might do well to examine how the transition to adolescence may operate as a risk factor for depression in young girls, thereby helping to clarify why the prepuberty antecedents of depressive symptoms differ from the postpuberty antecedents of depressive symptoms in women.

Direct comparisons of correlations between early personality characteristics and depressive symptoms at age 23 showed that preschool girls who later admitted to depressive symptoms at age 23 were considerably more mature, intellectually resourceful, interpersonally considerate, and overcontrolling of impulse than preschool boys who later admitted to depressive symptoms at age 23. Correlations between early CCQ evaluations (ages 3–4 and 7) and GBI Depression scores (at age 23) also showed that in childhood, depression-prone young women were likely to be more inner directed, socially avoidant, and intellectually resourceful than same-aged depression-prone young men, who tended to be more undercontrolling of impulse and more likely to engage in conflict-ridden social relations. These results suggest that the nature of the underlying vulnerability to depression is related to gender, and that psychological vulnerability accentuates different behavioral tendencies in boys and girls. With respect to aggressive behaviors, Ross (1974) suggested that there may be an optimal level of adaptation and that both overexpression and underexpression of aggressive behaviors may signal vulnerability. For example, "acting-out" behaviors (i.e., overexpression of aggression) may be more socially acceptable and more congruent with the socialization history of boys than of girls. Boys, in general, are also more likely than girls to rely on aggressive behaviors as a means to achieve ends and to engage in antagonistic relations with peers (e.g., Eron, 1980). For girls, by contrast, a more introverted, passive, and compliant behavior pattern (i.e., underexpression of aggression) may represent a more efficacious device for coping with psychological stress (J. H. Block, 1983). Maccoby (1986) has also argued that "a girl risks ostracism and the breaking off of highly valued friendships if she shows hostility or even disagreement too openly. The control of aggressive behaviors appears to be stronger in girls' groups than boys'" (p. 274). Furthermore, given that depression-prone girls are more intelligent than depression-prone boys (for a further discussion of this finding, see J. Block et al., 1991), it may be that these girls possess greater ability to monitor and control their behavior according to gender-specific role expectations, role expectations that stress compliance, inhibition, and dependence on others (J. H. Block, 1983). For these various reasons, it may be more difficult to detect early symptoms of vulnerability in girls than in boys.

Developmental psychopathologists propose that early adaptation failures defined in age-appropriate terms are important predictors of subsequent disorders (e.g., Masten & Braswell, 1990). My results indicate that early failures to thrive differed substantially for depression-prone boys and girls: Boys who relied on an outer-directed, allocentric mode of impulse expression and girls who relied on an inner-directed, autocentric mode of impulse direction were more at risk than their peers for developing later depressive symptoms. Interpersonal relations, intellectual resourcefulness, and impulse control appeared to play a central role in the origins of depressive symptoms for children of both sexes. Among boys, however, it was antagonism toward others, lack of intellectual resourcefulness, and undercontrol of impulse that anticipated later depressive symptoms. Among girls, by contrast, it was failure to engage the interpersonal world, relative intellectual resourcefulness, and overcontrol of impulse that related most strongly to later depressive symptoms. Hence, depression-prone individuals of both sexes appeared, albeit in markedly different ways, to have inadequately mastered during childhood important developmental tasks, such as impulse control and the establishment of adequate interpersonal relations. In general, these different early patterns of adaptational failures appear to be consistent with the socialization histories of boys and girls (e.g., J. H. Block, 1983) and with differences between the childhood cultures of boys and girls (Maccoby, 1986).

Although our results are fully prospective, they do not permit strong inferences about causality. In particular, we do not know whether prepuberty personality characteristics truly preceded the young adult's depressive experiences or whether individuals vulnerable to depressive mood at age 23 were already having depressive feelings when they were younger. Hence, we cannot say unequivocally that an outer-directed behavior pattern in boys and an inner-directed behavior pattern in girls are of causative and cardinal importance in the developmental course of depressive symptoms. We also cannot exclude the opposite possibility: that these psychological tendencies emerged during childhood in response to concurrently existing depressive experiences. The results do indicate, however, that depressive tendencies in young adults can be predicted from personality evaluations obtained early in life, that these prospective relations are stronger and emerge earlier for boys than for girls, and that their nature differs according to sex. The personality predictors of adulthood depressive symptoms were also longitudinally more consistent for boys than for girls. Hence, if one were to identify young children at risk for subsequent depressive mood, one may have to look for different behaviors in girls and in boys because each sex, our findings indicate, proceeds toward adult depressive symptoms along a different developmental pathway.

References

Akiskal, H. S., Hirschfeld, R. M., & Yerevanian, B. I. (1983). The relationship of personality to depressive disorders. *Archives of General Psychiatry, 40,* 801–810.

Arieti, S., & Bemporad, J. (1980). The psychological organization of depression. *American Journal of Psychiatry, 137,* 1360–1365.

Barnett, P. A., & Gotlib, I. H. (1988). Psychosocial functioning and depression: Distinguishing among antecedents, concomitants, and consequences. *Psychological Bulletin, 104,* 97–126.

Bemporad, J. (1980). The psychodynamics of mild depression. In S. Arieti & J. Bemporad (Eds.), *Severe and mild depression: The psychotherapeutic approach* (pp. 156–184). London: Tavistock.

Bemporad, J., Ratey, J. J., & Hallowell, E. M. (1986). Loss and depression in young adults. *Journal of the American Academy of Psychoanalysis, 14,* 167–179.

Bemporad, J., & Wilson, A. (1978). A developmental approach to depression in childhood and adolescence. *Journal of the American Academy of Psychoanalysis, 6,* 325–352.

Blatt, S. J. (1974). Levels of object representation in anaclitic and introjective depression. *Psychoanalytic study of the child* (Vol. 29, pp. 107–159). Madison, CT: International Universities Press.

Block, J. (1971). *Lives through time.* Berkeley, CA: Bancroft Books.

Block, J. (1978). *The Q-sort method in personality assessment and psychiatric research.* Palo Alto, CA: Consulting Psychologists Press. (Original work published 1961).

Block, J., & Block, J. H. (1980). *The California Child Q-Set.* Palo Alto, CA: Consulting Psychologists Press.

Block, J., Gjerde, P. F., & Block, J. H. (1991). Personality antecedents of depressive tendencies in 18-year-olds: A prospective study. *Journal of Personality and Social Psychology, 60,* 726–738.

Block, J. H. (1973). Conceptions of sex role: Some cross-cultural and longitudinal perspectives. *American Psychologist, 28,* 512–526.

Block, J. H. (1976). Issues, problems, and pitfalls in assessing sex differences: A critical review of "The psychology of sex differences." *Merrill-Palmer Quarterly, 22,* 283–308.

Block, J. H. (1979). Another look at sex differentiation in the socialization behavior of mothers and fathers. In J. Sherman & F. L. Denmark (Eds.), *Psychology of women: Future directions of research* (pp. 31–87). New York: Psychological Dimensions.

Block, J. H. (1983). Differential premises arising from differential socialization of the sexes: Some conjectures. *Child Development, 54,* 1335–1354.

Block, J. H., & Block, J. (1980). The role of ego-control and ego-resiliency in the organization of behavior. In W. A. Collins (Ed.), *The Minnesota Symposia on Child Psychology* (Vol. 13, pp. 39–101). Hillsdale, NJ: Erlbaum.

Blumberg, S. H., & Izard, C. E. (1985). Affective and cognitive characteristics of depression in 10- and 11-year-olds. *Journal of Personality and Social Psychology, 49,* 194–202.

Bowlby, J. (1988). Developmental psychiatry comes of age. *American Journal of Psychiatry, 145,* 1–10.

Caspi, A., & Moffitt, T. E. (1991). Individual differences are accentuated during periods of social change: The sample case of girls at puberty. *Journal of Personality and Social Psychology, 61,* 157–168.

Chodoff, P. (1970). The core problem in depression: Interpersonal aspects. In J. H. Masserman (Ed.), *Depression: Theories and therapies* (pp. 56–61). New York: Grune & Stratton.

Chodoff, P. (1972). The depressive personality. *Archives of General Psychiatry, 27,* 666–673.

Depue, R. A. (1987). *The General Behavior Inventory.* Unpublished manuscript, Department of Psychology, University of Minnesota, Minneapolis.

Depue, R. A., & Klein, D. (1988). Identification of unipolar and bipolar affect conditions by the General Behavior Inventory. In D. Dunner, E. Gerson, & J. Barrett (Eds.), *Relatives at risk for mental disorder* (pp. 257–282). New York: Raven Press.

Depue, R. A., Krauss, S., Spoont, M. R., & Arbisi, P. (1989). General Behavior Inventory identification of unipolar and bipolar affective conditions in a nonclinical university population. *Journal of Abnormal Psychology, 98,* 117–126.

Dweck, C. S., Davidson, W., Nelson, S., & Enna, B. (1978). Sex differences in learned helplessness: II. The contingencies of evaluative feedback in the classroom. III. An experimental analysis. *Developmental Psychology, 14,* 268–276.

Edelbrock, C., & Achenbach, T. M. (1980). A typology of child behavior profile patterns: Distribution patterns and correlates for disturbed children aged 6–16 years. *Journal of Abnormal Child Psychology, 8,* 441–470.

Eron, L. D. (1980). Prescription for reduction of aggression. *American Psychologist, 35,* 244–252.

Fredrichs, R. R., Aneshansel, C. S., & Clark, V. A. (1981). Prevalence of depression in Los Angeles County. *American Journal of Epidemiology, 113,* 691–699.

Gjerde, P. F. (1993). *Alternative pathways to depressive symptoms in young adults: Gender differences in psychological vulnerability.* Manuscript in review.

Gjerde, P. F., & Block, J. (1991). Preadolescent antecedents of depressive symptomatology in late adolescence: A prospective study. *Journal of Youth and Adolescence, 20,* 215–230.

Gjerde, P. F., Block, J., & Block, J. H. (1988). Depressive symptoms and personality during late adolescence: Gender differences in the externalization–internalization of symptom expression. *Journal of Abnormal Psychology, 97,* 475–486.

Hallowell, E. M., Bemporad, J., & Ratey, J. J. (1989). Depression in the transition to adult life. *Adolescent Psychiatry: Developmental and Clinical Studies, 16,* 175–188.

Hill, J. P., & Lynch, M. E. (1983). The intensification of gender-related role expectations during early adolescence. In J. Brooks-Gunn & A. Petersen (Eds.), *Girls at puberty: Biological and psychosocial perspectives* (pp. 175–201). New York: Plenum Press.

Hirschfeld, R. M. A., Klerman, G. L., Chodoff, P., Korchin, S., & Barrett, J. (1976). Dependency—self-esteem—clinical depression. *Journal of the American Academy of Psychoanalysis, 4*, 373–388.

Hirschfeld, R. M. A., Klerman, G. L., Clayton, P. J., Keller, M. B., McDonald-Scott, P., & Larkin, B. H. (1983). Assessing personality: The effects of the depressive state on trait measurement. *American Journal of Psychiatry, 140*, 695–699.

Hunt, J. V., & Eichorn, D. H. (1972). Maternal and child behaviors: A review of data from the Berkeley Growth Study. *Seminars in Psychiatry, 4*, 367–381.

Ingram, R. E., Cruet, D., Johnson, B. R., & Wisnicki, K. S. (1988). Self-focused attention, gender, gender role, and vulnerability to negative affect. *Journal of Personality and Social Psychology, 55*, 967–978.

Kovacs, M., Feinberg, T. L., Crouse-Novak, M. A., Paulauskas, S. L., Pollack, M., & Finkelstein, R. (1984). Depressive disorders in childhood: II. A longitudinal study of the risk for a subsequent major depression. *Archives of General Psychiatry, 41*, 636–644.

Lewis, M., Feiring, C., McGuffog, C., & Jaskir, J. (1984). Predicting psychopathology in six-year-olds from early social relations. *Child Development, 55*, 123–130.

Looney, J. G. (1989). Editor's introduction. *Adolescent Psychiatry: Developmental and Clinical Studies, 16*, 121–126.

Maccoby, E. E. (1986). Social groupings in childhood: Their relationship to prosocial and antisocial behavior in boys and girls. In D. Olweus, J. Block, & M. Radke-Yarrow (Eds.), *Development of prosocial and antisocial behavior* (pp. 263–284). San Diego, CA: Academic Press.

Masten, A., & Braswell, L. (1990). Developmental psychopathology: An integrative framework for understanding behavior problems in children and adolescents. In P. R. Martin (Ed.), *The handbook of behavior therapy and psychological science: An integrative approach* (pp. 35–56). Elmsford, NY: Pergamon Press.

McCranie, E. J. (1971). Depression, anxiety, and hostility. *Psychiatric Quarterly, 45*, 117–133.

McGrath, E., Keita, G. P., Strickland, B. R., & Russo, N. F. (1990). *Women and depression.* Washington, DC: American Psychological Association.

McNemar, Q. (1969). *Psychological statistics.* New York: Wiley.

Nolen-Hoeksema, S. (1987). Sex differences in unipolar depression: Evidence and theory. *Psychological Bulletin, 101*, 259–282.

Ostrov, E., Offer, D., & Howard, K. I. (1989). Gender differences in adolescent symptomatology: A normative study. *Journal of the American Academy of Child and Adolescent Psychiatry, 28*, 394–398.

Panter, A. T., & Tanaka, J. S. (1987, August). *Cognitive "activity" and dysphoric affect: Gender differences in information processing.* Paper presented at the 95th Annual Convention of the American Psychological Association, New York.

Petersen, A. C., Sarigiani, P. A., & Kennedy, R. E. (1991). Adolescent depression: Why more girls. *Journal of Youth and Adolescence, 20,* 247–271.

Puig-Antich, J. (1982). Major depression and conduct disorder in prepuberty. *Journal of the American Academy of Child Psychiatry, 21,* 118–128.

Radloff, L. S. (1977). The CES-D Scale: A self-report depression scale for research in the general population. *Applied Psychological Measurement, 3,* 385–401.

Robins, L., & Rutter, M. (1990). *Straight and devious pathways from childhood to adulthood.* New York: Cambridge University Press.

Ross, A. O. (1974). *Psychological disorders of children: A behavioral approach to theory, research, and therapy.* New York: McGraw-Hill.

Rutter, M. (1986). The developmental psychopathology of depression: Issues and perspectives. In M. Rutter, C. E. Izard, & P. B. Read (Eds.), *Depression in young people* (pp. 3–32). New York: Guilford Press.

Rutter, M. (1988). Longitudinal data in the study of causal processes: Some uses and some pitfalls. In M. Rutter (Ed.), *Studies of psychosocial risk* (pp. 1–28). Cambridge, England: Cambridge University Press.

Rutter, M., & Garmezy, N. (1983). Developmental psychopathology. In P. Mussen (Ed.), *Handbook of child psychology* (4th ed., Vol. 4, pp. 775–911). New York: Wiley.

Salzman, L. (1975). Interpersonal factors in depression. In F. F. Flack & S. C. Draghi (Eds.), *The nature and treatment of depression* (pp. 43–56). New York: Wiley.

Sroufe, L. A., & Rutter, M. (1984). The domain of developmental psychopathology. *Child Development, 55,* 17–29.

Stapley, J. C., & Haviland, J. M. (1989). Beyond depression: Gender differences in normal adolescents' emotional experiences. *Sex Roles, 20,* 295–308.

Stein, N. L., & Levine, L. J. (1987). Thinking about feelings: The development and organization of emotional knowledge. In R. E. Snow & M. J. Farr (Eds.), *Aptitude, learning, and instruction: Vol. 3. Conative and affective process analyses* (pp. 165–197). Hillsdale, NJ: Erlbaum.

CHAPTER 13

Child-Rearing Antecedents of Suboptimal Personality Development: Exploring Aspects of Alice Miller's Concept of the Poisonous Pedagogy

David M. Harrington

I n his address to the 99th Annual Convention of the American Psychological Association in August 1991, on the occasion of his receiving the G. Stanley Hall Award, Jack Block observed with approval that laypeople expect psychologists to address what he termed *homely human*

The study was supported by National Institute of Mental Health Grant MH 16080 to Jack Block and Jeanne H. Block.

This chapter is based on a presentation given at "Lives Through Time: Assessment and Theory in Personality Psychology from a Longitudinal Perspective," a research conference with special guest of honor, Jack Block, held in Palm Springs, California, in November 1991.

I would like to thank Cam Leaper and Per Gjerde for helpful consultations regarding this project. In addition, I thank Anne Roesler for her extensive and multifaceted assistance with this project in its early and fragile stages as well as Frances Hatfield, Cynthia McCabe, Rose Perrine, and Paul Sanders for their excellent work as judges and translators in this project. Athena Kalandros and Jennifer Schultz also facilitated this research in several important ways.

concerns (J. Block, 1991). In particular, Block noted, laypeople wish to know why people turn out the way they do, want to know how and whether child-rearing practices shape human development, and expect scientific psychology to shed some light on these matters of enduring and everyday human concern. It is clear from his comments and from his life's work that Jack Block shares and endorses that expectation.

Partially in the spirit of that enterprise, though also in the spirit of sheer curiosity, I have undertaken a series of analyses designed to explore Alice Miller's (1983) concept of the "poisonous pedagogy" (PP)—a constellation of child-rearing practices and attitudes by means of which, according to Miller, much of the psychological pain and psychological ill-health of one generation is transmitted to the next. In order to bring systematic empirical evidence to bear on Miller's general hypothesis that exposure to PP in childhood decreases the likelihood of optimal personality development, I have turned to data drawn from the J. H. Block and Block (1980) longitudinal study of personality and cognitive development. Using those data, I have developed indexes of the degree to which parents in the Block & Block study displayed aspects of the PP when dealing with their preschool children and have correlated those indexes of preschool PP with personality descriptions of the children obtained 15–20 years later when the children were approximately 18 and 23 years old.

Alice Miller is a Swiss psychologist, psychotherapist, and author of several books, including *Prisoners of Childhood: The Drama of the Gifted Child* (Miller, 1981) and *For Your Own Good: Hidden Cruelty in Child-Rearing and the Roots of Violence* (Miller, 1983). It was in *For Your Own Good* that Miller first presented her concept of the PP. *For Your Own Good* is an ambitious, polemical, and passionately argued book. On the basis of her own clinical experiences and her study of central European child-rearing practices of the past two centuries, Miller asserted that much of the violence that people see around them, and a significant portion of the psychological pain as well, is traceable to the psychological suffering and deprivation that she believed many experience as young children. Furthermore, Miller believed much of this childhood suffering is the product of PP.

In practice, PP involves the weakening of the child's self-confidence and curiosity, the ridiculing of the child's lack of competence, the suppression of crying, the ridiculing and suppression of feelings in general, the early teaching of self-renunciation, the attacking and suppression of the child's exuberance, the suppression of the child's life-affirming feelings and impulses, and a belief that a child's will must be "broken" as early as possible (Miller, 1983, pp. 21–33).

Miller believed that PP undermines the growing child's capacity to know, express, and act appropriately on his or her own feelings, a developmental handicap of immense ramifications. She also believed that PP undermines the capacity for the full development of empathy, creativity, and effective intelligence. Miller (1984) argued that PP fosters feelings of "anger, helplessness, despair, longing, anxiety and pain" and believed that such feelings predispose adults to behave in unconsciously rageful and violent ways toward others and themselves. She also asserted that PP in extreme form leads to "drug addiction, alcoholism, prostitution, psychic disorders [and] suicide" (Miller, 1984, Afterword to the Second Edition).

In Miller's view, parents who use the PP do so out of a *conscious* and understandable desire to accelerate their children's development and to help their children move as quickly as possible from vulnerable states of childhood helplessness, incompetence, and dependence to safer states of adult competence, independence, self-sufficiency, and power. Miller also believed that parents are driven to apply PP as an *unconscious* reaction to the emotional damage they have suffered as a consequence of having been subjected to PP by their own parents. According to Miller, parents who were subjected to PP as children are apt to be driven by several unconscious needs, including the need to defend themselves against the reappearance in their own children of that which was repressed in themselves and around which they have so much unconscious pain, rage, and shame and by the unconscious need to manipulate their children as outlets for their own repressed rage and grief at the manner in which they were treated as children (Miller, 1983, pp. 97–98).

Miller's (1983) theory is profoundly intergenerational in character. By describing a mechanism for the transmission of the PP from one generation to the next and by presenting this alleged mechanism to both professional and lay audiences, Miller was explicitly attempting to break what she saw as a tragic intergenerational connection.

Miller's (1983) concept has received considerable attention from a large lay readership, from other social scientists (e.g., Montagu, 1983; Pharis, 1984), and from the world of self-help psychology (e.g., Bradshaw, 1988; Steinem, 1992; Whitfield, 1989). Although PP might not yet have achieved the status of a household phrase, it has certainly attracted considerable attention as a concept that addresses some of those "homely human concerns" about which laypeople are so legitimately curious.

As far as I have been able to determine, however, Miller's (1983) concept has received little or no systematic empirical evaluation beyond case studies. The study described here represents an attempt to bring Miller's concept into the realm of systematically studied child-rearing practices.

Research Overview

The research reported here relates indexes of Miller's (1983) concept of PP to data that have been collected over the nearly 20-year span of J. H. Block and Block's (1980) ongoing longitudinal study of personality and cognitive development. Indexes of parental PP based on direct observations of parent–child interactions when the children were in preschool, and based on parents' self-reports of their own child-rearing attitudes and practices, were developed and then correlated with completely independent personality descriptions of the children when they were 18 and 23 years old. These correlations, spanning between 15 and 20 years' time, constituted the empirical heart of this study.

All of the empirical research I am presenting here rests on the splendid groundwork laid by Jack Block and Jeanne Block, who created and sustained the longitudinal study from which these data were drawn (J. H. Block & Block, 1980); who developed assessment instruments flexible and broad-band enough to capture constructs formulated years after they were created; and who assembled and supervised a large team of psychologists, research assistants, teachers, and staff members who gathered, created, and organized these data over two decades. I am also indebted, of course, to this large research team, which has spanned two decades. In carrying out and reporting these analyses, I often felt that I was riding on the back of a large but surprisingly agile elephant.

Method

Subjects

Data were derived from approximately 100 families who are still, as of this writing, participating in the ongoing longitudinal study of ego and cognitive development initiated by Jack Block and Jeanne H. Block in 1968 (see J. H. Block & Block, 1980, for an extensive description of the project). Most families entered the study when their children were enrolled as 3-year-olds in one of two nursery schools associated with the Harold E. Jones Child Study Center at the University of California, Berkeley. Some joined when their children were enrolled as 4-year-olds. My analyses involved 52 females and 48 males. Because of missing data at various points, however, the effective working samples were often closer to 70 or 80 families for many of the analyses reported here. Approximately two thirds of the children were White, about one fourth were African American, and about one twelfth were Asian.

The average Wechsler Preschool and Primary Scale of Intelligence (WPPSI) Full Scale IQ score for these children at age 4 years was 118.3 ($SD = 11.9$, range $= 89–147$).

Although the parents had an average of more than 4 years of college and were generally well employed, their socioeconomic and educational range was moderately wide. Specifically, their average education when their children were in preschool was 15.6 years ($SD = 2.33$, range $= 7–20$) for the mothers and 17.9 years ($SD = 2.55$, range $= 13–19$) for the fathers. The average socioeconomic status (SES), as reflected in Duncan's (1961) index, was 17.9 ($SD = 1.75$, range $= 13–19$).

These children were studied by numerous examiners administering wide-ranging batteries of assessment procedures at ages 3, 4, 5, 7, 11, 14, 18, and 23 years. The analyses reported here involved data gathered between the ages of 3 and 5 and again at ages 18 and 23 years.

Parental PP Indexes

Self-Reported Child-Rearing Practices and Attitudes

During the first year the families joined the study in the late 1960s, the mothers and fathers independently described their child-rearing practices and attitudes using the Child-Rearing Practices Report (CRPR), a 91-item Q-set (J. H. Block, 1965, 1984; see also J. H. Block, cited in Johnson, 1976).

To make possible a comparison of the parents' self-reported child-rearing practices and attitudes to Miller's (1983) description of the PP, six judges (one psychologist, one graduate student, and four older undergraduate psychology majors who were also parents) were asked to translate Miller's concept into the vocabulary of the CRPR. Each judge read a 4-page summary of Miller's description of the PP (including extensive quotes) and then arranged the CRPR items in a nine-step rectangular distribution reflecting the degree to which each item matched Miller's description of the PP. The 10 CRPR items most descriptive of the PP were placed in Pile 9, the 10 items least characteristic of the PP were placed in Pile 1, and so on. The judges' independent ratings were then averaged to form a composite prototype of the construct. The judges agreed very well in identifying items that characterized the PP; the interjudge reliability of the CRPR PP prototype was .96. Indexes of the degree to which the parents exhibited PP in their self-reported child-rearing practices and attitudes were then generated by computing the Pearson product–moment correlations between each parent's CRPR and the CRPR prototype of Miller's PP. The mothers' average CRPR PP index was $-.50$ ($SD = .15$, range $= -.61$ to .12). The fathers' average CRPR PP index was $-.54$ ($SD = .20$, range $= -.76$ to .39). Of course, in the absence of CRPR PP data for norm-providing samples, it was not possible to know whether this group of parents was unusually high or low with respect to self-reported PP, nor was it possible to say how extremely "poisonous" parents would actually score on this index.

CRPR items judged to be the most and least characteristic of PP are presented in Table 1.

As seen in Table 1, the CRPR PP scale contains at its poisonous end items involving the suppression of the child's feelings, strict maintenance of parental authority, fear that affection may weaken a child, and a certain element of parental hostility. At the nonpoisonous end are items that involve the easy and physical expression of parental affection, parental responsiveness to the child's signals of distress, encouragement of the child's expression of his or her opinions, and a taking into account of

TABLE 1
Child-Rearing Practices Report (CRPR) Items Judged Most and Least Descriptive of Miller's (1983) Poisonous Pedagogy

---

Items judged to be the most characteristic of the poisonous pedagogy
- I do not allow my child to get angry with me.
- I believe that too much affection and tenderness can harm or weaken a child.
- I sometimes tease and make fun of my child.
- I do not allow my child to question my decisions.
- I think children must learn early not to cry.
- I teach my child to keep control of his [or her] feelings at all times.
- I believe that a child should be seen and not heard.
- I believe that scolding and criticism make my child improve.

CRPR items judged to be the least characteristic of the poisonous pedagogy
- I express affection by hugging, kissing, and holding my child.
- My child and I have warm, intimate times together.
- I respect my child's opinions and encourage him [or her] to express them.
- I feel a child should be given comfort and understanding when he [or she] is scared or upset.
- I usually take into account my child's preferences in making plans for the family.
- I believe in praising a child when he [or she] is good and think it gets better results than punishing him [or her] when he [or she] is bad.
- I encourage my child to be curious, to explore and question things.

---

those opinions and preferences. Parents who endorsed items such as those in the top half of Table 1 obtained relatively high PP scores; parents who endorsed items such as those in the bottom half of Table 1 obtained relatively low (i.e., nonpoisonous) PP scores.

Parent–Child Interactions in a Teaching Situation
When the children were approximately 4.5 years old, their mothers and fathers individually taught them a battery of two divergent thinking tasks and two convergent thinking tasks in a standardized situation (for more details, see Harrington, Block, & Block, 1978). An observer of these parent–child interactions immediately described them using the 49-item Parent–Child Interaction Q-Set (PCIQ).[1] Later, other judges observed vid-

---

[1]Also referred to as the Teaching Strategies Q-Set in some previous reports from this project.

eotapes of the interactions and described those interactions using the 19-variable Teaching Strategies Rating Form (TSR).

Prototypic descriptions of PP in the teaching situation were developed in a manner analogous to that used to develop the PP prototype for the CRPR. The same six people who translated the PP into the CRPR also translated Miller's (1983) concept into the vocabularies of the PCIQ and the TSR. Again, these independent translations were averaged to form composite prototypes, and again the judges agreed strongly in their identification of items reflecting high or low PP. The internal reliability of the PCIQ and TSR PP prototypes were .96 and .98, respectively. PCIQ and TSR items judged to be the most and least characteristic of PP are presented in Table 2.

As can be seen in Table 2, the PCIQ and TSR PP scales contained at their poisonous ends items involving parental control of the tasks and overcontrol of their own feelings and an ashamed, critical, rejecting, and

TABLE 2

Parent-Child Interaction Q-Set Items and Teaching Strategy Rating Form Items Judged Most and Least Descriptive of Miller's (1983) Poisonous Pedagogy

---

Items judged to be the most characteristic of the poisonous pedagogy
    Parent was critical of child; rejected child's ideas and suggestions.
    Parent tended to control the tasks.
    Parent tended toward overcontrol of own needs and impulses.
    Parent appeared ashamed of child; lacked pride in child.
    Parent pressured child to work at the tasks.
    Parent was impatient with the child.
    Parent tended to reject inadequate solutions.

Items judged to be the most uncharacteristic of the poisonous pedagogy
    Parent was responsive to child's needs from moment to moment.
    Parent was supportive and encouraging of child in the situation.
    Parent was warm and supportive.
    Parent praised the child.
    Parent reacted to the child in an ego-enhancing manner.
    Parent encouraged the child.
    Parent surrendered control of the situation to the child.
    Parent encouraged the child to proceed independently.
    Parent valued the child's originality.

---

impatient parental posture with respect to the child and his or her ideas. On the nonpoisonous end of the scales, on the other hand, were items involving parental warmth and encouragement, granting of task control to the child, parental responsiveness to the child's signals for help, valuing of the child's independence and originality, and enhancement of the child's ego. Parents who were described as exhibiting behaviors such as those listed in the top half of Table 2 obtained relatively high PP scores in the teaching situation; parents who were seen exhibiting behaviors such as those described in the bottom half of Table 2 obtained relatively low (i.e., nonpoisonous) PP scores.

Two indexes of the degree to which each parent exhibited PP in the teaching situation were then generated by the same method used with the CRPR. One index was based on the PCIQ and one on the TSR. The mothers' PP index averaged $-.26$ on the PCIQ ($SD = .35$, range $= -.74$ to .52) and averaged $-.05$ on the TSR ($SD = .50$, range $= -.77$ to .85). The fathers' PP index averaged $-.24$ on the PCIQ ($SD = .32$, range $= -.70$ to .52) and $-.04$ on the TSR ($SD = .45$, range $= -.81$ to .88). Again, without normative data, it was not possible to determine whether these parents were unusually high or low with respect to observed PP in this culture. The PCIQ and TSR indexes (which correlated .68 with one another among the mothers and .66 among the fathers) were then standardized and averaged to form a single index of each parent's PP in the teaching situation.[2]

Residualized Indexes of PP by Sex

The indexes of parental PP correlated negatively—and highly negatively in some cases—with indexes of parental education and with a WPPSI Full Scale IQ score that was available for the children at 4 years of age. In order to remove the impact of parental education and child's preschool intelligence from the indexes of parental PP as much as possible, I also computed residualized forms of the four PP indexes. I did this by subtracting from each raw PP score that portion which was linearly pre-

---

[2]If information from the Parent–Child Interaction Q-Set or the Teaching Strategies Rating Form was missing, a linear-regression-based prediction from the available piece of data was substituted for the missing data in the averaging process.

dictable from an index of parental education and the WPPSI Full Scale IQ index of childhood IQ at 4 years of age.[3]

It is important to note that because the parental education and WPPSI Full Scale IQ scores correlated substantially more negatively with raw PP indexes for boys than for girls (e.g., the raw index of mothers' PP in the teaching situation correlated $-.60$ with parental education among the boys and $-.16$ with parental education among the girls), I created three different sets of residualized PP indexes: one set each for the total sample, boys, and girls. The analyses reported in this chapter involved these double-residualized indexes: indexes of PP that were constructed to correlate exactly zero with parental education and with IQ at age 4 years in the total, male, and female samples separately.

It should be noted carefully and clearly that this process of statistically removing the linear impact of parental education and child's IQ on the PP indexes worked *against* Miller's (1983) hypotheses by *reducing* the number and strength of the relationships subsequently found between PP indexes and measures of personality in young adulthood. Had raw PP scores been used in these analyses, rather than double-residualized indexes, the results would have been much stronger, although they would have been seriously contaminated by parental education and SES and by the child's IQ. The hundreds of item-level path analyses that would have illuminated these complex relationships were beyond the scope of this chapter.

Personality Descriptions at Ages 18 and 23 Years

When the subjects were 18 years old, they interacted with four examiners, each of whom individually administered a variety of psychological assessment procedures to each subject in sessions typically lasting 2–3 hours. At the conclusion of these interactions, the four examiners independently described each subject by placing the 100 items of the California

---

[3]The parental education index was constructed by averaging the standardized years of education for mothers and fathers. If level of education was unavailable for one parent, a linear regression prediction of the missing educational data was made based on Duncan's (1961) socioeconomic status (SES) index. The regression-based prediction was then substituted for the missing educational information in the averaging process. The resulting index of parental education correlated .88 with years of mothers' education, .91 with years of fathers' education, and .82 with the SES index.

Adult Q-Set, Form III (CAQ; J. Block, 1961; Block, 1962) in a forced nine-step distribution reflecting the salience and applicability of each item to the subject being described. The CAQ contains 100 items, each describing an aspect or quality of adult personality. The four examiners' completely independent ratings were then averaged to yield "scores" for each subject on each of the 100 CAQ items at 18 years of age.

When the subjects were 23 years old, they interacted with a completely new and independent set of four examiners, who individually administered a new set of procedures and who also independently described the subjects using the CAQ. These independent ratings were also averaged to yield scores for each subject on each of the 100 CAQ items at age 23 years. For some analyses, the 18- and 23-year-old CAQ items were also standardized and composited to form 100 CAQ items at 18 and 23 years of age.

Global Indexes of Optimal Psychological Adjustment at Ages 18 and 23 Years

A global index of healthy psychological functioning was needed to test Miller's (1983) prediction that PP impedes optimal psychological development. It just so happened that Jack Block had developed just such an index about 30 years ago (see J. Block, 1961, Appendix D) and had used it successfully in some important studies of personality development (J. Block, 1971; J. H. Block, Block, Siegelman, & von der Lippe, 1971; and Siegelman, Block, Block, & von der Lippe, 1970 [in slightly abbreviated form]). To generate this index, Block asked nine experienced clinical psychologists to independently describe the optimally adjusted individual using the 100-item CAQ and then averaged their descriptions to generate a composite and internally highly reliable description of the optimally adjusted person.

The CAQ Optimal Adjustment Index involves, at its positive end, elements such as the capacity for close relationships; forthrightness in dealing with others; social perceptivity; ethically consistent behavior; valuing of independence; and an ability to see to the heart of important problems, to be productive, and to have insight into one's own motives and behaviors. The index is negatively anchored by items involving a

brittle ego-defense system; the prevalence of repressive defense mechanisms; the tendency to avoid close interpersonal relationships; fearful,
anxious, self-pitying, negativistic, and self-defeating feelings and attitudes;
deceitful and manipulative postures with respect to others; and a lack of
personal meaning in life. Optimal Adjustment Index scores for this study
were calculated by computing the Pearson product–moment correlation
between each subject's 100-item CAQ description and the 100-item prototypic description of the optimally adjusted person. Optimal Adjustment
Index scores were computed separately at ages 18 and 23 years and were
correlated .58 with one another.

Creative Personality at 18 and 23 Years of Age

Because Miller (1983) hypothesized that PP inhibits the full development
of human creativity, I also included two indexes of creative personality
at ages 18 and 23 in these analyses.

The CAQ–IPAR Creative Personality Scale

The CAQ–IPAR Creative Personality Scale contains 19 CAQ items that
had correlated significantly with real-world indexes of creativity or had
been extremely characteristic or uncharacteristic of creative architects
(MacKinnon, 1962, 1965, 1966), creative writers (Barron, 1969), or creative
undergraduate women (Helson, 1967, 1985) who had been studied at the
University of California's Institute of Personality Assessment and Research (IPAR).

The Creative Personality Scale is defined at the positive end by items
involving a wide range of interests, high intelligence, productive manner,
unconventional thought processes, aesthetic reactivity, high aspiration
level, concern with one's own adequacy as a person, ethically consistent
behavior, valuing of independence, being an interesting person, and being
interested in philosophical issues. The scale is defined at the negative
end by items having to do with being uncomfortable with uncertainties
and complexities, self-pitying and self-defeating attitudes and behaviors,
flattened affect, reluctance to commit self to action and heightened read-
iness to withdraw from action in the face of adversity, and a lack of

personal meaning in life (for a fuller description, see Harrington, Block, & Block, 1987). The CAQ–IPAR indexes of creative personality at ages 18 and 23 correlated .55 with one another.

The Creative Female Careerist Scale

To help ensure adequate assessment of personality characteristics associated with creative potential and creative performance in young women, I developed an additional creative personality scale based on Helson's (1967, 1985) pioneering work with creative undergraduate women. The Creative Female Careerist Scale consists of 14 CAQ items that significantly differentiated Mills College women who had been nominated by the Mills faculty as showing unusual creative potential and who also went on to creative careers from Mills seniors who had been nominated by the Mills faculty as showing unusual creative potential but who did not enter creative careers (Helson, 1967, 1985).

The Creative Female Careerist Scale is defined at the positive end by high aspiration; concern with philosophical problems; a tendency to interpret simple situations in complicated ways; skill in the social techniques of imaginative play, expressiveness, and talkativeness; a generally self-dramatic manner; and a tendency for tension to manifest itself as bodily symptoms. The scale is negatively anchored by items involving discomfort with complexity, overcontrol, flattened affect, a bland calmness, reluctance to commit to action, and a hyperreadiness to withdraw from action in the face of adversity.

The Creative Female Careerist Scale scores at 18 and 23 years of age correlated .58 with one another. The Creative Female Careerist Scale scores were also sufficiently independent of the CAQ–IPAR Creative Personality Scale scores obtained at the same time (rs = .51 and .67 at 23 and 18 years of age, respectively) to justify their inclusion in subsequent analyses. The Creative Female Careerist Scale seemed especially appropriate for this investigation because it was derived from assessments originally made of Mills College women when they were approximately the age of J. H. Block and Block's (1980) subjects at their 23-year-old assessment.

Results

Sex Differences

Scattered and Inconsequential Mean Sex Differences

There were no significant sex differences with respect to mean scores. Indeed, the only significant mean differences involved the CAQ–IPAR Creative Personality Scale, on which the women scored higher than the men at 18 and 23 years ($p < .05$).

Substantial and Consequential Sex Differences Involving Correlational Patterns

As noted earlier, the correlations between WPPSI Full Scale IQ at age 4 and parental education on the one hand, and raw indexes of PP and several outcome variables on the other, were substantially different for boys and girls. For example, mothers' observed PP correlated $-.53$ with boys' WPPSI IQ but only $-.20$ with girls' WPPSI IQ. It was such correlational differences that led to the construction of three separate sets of double-residualized PP indexes for the total, male, and female samples separately.

Distributional Properties of the Central Variables

The distributions of most variables used in this study were sufficiently normal to justify the routine use of Pearson product–moment correlations, linear regressions, t tests, and analyses of variance. Four variables, however, were sufficiently skewed to suggest the use of analytic techniques based on rank order alone.

Skewed Indexes of Self-Reported PP and Optimal Adjustment

The residualized indexes of PP based on parents' CRPR self-reports (although not those based on observers' descriptions of actual parent–child interactions) were substantially positively skewed. On the other hand, the Optimal Adjustment Index scores at age 18 and, to a lesser extent, at age 23, were substantially negatively skewed. As a consequence of their skewed distributions, correlations involving the two self-reported indexes of PP and the Optimal Adjustment Index scores at 18 and 23 years of age were calculated in terms of Spearman rank order coefficients rather than Pearson product–moment coefficients unless otherwise specified.

Correlations Among the PP Indexes

As seen in Table 3, correlations among the four residualized indexes of PP were modest.

The within-sex correlations between self-reported and observed PP did not exceed .20 for mothers and were .30 and .42 for fathers of girls and boys, respectively. These within-parent correlations, along with the cross-parent correlations, suggested that the four PP indexes captured substantially different aspects of parental PP. As a consequence, all four residualized indexes of PP were carried on for further analyses and no additional PP composites were constructed.

Parents' PP Indexes and Children's Personality and Behavior

Of the four PP indexes examined in this study, the index of the mothers' PP in the preschool teaching situation yielded by far the strongest pattern of correlations with indexes of the children's personalities and behaviors almost 15–20 years later. Of the 18 correlations computed between the index of observed maternal PP and the six outcome measures within the total, male, and female samples separately, 69% were significant at or beyond the 5% level, and 79% were significant at or beyond the 10% level of significance. All of these significant and marginally significant corre-

TABLE 3

Spearman Correlations for the Residualized Indexes of Poisonous Pedagogy (PP)

	Observed maternal PP	Self-reported maternal PP	Observed paternal PP	Self-reported paternal PP
Observed maternal PP	—	.00	.15	.27
Self-reported maternal PP	.20	—	.05	.22
Observed paternal PP	.35*	.12	—	.42*
Self-reported paternal PP	.10	.29	.30	—

Note. Correlations for parents of boys (36 mothers and 31 fathers) are above the diagonal, and those for parents of girls (40 mothers and 38 fathers) are below the diagonal.
*p < .05.

lations were in the theoretically predicted direction. By contrast, only 6% of the correlations computed between the other three indexes of PP and the outcome measures were significant at or beyond the 5% level, and only 13% were significant at or beyond the 10% level. I therefore present only the results involving the index of maternal PP observed in the teaching situation.

Mothers' PP and Children's Personality and Behavior

Negative Correlations With Indexes of Optimal Adjustment and Creative Personality

As can be seen in Table 4, maternal PP in the preschool interaction was significantly negatively predictive of Optimal Adjustment at ages 18 ($r = -.45, p < .001$) and 23 ($r = -.32, p < .01$), Creative Personality at ages 18 ($r = -.33, p < .01$) and 23 ($r = -.26, p < .05$), and Creative Female Careerist at age 23 ($r = -.32, p < .01$) in the total sample.

TABLE 4

Correlations Between the Index of Mothers' Observed Preschool Poisonous Pedagogy and Measures of Their Children's Personality at Ages 18 and 23 Years

Personality and behavior indexes	Pearson correlations[a]		
	Boys[b]	Girls[c]	Total
Optimal adjustment indexes			
At age 18	−.33**	−.47***	−.44****
At age 23	−.30*	−.34*	−.35***
Creative personality indexes			
Creative personality at age 18	−.12	−.50***	−.33***
Creative personality at age 23	−.21	−.29*	−.26*
Creative female careerist at age 18	.05	−.46***	−.22*d
Creative female careerist at age 23	−.11	−.45***	−.32***

[a]Pearson product–moment correlations for creative personality indexes; Spearman *rhos* for optimal adjustment indexes.
[b]The number of boys in the sample ranged from 33 to 36.
[c]The number of girls in the sample ranged from 38 to 39.
[d]Significant sex difference ($p < .05$) in regression slopes as tested in multiple regression analyses in which variables were entered in the following order: sex, IQ at age 4, parental education, Sex × IQ, Sex × Parental Education, PP index, and Sex × PP Index.
*$p < .10$. **$p < .05$. ***$p < .01$. ****$p < .001$. All tests are two-tailed.

The correlations involving optimal adjustment were significant for both sexes separately. The correlations involving the two creative personality indexes were generally significant among young women but not significant among young men, although a significant sex difference in regression slopes was detected only for the Creative Female Careerist Scale at age 23 years. These statistically significant correlations involving optimal adjustment and creative personality were all in the direction predicted by Miller's (1983) theory.

Mothers' Observed PP and Individual CAQ Items

To examine the results in finer detail, the index of mothers' observed PP was also correlated with the 100 CAQ items at ages 18 and 23 and with the standardized composite of the 18- and 23-year-old descriptions. Although the 18-year-old and 23-year-old CAQ results differed slightly from one another, the same underlying themes emerged in both years and were well reflected in the correlational pattern obtained with the 18- and 23-year-old composite descriptions. Therefore, to simplify presentation and facilitate understanding of these item-level correlations, I present only the results involving the 18- and 23-year-old composite items.

To further simplify this presentation and to avoid presenting results that involved substantial sex differences, the 18- and 23-year-old items had to (a) correlate significantly with the index of maternal PP in the teaching situation for the total sample, (b) generate correlations whose absolute values exceeded .20 within both the male and female samples separately, and (c) not exhibit significantly different regression slopes in the male and female samples. Items passing all three tests are presented in Table 5.

The picture that emerged from an analysis of the item-level personality correlates at 18 and 23 years of age was consistent with the theoretical expectation that PP in childhood tends to be followed by substantially suboptimal personality development.

The subjects raised by mothers who exhibited relatively high degrees of PP in the preschool teaching situation were seen as being significantly more brittle and easily disorganized by stress, more fearful, anxious, thin-skinned, self-defensive, concerned with their own adequacy, negativistic,

TABLE 5

Personality Characteristics[a] at Ages 18–23 Years Associated[b] With Mothers' Poisonous Pedagogy (PP) in the Teaching Situation at 4.5 Years

Personality characteristics	rs
Positive	
Has a brittle ego-defense system; has a small reserve of integration; would be disorganized and maladaptive when under stress.	.37***
Is vulnerable to real or fancied threat; generally fearful.	.36**
Keeps people at a distance; avoids close interpersonal relationships	.36**
Gives up and withdraws where possible in the face of frustration and adversity.	.34**
Is basically anxious.	.34**
Is thin-skinned, sensitive to anything that can be construed as criticism or an interpersonal slight.	.33**
Concerned with own adequacy as a person.	.33**
Tends to be self-defensive.	.32**
Feels cheated and victimized by life, self-pitying.	.31**
Seeks reassurance from others.	.29*
Anxiety and tension find an outlet in bodily symptoms.	.28*
Feels a lack of personal meaning in life.	.28*
Is basically distrustful of people in general.	.26*
Is subtly negativistic; tends to undermine and obstruct or sabotage.	.25*
Negative	
Is turned to for advice and reassurance.	− .35**
Appears straightforward, forthright, candid.	− .35**
Responds to humor.	− .32**
Is personally charming.	− .32**
Has warmth; has the capacity for close relationships; compassionate.	− .31**
Has social poise and presence; appears socially at ease.	− 31**
Is socially perceptive of a wide range of interpersonal cues.	− .30**
Tends to arouse liking and acceptance in people.	− .28*
Able to see to the heart of important problems.	− .28*
Emphasizes being with others; gregarious.	− .26*
Is cheerful.	− .24*

Note. $n = 76$.

[a]Independent California Adult Q-Set (CAQ) descriptions at ages 18 and 23 years were standardized and averaged to form the composites used in these analyses. CAQ items are presented here in abbreviated form.

[b]Listed here are those items that yielded (a) a significant correlation with mothers' observed PP in the total sample ($p < .05$, two-tailed), (b) correlations whose absolute values equaled or exceeded .20 within each of the single-sex samples, and (c) no significant sex difference in terms of regression slopes.

*$p < .05$.   **$p < .01$.   ***$p < .001$. All tests are two-tailed.

unincisive in their analysis of problems, and apt to give up and withdraw in the face of adversity compared with young adults raised by mothers who used relatively little PP. These children of comparatively high PP mothers were also described as experiencing an unusual lack of personal meaning in their lives, appeared to feel cheated and victimized, and were comparatively cheerless.

Interpersonally, the children of relatively high PP mothers were described as being comparatively avoidant, distancing, and ungregarious. They sought reassurance from others but others did not turn to them for reassurance or advice. They were comparatively ill at ease socially, were socially unperceptive, and were relatively unresponsive to humor. Compared with their more fortunate peers, they were seen as lacking personal warmth and the capacity for close relationships, they aroused less liking and acceptance in others, and were described as less charming than their peers. They were seen as being more distrustful of others and less straightforward and candid with others than were those raised by more supportive mothers.

Comparatively speaking, then, children raised by mothers who exhibited considerable PP in the preschool teaching situation appeared to be significantly less psychologically healthy in young adulthood than did their peers who were raised by mothers who exhibited lower levels of PP 15–20 years earlier.

Discussion

Several points should be made regarding the data and this study.

1. Longitudinal studies involving early parent–child interactions and subsequent personality development cannot disentangle causal chains. Although early child-rearing practices may influence personality development, it is also possible that child-rearing practices themselves are partly shaped by children's characteristics or by genetically influenced parental characteristics, either or both of which may influence children's later personality development. As a consequence, caution must be exercised in drawing causal inferences from these data.

2. The indexes of PP used here were new and certainly imperfect. Until the construct validity of these indexes is more firmly established, interpretative caution should be exercised.

3. As always, generalizing these results to populations, times, or settings other than those studied here should be done cautiously, if at all (Campbell & Stanley, 1963). Whether the child-rearing practices characterized as "poisonous" by Miller (1983) and apparently an antecedent of suboptimal personality development in this sample of predominantly middle-class, White families whose children attended Berkeley preschools in the late 1960s are psychologically harmful to children in other circumstances is a question that, like many others in developmental psychology (e.g., Maccoby & Martin, 1983), must await the outcome of careful empirical studies conducted within a wide variety of other contexts.

4. Having acknowledged these standard methodological limitations, it seems fair to say that the data involving the mothers' observed PP in the parent–child interactions were significantly consistent with and supportive of Miller's (1983) belief that PP is psychologically harmful. As young adults, the children raised by mothers who appeared to use relatively high levels of PP in the preschool teaching situation were seen as being significantly less psychologically healthy, less comfortable with themselves and others, and more vulnerable to stress than peers who were raised by mothers who exhibited lower levels of preschool PP. These results seem to justify further empirical study of Miller's (1983) construct.

5. The predictive correlations involving the fathers' PP were considerably weaker than those involving the mothers' PP.[4] This comparative weakness may be attributable to the fact that the mothers in this sample were typically more involved with their preschool children than were the fathers. The mothers' interactions with the children might therefore have been more frequent and influential than the fathers'.

6. The predictive correlations involving self-reported PP were also much weaker than those involving observed PP. The relative weakness of the data involving self-reported PP may have been caused by two factors. First, the parental self-reports might have been influenced substantially by conscious and unconscious impression management. Second,

---

[4]In fact, the poisonous pedagogy (PP) indexes based on self-reports and the indexes of fathers' PP did yield some interesting patterns of correlations at the level of individual California Adult Q-Set items at ages 18 and 23. Compared with the index involving mothers' observed PP in the teaching situation, however, these item-level correlations were weaker and less consistent over time.

it seems possible that the parents varied widely in their interpretations of particular CRPR items and in the frames of reference they brought to this self-descriptive task. Most parents, after all, have had limited and idiosyncratic opportunities to observe other parents' child-rearing practices over sustained periods of time. Indeed, many parents have probably really seen only their own parents' child-rearing practices (through their childhood and memory-transmuted eyes) in addition to their own. As a consequence, parents probably bring widely varying frames of reference to bear as they describe their own child-rearing practices using the CRPR. This second factor could obviously introduce a form of error into the CRPR data that is not present in the observer-based PCIQ and TSR reports.

7. There were sex differences observed in the correlational patterns involving PP that deserve greater attention than they were given here. In general, for example, the index of maternal PP in the teaching situation was more strongly correlated with personality descriptions involving emotional overcontrol and restriction in the young women at ages 18 and 23 than in the young men. A fuller analysis of these sex-related correlational differences must await another occasion.

8. The substantial negative correlations observed between parental education and PP directed toward the preschool boys in this sample are also worthy of further study in their own right. As Miller (1983) herself has clearly suggested, child-rearing practices are often deeply imbedded in cultural systems. And as many others (e.g., Baumrind, 1992) have also noted, child-rearing practices are also functionally related to the physical and social realities dealt with by those cultural systems in the past or currently. Ways in which elements of Miller's PP may be related to such social and physical realities deserve careful and culturally respectful study.

9. In many respects, this study is a testament to the value and flexibility of well-designed Q-sets. For example, the existence and prior use of the CAQ made it possible to connect independent formulations of optimal psychological adjustment, empirical studies of creative adults conducted at the IPAR, Ravenna Helson's ongoing longitudinal study of creative women, and the personal characteristics of the subjects in this study and to bring these disparate lines of inquiry to bear on one another

in mutually illuminating ways. Additionally, the existence of the PCIQ and the CRPR made it possible to bring Alice Miller's theoretical formulations to bear on a study designed years before her ideas were known to those involved with this project.

10. The child-rearing practices indicated and contraindicated by the PP are similar to those explicitly or implicitly identified as consequential by a number of theorists, including Otto Rank, Karen Horney, Erik Erikson, Carl Rogers, and Donald Winnicott, among others. Inspection of the defining PP items suggested that the PP scales used here conflated at least two robust, but variously labeled, dimensions of child rearing. The high end of the PP indexes appeared to be located in the "hostile" and "controlling" region of Schaefer's (1959) circumplex; the "demanding, controlling, rejecting, unresponsive, parent-centered" quadrant of Maccoby and Martin's (1983) fourfold typology; and Baumrind's (1991) "authoritarian" prototype. The low end of the PP indexes appeared to be anchored in Schaefer's warm and autonomous zone; in Maccoby and Martin's undemanding, low-controlling, accepting, responsive, child-centered quadrant; and within Baumrind's "permissive" prototype. There are, in short, a variety of theoretical perspectives within which to frame these PP data.

I believe research psychologists can provide a useful social service by explicating and describing the connections between and among alternative ways of organizing and describing complex domains such as child-rearing practices. I particularly believe researchers can provide a useful social function by including in those analyses global constructs such as the PP—constructs that speak in languages that resonate with and have thereby attracted the serious attention of lay audiences.

Conclusions

Of course, many important questions regarding PP were not addressed in this preliminary investigation. The most provocative psychodynamic aspects of Miller's (1983) theory involving the allegedly unconscious motives underlying PP, for example, were not and cannot be addressed with these data.

Although the intergenerational component of Miller's theory was not addressed here, it may be possible to shed empirical light on this issue in a few years if the J. H. Block and Block (1980) study is continued long enough that these subjects, now in their mid-20s, can be studied as parents. Is Alice Miller correct in her prediction that children who have been raised in environments of PP tend to use PP with their own children? In another decade or so, the Block and Block study may be able to address that question.

And if poisonous pedagogy is in fact transmitted intergenerationally, several additional questions arise. Is it true, for example, as Alice Miller and some therapists believe (Miller,1990, pp. vii–ix), that therapeutic interventions can disrupt the causal paths by which these particular forms of childhood pain and adult dysfunction are allegedly passed from one generation to the next? And is it also true, as many laypeople currently hope and believe, that various self-help programs designed to address adult dysfunction and psychological pain can also help break these allegedly tragic causal chains? These questions, too, address homely human concerns and therefore deserve our future attention and respect.

References

Barron, F. (1969). *Creative person and creative process.* New York: Holt, Rinehart & Winston.

Baumrind, D. (1991). Parenting styles and adolescent development. In J. Brooks, R. Lerner, & A. C. Peterson (Eds.), *The encyclopedia on adolescence* (pp. 758–772). New York: Garland.

Baumrind, D. (1992). *The average expectable environment is not good enough: A response to Scarr.* Unpublished manuscript, Institute of Human Development, University of California, Berkeley.

Block, J. (1961). *The Q-sort method in personality assessment and psychiatric research.* Springfield, IL: Charles C Thomas.

Block, J. (1962). *The California Q-Set.* Palo Alto, CA: Consulting Psychologists Press.

Block, J. (1971). *Lives through time.* Berkeley, CA: Bancroft Books.

Block, J. (1991, August). *Studying personality the long way.* G. Stanley Hall Award address presented at the 99th Annual Convention of the American Psychological Association, San Francisco.

Block, J. H. (1965). *The Child-Rearing Practices Report: A set of Q items for the description of parental socialization attitudes and values.* Unpublished manuscript, Department of Psychology, University of California, Berkeley.

Block, J. H. (1984). *The Child-Rearing Practices Report: A bibliography of research using the CRPR.* Unpublished manuscript, Department of Psychology, University of California, Berkeley.

Block, J. H., & Block, J. (1980). The role of ego-control and ego-resiliency in the organization of behavior. In W. A. Collins (Ed.), *Minnesota Symposia on Child Psychology* (Vol. 13, pp. 39–101). Hillsdale, NJ: Erlbaum.

Block, J. H., Block, J., Siegelman, E., & von der Lippe, A. (1971). Optimal psychological adjustment: Response to Miller's and Bronfenbrenner's discussions. *Journal of Consulting and Clinical Psychology, 36,* 325–328.

Bradshaw, J. (1988). *The family.* Deerfield Beach, FL: Health Communications.

Campbell, D. T., & Stanley, J. C. (1963). *Experimental and quasi-experimental designs for research.* Chicago: Rand McNally.

Duncan, O. (1961). A socioeconomic index for all occupations. In A. J. Reiss, Jr. (Ed.), *Occupations and social status* (pp. 109–138). New York: Free Press.

Harrington, D. M., Block, J. H., & Block, J. (1978). Intolerance of ambiguity in preschool children: Psychometric considerations, behavioral manifestations, and parental correlates. *Developmental Psychology, 14,* 242–256.

Harrington, D. M., Block, J. H., & Block, J. (1987). Testing aspects of Carl Rogers's theory of creative environments: Child-rearing antecedents of creative potential in young adolescents. *Journal of Personality and Social Psychology, 52,* 851–856.

Helson, R. (1967). Personality characteristics and developmental history of creative college women. *Genetic Psychology Monographs, 76,* 205–256.

Helson, R. (1985). Which of those young women with creative potential became productive? I. Personality in college and characteristics of parents. In R. Hogan & W. Jones (Eds.), *Perspectives in personality: Theory, measurement, and personality dynamics.* (Vol. 1, pp. 49–80). Greenwich, CT: JAI Press.

Johnson, O. G. (Ed.). (1976). *Tests and measurements in child development: Handbook II* (Vol. 1). San Francisco: Jossey-Bass.

MacKinnon, D. W. (1962). The nature and nurture of creative talent. *American Psychologist, 17,* 484–495.

MacKinnon, D. W. (1965). Personality and the realization of creative potential. *American Psychologist, 20,* 273–281.

MacKinnon, D. W. (1966). *Illustrative material for some reflections on the current status of personality assessment with special references to the assessment of creative persons.* Lecture given to graduate students, Department of Psychology, University of Utah, Salt Lake City.

Maccoby, E. E., & Martin, J. A. (1983). Socialization in the context of the family: Parent-child interaction. In P. H. Mussen (Ed.), *Handbook of child psychology* (Vol. 4, pp. 1–101). New York: Wiley.

Miller, A. (1981). *The drama of the gifted child.* New York: Harper & Row.

Miller, A. (1983). *For your own good: Hidden cruelty in child-rearing and the roots of violence.* New York: Farrar, Straus & Giroux.

Miller, A. (1984). *For your own good: Hidden cruelty in child-rearing and the roots of violence* (2nd ed.). New York: Farrar, Straus & Giroux.

Miller, A. (1990). *For your own good: Hidden cruelty in child-rearing and the roots of violence* (3rd ed.). New York: Farrar, Straus & Giroux.

Montagu, A. (1983, May). Poisonous pedagogy. *Psychology Today,* pp. 80–81.

Pharis, M. E. (1984). Review of *For your own good. Social Work, 29,* 412.

Schaefer, E. S. (1959). A circumplex model for maternal behavior. *Journal of Abnormal and Social Psychology, 59,* 226–235.

Siegelman, E., Block, J. H., Block J., & von der Lippe, A. (1970). Antecedents of optimal psychological adjustment. *Journal of Consulting and Clinical Psychology, 35,* 283–289.

Steinem, G. (1992). *Revolution from within.* New York: Little, Brown.

Whitfield, C. L. (1989). *Healing the child within.* Deerfield Beach, FL: Health Communications.

CHAPTER 14

Individuals in Relationships: Development From Infancy Through Adolescence

L. Alan Sroufe, Elizabeth Carlson, and Shmuel Shulman

I n the past two decades a number of fruitful solutions have been offered to the problem of the coherence of personality and its unfolding over time. These solutions have included thoughtful selection of robust constructs (J. H. Block & Block, 1980); aggregation of data (J. H. Block & Block, 1980; Epstein, 1979); and configural, "person" approaches to assessment (Magnusson & Bergman, 1990). In our research we have drawn on each of these approaches and combined them in a longitudinal study of individual development from birth through adolescence.

In addition, we used two other strategies to demonstrate continuity in individual development from the infancy period through the childhood years. The first of these involved a focus on and assessment of the infant caregiving system in the early years as the matrix out of which the personality forms (Ainsworth, Blehar, Waters, & Wall, 1978; Bowlby, 1973;

This research has been supported by National Institute of Mental Health Grant MH 40864-05.

Sander, 1975). The second, which also has a rich tradition (e.g., Havighurst, 1948), was to use assessments that were centered on adaptation with respect to salient developmental issues (Sroufe, 1979). Thus, diverse arenas and domains were the contexts for assessment across ages, such as attachment–exploration balance in infancy, curiosity, self-management and social engagement in preschool, and formation of loyal friendships and effective peer-group functioning in middle childhood. Following J. Block (1991), the quest was for coherence in individual development, not for continuity in the sense of the same behavior being manifested over time.

The approach is conceptually straightforward but challenging to carry out. Individuals are assessed in terms of the quality of adaptation with respect to the salient issues of a given developmental period. These individual differences, then, are hypothesized to spring from variation in earlier developmental periods and to forecast variation in later periods, however different appropriate contexts and developmental assessments may be. Our research was conducted in the home, the laboratory, the nursery school, the playground, the elementary school, and the summer camp. Assessments ranged from the frequency of sitting next to a teacher to molar assessments of broad, integrative concepts. At times, assessments were aimed at the level of the individual and at times at the quality of the individual's social relationships. In so doing, we were able to demonstrate not only coherence of individual development over time but also continuity in social relationships in particular, across partners as well as ages. We have also shown that qualities of early primary relationships predict patterns of individual adaptation across the childhood years, even outside of the family context.

The focus of this chapter is on the coherence of individual behavior in middle childhood and its logical ties to early development. Although beyond the scope of this chapter, we point out that this approach also lends itself to studying the coherence of change. In other articles we have shown that change in individual adaptation is lawful and apparently mediated by the same factors that are central to studying individual differences in the first place. For example, mothers of children whose adjustment in one period was better than would have been predicted from prior assessments more likely had formed stable partnerships in the intervening years, or had experienced greater reductions in life stress, than mothers of children whose adjustment remained comparably poor (Egeland, Kalkoske, Gottesman, & Erickson, 1990; Erickson, Sroufe, & Egeland, 1985). We have also found evidence that prior adaptation and history are not "erased" by change (Sroufe, Egeland, & Kreutzer, 1990). Earlier patterns may be reactivated, and early history adds to current circumstances in predicting current adaptation.

History of the Minnesota Parent–Child Project

In 1974–1975 we recruited 267 women in the third trimester of their first pregnancy. All of the women were receiving public assistance for their prenatal care and were representative of a Twin Cities urban poor population at that time; that is, the mothers were young (M = 20.52 years), 62% were single, and 40% had not completed high school. Eighty percent were White, 14% were Black, and 6% were Native American or Hispanic. (See Egeland & Brunnquell, 1979, for an early report.) Although all of the mothers were poor at the time of the infant's birth, by the time the children were 11 years old there was some socioeconomic status (SES) spread: Twenty percent of the heads of household in the subsample had professional, technical, or managerial jobs; 62% were in clerical, craftsperson, service, or labor jobs; 16% were unemployed; and 2% were students.

The study has been comprehensive and detailed. Infants and caregivers were seen seven times in the first year, twice in each of the next 3 years, and yearly through Grade 7. Assessments included neonatal neurological status; motor, cognitive, and intellectual development; maternal personality and IQ; parent–child interaction; temperament; peer relationships; and personality development. Contextual variables such as life stress and social support were assessed regularly. Children were observed in the home, laboratory, and school.

We experienced some subject attrition early in the study. This was a highly mobile sample, and it took us some time to build up a contact network. By 18 months the sample size was 190, and chaotic families were disproportionately represented in our losses (which likely would diminish effect sizes in later years). In the following 13 years, however, attrition was only 6%.

Over the years, a subsample of these subjects has been studied in great detail, including observations in a weekend retreat at age 15, a 4-week summer camp at age 10, and a semester-long nursery school program; 27 children were in all 3 programs and 41 were in the camp and retreat. The subjects in these special programs were representative of the sample at large (e.g., slightly more than half had been securely attached in infancy). These observational experiences allowed us to examine closely the links between early care and later social relationships, which has been a key goal of the project.

Adaptation in Infancy

Ainsworth, drawing on Bowlby's theory, provided an assessment scheme ideally suited to the problem addressed in our research (Ainsworth et al., 1978; Bowlby, 1969/1982). First, Ainsworth's assessment of the attachment relationship was centered on the most salient issues of the infant developmental period; specifically, achieving a balance among the attachment, exploratory, affiliative, and fear behavioral systems. Second, her assessment procedure (see the next paragraph) yielded groupings of individuals in terms of behavioral patterns. Finally, by examining the organization of behavior with respect to the primary caregiver, a stability of patterning may be tapped well before it could be assessed with reliability and validity in other contexts. Thus, Ainsworth's approach offered the promise of predicting later personality organization from an earlier time than previously possible. In addition, as an early relationship assessment, it provided an opportunity to examine coherence at the relationship level.

Ainsworth's (1978) laboratory assessment, known as the Strange Situation, is a 20-minute procedure involving a series of episodes with primary caregiver and infant in a playroom, joined by a stranger who ultimately initiates a brief interaction with the baby, followed by two brief separations and reunions with the caregiver, with the infant left entirely alone during the second separation. The predictive power of such a brief separation draws on two factors: (a) the salience of separations from the caregiver for the 12- to 18-month-old infant and (b) the anchoring of these assessments to hundreds of hours of home observation of attachment–exploration balance and crying in the home.

Three patterns of behavior were described by Ainsworth (1978). The modal pattern, which Ainsworth labeled *secure attachment,* was manifest in two basic forms. All secure cases have in common the use of the caregiver as a secure base for exploration. However, in some cases, this is manifest primarily through "affective sharing" (Waters, Wippman, & Sroufe, 1979) and positive greetings and interaction with the caregiver upon reunion. In other cases, secure base behavior is manifest by ease of settling upon reunion in infants distressed by separation. In both cases, the infants take active initiative in seeking contact (or interaction) with the caregiver following reunion, and such efforts support a return to play and exploration. It is postulated that all infants judged as having secure relationships are confident of the accessibility and responsiveness of the caregiver and that such confidence mediates their reunion behavior. Indeed, Ainsworth's research and numerous replications (see Sroufe, 1985, for a review) confirm that these secure patterns are predicted by observations of sensitive responsiveness in interactions earlier in the first year.

A second pattern described by Ainsworth (1978) was termed *anxious/resistant attachment.* These infants (roughly 10% of all cases) have difficulty exploring even in the early episodes of the Strange Situation. They often are wary of the stranger and become upset by both separations. Some secure cases show parts of this pattern. However, in contrast to secure cases, these infants show great difficulty settling upon reunion, even when given contact. Indeed, they often mix contact seeking with contact "resistance," pushing away, squirming to be put down (only to want to be picked back up again), batting away offered toys, and the like. As a result, they do not return to active play and exploration during the 3-minute reunion.

The last pattern is called *anxious/avoidant attachment* (20% of all cases). These infants commonly become engaged with the toys during the early episodes, are accepting of the stranger, and show little distress during the separations, especially when left with the stranger. Again, some secure cases show somewhat similar behavior up to this point. Strikingly, however, upon reunion, these infants ignore, turn or move away from, or show abortive approaches to their caregivers. Such avoidance typically increases at the second reunion, when presumably they are more stressed and often had been crying. This is the exact opposite of secure infants, who seek increased contact or interaction following the stress of the second separation. Like resistance, such avoidance interferes with a return to play. Anxiously attached pairs have in common the ineffectiveness of the dyadic system in serving the infant's exploration and mastery of the environment.

Again, Ainsworth's (1978) work has suggested that anxiously attached infants have evolved expectations regarding the caregiver based in the history of interaction. Mothers of both groups were observed to be less sensitive and responsive to their infants in earlier home observations. One interpretation is that caregivers of avoidant infants have consistently rebuffed their infants when they sought contact or reassurance. Indeed, failure to pick up the baby when she or he sought to be picked up specifically discriminated this group. Not surprisingly, then, when attachment feelings are aroused in the Strange Situation, these infants specifically block off approach behaviors at that time. The resistant pattern appears to be associated with inconsistent, hit-or-miss, or chaotic care. Thus, these infants have difficulty being firmly reassured, although they continue to (even continually) seek contact.

In an early research project, Matas, Arend, and Sroufe (1978) showed that these attachment assessments predicted individual differences in the subsequent toddler period, when movement toward autonomy may be considered a salient developmental issue. In a tool problem situation, toddlers who had been securely attached, in contrast to those who had been anxiously attached, showed more enthusiasm in engaging the problems, were more persistent, and more independent; yet they turned to their caregivers when their own resources were exhausted, and they complied with the caregiver's directives. They also were more affectively positive and less affectively negative, all rated by coders who were unaware of the subjects' developmental history. Mothers were independently rated as showing more emotional support and a higher quality of assistance.

Two features are especially noteworthy in these results. First, the 20-minute attachment assessment was predictive of a later assessment in a new context, which again was anchored to a salient developmental issue. Second, attachment assessments predicted the mother's behavior as well as the child's. This supports the contention that relationships are captured by Ainsworth's procedure, even though infant behavior is the focus of the attachment assessments. Later research has shown that attachment assessments with one child also predict mother's behavior with a second child and the quality of that relationship (Ward, Vaughn, & Robb, 1988).

It could be argued that the continuity just described hinged entirely on the caregiver's behavior because she was present in both settings. Subsequent research, however, involved procedures in which mother was not present and included settings beyond the laboratory. Thus, differences in confidence, curiosity, and positive affectivity were shown in solitary problem-solving situations (e.g., Arend, Gove, & Sroufe, 1979), and a host of meaningful individual differences were predicted in the social world of a laboratory preschool.

Adaptation in the Preschool Years

Associations between attachment assessments in infancy and individual differences in social and emotional behavior in the preschool years are numerous and have been summarized in several publications (e.g., Erickson et al., 1985; Sroufe, 1983, 1988; Sroufe & Fleeson, 1988; Troy & Sroufe, 1987). Here, we present only highlights of special importance to the problem of coherence in personality. As at other age periods, assessments were keyed to salient developmental issues; here, assessments were made of the growth of self-reliance and self-management, internalization of controls and standards of behavior, entrée into the peer group, and broadening of relationships outside of the family.

Having our own preschool allowed extensive observation in a "standard" environment with constant teachers. We were also able to experimentally pair children with different attachment histories in special play sessions to supplement naturalistic observation of social relationships. All of this, plus standard sociometrics, provided converging data on the issues at hand.

Of special interest from Bowlby's (1969/1982) theory was the prediction that secure attachment would promote later self-reliance. This prediction is important because it is theory specific (and nonobvious from competing theories) and because it illustrates the importance of the concept of coherence (vs. simple continuity). Infants are deemed to be secure in their attachments because they effectively seek contact with their caregivers and use the fact or possibility of such contact as a source of reassurance. From some points of view, this seeking of contact and parental responsiveness to contact seeking might support dependency (e.g., Gewirtz, 1972) or lead to spoiling the child. Similarly, those showing avoidant attachment might be viewed as precociously independent (Clarke-Stewart & Fein, 1983) or temperamentally bold (Kagan, 1982). Bowlby and Ainsworth's positions, however, strongly predict greater dependency in those who have been anxiously attached, including the avoidant group. Those with secure attachments are predicted to later be more self-reliant. Having experienced responsive care, such infants do not learn to be spoiled but that care is available when needed. They need not constantly seek contact or reassurance because they believe that such contact will be readily available if needed. Moreover, in developing a representation of the caregiver (and, ultimately, others) as available, the child inevitably, as a matter of course, evolves a complementary representation of the self as effective in eliciting care and, by extension, of having potency in the environment.

The data come out strongly and consistently in the direction predicted by Bowlby (1969/1982), on the basis of blind ratings and rankings made by teachers and by direct observation of the quantity and quality of contact between children and teachers (Sroufe, Fox, & Pancake, 1983). Those with avoidant histories might have been more indirect in seeking contact, but they spent more time interacting with and being in physical contact with teachers than those with secure histories and just as much as those with resistant histories. Teachers rated both the resistant and avoidant groups as being highly dependent.

The construct of ego-resiliency also was of special interest in this research for several reasons. Flexible management of impulses, desires, and behavior is an ascendant issue during the preschool period, and it is central to the definition of ego-resiliency (J. H. Block & Block, 1980). Moreover, ego-resiliency has been shown to be a robust variable from the preschool period throughout childhood and adolescence (J. Block, 1991). If we were able to predict individual differences in ego-resiliency in the preschool period, we could link up with the compelling work of Block and Block. Again, there was a strong theoretical basis for such a prediction. Some children have been part of a well-regulated dyadic system, wherein variation in arousal was tolerated, sharp swings in arousal largely precluded, and excessive arousal modulated. Such children should bring forward the capacity for self-regulation and confidence in their regulatory capacity (Sroufe, 1990). Smooth dyadic regulation of affect and arousal is central to the definition of secure attachment. Once again, the empirical data overwhelmingly supported the hypothesis (Sroufe, 1983). Using California Q-Sorts, composited across four preschool teachers, correlations with the resiliency criterion were significantly higher for those with secure histories. Comparing the avoidant group, with the secure group, there was virtually no overlap. All of the secure cases showed positive correlations with the resiliency criterion, whereas 13 of 15 avoidant cases showed negative correlations. This association between attachment history and ego-resiliency persisted into middle childhood. The correlation between an attachment security variable (0, 1, or 2 times secure across two assessments in infancy) and ego-resiliency at ages 10–11 years at summer camp was .32 ($p < .02$).

Numerous aspects of relationships with peers in the preschool setting were also significantly related to attachment history. Those with secure histories, compared with the two anxious groups, participated more actively in the peer group, were more affectively positive and less affectively negative in their encounters, and were more popular (Sroufe, 1983; Sroufe, Schork, Motti, Lawroski, & LaFreniere, 1984). In general, whether rated by teachers, assessed by coders using a variety of objective procedures, or judged by the other children themselves through sociometrics, those with secure histories were more competent with their preschool peers. Thus, early assessments of attachment were shown to be linked to another salient developmental issue.

Beyond these associations with peer competence, early attachment history also predicted qualities of later interpersonal relationships, at times with extraordinary specificity. For example, from attachment–relationship theory, one could posit that secure infants, having experienced and therefore internalized a responsive relationship, later would be more empathic. Participating in a relationship system in which one is routinely treated empathically, one would not only come to expect such treatment but would learn more generally that this is the way relationships work. With such an understanding, along with corollary feelings of self-worth, one is primed to be empathically responsive to others when cognitive advances allow sufficient perspective taking. Indeed, both teacher judgments (extracted from the Q-sorts via J. H. Block & Block's, 1980, Empathy Scale) and videotaped records from the classroom showed that those with secure histories were more empathic than those with anxious histories (Kestenbaum, Farber, & Sroufe, 1989; Sroufe, 1983). In addition, those with avoidant histories, presumed to experience chronic rebuff when needs for tender care were expressed, were significantly more likely than both other groups to show "antiempathy"; that is, at times when another child was distressed, they behaved in a manner that would make the distress worse (e.g., taunting the crying child). Those with resistant histories behaved as though the distress were their own, blurring the boundary between self and other.

In our intensive study of play pairs at the preschool, we found that the pairs containing at least one avoidant member formed relationships that were less deep (i.e., less characterized by mutuality, responsiveness, and affective involvement) and more hostile than other pairs (Pancake, 1988). (Avoidant children were also observed to be more aggressive in the classroom.) In addition, 5 of 19 dyadic relationships studied were characterized by "victimization," a repetitive pattern of physical or verbal exploitation or abuse by one child of the other (Troy & Sroufe, 1987). In each case, the "exploiter" was a child with an avoidant history and the victim was another anxiously attached child (avoidant or resistant). Moreover, there had only been 5 such possible pairings. Those with secure histories never victimized and never were victims. These results, like all other data reported, were based on independent raters who had no knowledge about the children.

Data on child–teacher relationships likewise revealed the coherence of relationships over time (Sroufe & Fleeson, 1988). Coders rated videotapes of 50 randomly sampled interactive episodes of both main teachers with each child. With children having secure histories, teachers were judged to be warm and straightforward in their engagement of these children, to hold out age-appropriate standards for them, and to expect self-direction and compliance with classroom rules. With children from the resistant group, teachers were unduly nurturant and caretaking, were controlling, had low expectations for compliance, and were quite tolerant of minor violations of classroom rules. (This pattern may be summarized by saying teachers "infantalized" them.) Finally, teachers' relationships with children with avoidant histories were controlling and, at rare times, even angry. With these children, they had low expectations for compliance and little tolerance for violations. To some extent, the rejecting relationships of the avoidant child's early years were recapitulated in the preschool classroom and not for mysterious reasons. These children often engaged in hostile or defiant behavior that alienated teachers as well as children, although they had, of course, been capable of no such behavior in early infancy.

It has sometimes been argued that there is no continuity from infancy on because children are elastic (Kagan, 1984) or that any continuity is due simply to continuity in the environment (Lamb, 1984). Our findings of clear coherence of individual behavior over time and active engendering of perpetuating environmental circumstances show that such arguments are simplistic. Children actively create their environments based on their history of experiences (Sroufe & Egeland, 1991).

Finally, on the basis of a variety of theoretical considerations, we outlined a number of profiles of adaptation in the preschool years that we thought might differentiate between the three patterns of attachment outlined by Ainsworth et al. (1978; see Table 1). Clinical judges then took the most characteristic and least characteristic Q-sort items for each child and classified them into one of these hypothetical patterns. The overall

TABLE 1
Hypothetical Profiles

Group	Description
A	
A_a	Hostile and mean, aggressive, antisocial (lying, stealing, devious)
A_b	Emotionally insulated, asocial, isolated
A_c	Disconnected, spaced out, psychoticlike; may be oblivious or bizarre or just unaware of what is going on
C	
C_a	Overstimulated (hyper), easily frustrated, tense or anxious, impulsive, flailing out rather than hostile
C_b	Dependent, passive, weak, helpless, teacher oriented

match with actual attachment history was highly significant (Sroufe, 1983).

Adaptation in the Middle Childhood Years

With each subsequent phase of development, it becomes increasingly difficult to summarize the period with a small number of issues. Nonetheless, there is broad consensus that the following are among the most salient in middle childhood:

1. There must be achievement of competence in the concrete, everyday world. In most traditional cultures, this has included acquiring the skills to be used for sustenance and survival (gathering foods, catching fish, making baskets). In Western culture, formal schooling is included. In general, however, this is an age in which the child is expected to show an increased sense of responsibility, purposefulness, and agency (Shapiro & Perry, 1976) or what Erikson (1963) called "industry"—being a capable and hard worker.

2. Related to the first issue, the child is expected to show a growing independence from adult supervision and support, operating in arenas outside of adult overview and directing his or her own activities.

3. During middle childhood, the child is expected to consolidate a sense of self by integrating various threads of self-development, devel-

oping a comfort and confidence in one's body, and developing pride in one's sex, all based on favorable social comparison. This issue, focusing largely on self-attitudes, is discussed in a later section dealing with mechanisms and processes underlying continuity.

4. A major issue for this period is advanced development of competence with peers. Peer competence at this age is a complex matter, actually including twin tasks that a child must integrate: (a) At this age, the child is expected to form an emotionally close, loyal friendship with at least one other person, something Sullivan (1953) called a "chumship." (b) At the same time, the child must function effectively in the same-sex peer group, adhering to its norms, finding acceptance, and capitalizing on all of the opportunities for learning about negotiation and other aspects of group functioning. Each of these has multiple aspects, and additional challenge derives from the requirement of balancing loyalty to one's friends and effective participation in the larger group.

The peer issue is the primary focus in the following discussion for several reasons: Not only does it illustrate the increasing complexity of assessing adaptation with respect to developmental issues, but it is a broad, integrative issue. Successful functioning in the peer group calls on the consolidating sense of self, the child's advancing moral capacity (as in the sense of fairness and reciprocity, understanding and adherence to social norms, etc.), and the capacity for role flexibility (leadership and initiative vs. accommodation). It also is a suitable arena for examining continuity at both the individual and relationship levels.

Description of the Minnesota Summer Camp Study

Most of the results presented in this section were derived from counselor ratings and observations made at a series of three summer day camps. Across the camps, which each lasted 4 weeks, a total of 47 children from our longitudinal study were observed. Approximately equal numbers of children with histories of secure and anxious attachment were included, and the attachment groups were not different on ethnicity or IQ. There were 24 girls and 23 boys (1 boy moved at the beginning of his camp). The children were aged 10 and 11, with no more than 1-year age range in any camp.

Assessments

As in the nursery school study, assessments were carried out at different levels from broadband to the highly specific, and we used a variety of methods. We obtained information from independent ratings, rankings, Q-sorts, and nominations of four counselors; child interview-based measures of acceptance, rejection, popularity, and friendship; and direct behavioral observations of child social contact using child-sampling and event-sampling techniques. In addition, some behavioral analyses involved hundreds of hours of videotape.

In general, ample evidence of convergence was obtained from these independent sources. For example, counselor judgment of friendship pairs, reciprocal nomination of best friend from child interviews, and a behavioral friend index (the proportion of interactions with the child's most frequent partner) were in strong accord. Other examples are discussed later (e.g., correlations between the frequency of observed child–counselor contact and counselor ratings of dependency). All people contributing data had no knowledge of the children's attachment history or other information.

Instrumental Competence and Effectance

Composited rankings and ratings by the four counselors at each camp revealed significant associations between attachment history (secure vs. anxious attachment) and agency/self-confidence and self-esteem. All correlations on these and related variables were in the .30s and were significant beyond the .02 level of confidence. These ratings were supported by observational assessments of efficiency of goal accomplishment by teams of secure or anxious children. When given tasks such as getting all members of the team over a barrier or coordinating efforts to traverse a course on four-person skis, the secure groups showed a smoother process with fewer false starts and faster completion of the tasks. Individuals in the secure groups also showed a higher degree of physical coordination. Children with secure histories were also observed to set higher personal goals (e.g., during crafts or carpentry time) and to persist to completion of those goals.

Thus, in their behavior, as both judged by counselors and as revealed by videotape-based observation, children with secure histories conveyed a sense of self-confidence, purposefulness, and industry that surpassed those with histories of anxious attachment, 9–10 years after the infant assessment.

A related finding from the larger study concerned achievement in school. As is common, we found high correlations between IQ and achievement assessments (.70). However, when IQ was entered first in a regression analysis, followed by an attachment variable (0, 1, or 2 depending on the number of times the attachment had been assessed as secure across the 12- to 18-month assessments), attachment history added significant predictive power (Mathieu, 1990).

Self-Reliance Versus Continued Dependency

The summer camp data revealed that at age 10 strong differences in dependency continued to be shown by the different attachment groups. Counselor ratings again showed both the avoidant and resistant groups to be more dependent than those with secure histories. Behavioral observations confirmed these differences. Children in both anxious groups spent significantly more time interacting with counselors than did the children with secure histories. Interestingly, and reminiscent of the nursery school findings reported earlier, counselors were observed to clearly initiate contact more often with those having resistant histories than even those with avoidant histories, although the amount of contact between adult and child was not different (Urban, Carlson, Egeland, & Sroufe, 1991).

Peer Competence and Peer Relationships

At the most molar level, counselor judgments of social competence and social skill again significantly differentiated between those with secure and anxious histories. Table 2 summarizes the correlations between these and other summer camp variables and the infant security variable, as well as central variables from the toddler tool-problem assessment. Links between our assessments in the first 2 years and the molar social competence variables at ages 10–11 were consistent and substantial, especially

TABLE 2

Correlations Between Attachment Security and Adaptation at Age 2 Years With Summer Camp Ratings in Middle Childhood

	Camp ratings									
	Emotional health		Self-confidence		Social competence		Social skills		Ego-resiliency	
Variable	r	p	r	p	r	p	r	p	r	p
Attachment security at 12–18 months	.35	.011	.34	.012	.36	.007	.33	.013	.32	.019
Overall experience in the session at 24 months	.36	.007	.42	.002	.41	.003	.42	.002	.25	.047
Coping 24 months	.44	.001	.41	.002	.42	.002	.46	.001	.38	.005
Anger at 24 months	−.41	.003	−.43	.002	−.46	.001	−.51	.000	−.29	.027
Enthusiasm at 24 months	.23	.061	.31	.018	.29	.025	.32	.017	.27	.040

Note. The number of subjects ranged from 44 to 47.

considering the developmental span covered. Moreover, as we have reported elsewhere, the counselor ratings had discriminant validity rather than simply reflecting halo from one variable to another (Elicker, Englund, & Sroufe, 1992; Urban et al., 1991). For example, the social competence ratings correlated most highly (negatively) with observations of social isolation, and the dependency ratings correlated most highly with observations of time with counselors.

Children with secure histories were also more likely to form a friendship during the camp, regardless of whether they were assessed by counselor nomination, mutual child nomination, or objective observation of time in association with a particular partner (Elicker et al., 1992). Moreover, friendships tended to form along attachment lines, with secure–secure pairs being the dominant pattern, even correcting for the simple probability of making a friend.

At the same time, children with secure histories were observed to spend more time in group activities, and activities dominated by secure members were more complex. Rarely was a group (3 or more) made up of only children with anxious histories, whereas groups made up of only children with secure histories and groups including only 1 child with an anxious history were common. This was especially true for boys. Apparently, the coordination, give-and-take, and arousal modulation required for group functioning was beyond the resources of many of the children with anxious attachment histories. When anxiously attached children were strongly or solely represented in a group, activities either were structured by counselors or were simple (e.g., playing on the swings vs. setting up a macramé shop or building a fort). Playing on swings, although providing a context for social exchange, in many ways resembles the parallel play characteristic of the preschool period. Joint construction of a physical structure or a "business" (e.g., a macramé concession) involves a great deal of coordination, negotiation, conflict resolution, and other aspects of social reciprocity; such activities were common for the secure groups.

The importance of these differences can be seen when one considers the function of group participation developmentally. Young children's groups meet on a momentary basis for the sake of a clear task, for play, or for a game (Hartup, 1983). Adolescent groups reflect more stable and advanced interpersonal processes, in which issues of hierarchy and dominance are to be negotiated (Savin-Williams, 1979). Preadolescence marks an important transition, and for some children, those with secure histories, a successful one. When 10- to 11-year-olds with anxious histories join groups to participate in a clearly defined activity, there is hardly any need to negotiate one's place in the groups or issues of dominance. There is little need for negotiation of one's status when sitting with some other youngsters on parallel swings. Preadolescents with secure histories are more comfortable negotiating issues of status and role and therefore participate in complex activities. In turn, such participation better prepares them for the increased complexity of adolescent peer-group functioning.

More impressive than all of these findings was the capacity of secure children to coordinate friendships and group functioning. This was revealed by detailed, qualitative study of friendship pairs. Secure pairs were able to maintain their friendships in the context of group functioning. (In fact, they inspired a new behavioral code that we are now using in our adolescent follow-up: "pair, in group".) That they were friends remained apparent in group contexts, and they enjoyed group activities. Moreover, such friends often played in the vicinity of others, invited others to join in their activities, and were not threatened by their partners engaging other individuals. They might be described as having a semipermeable membrane. Those with resistant histories had great difficulty sustaining their relationship, especially in the context of group functioning, in which one or another child might be absorbed by the group, leaving the other behind, or one or both might become overwhelmed by the complexity of coordinating multiple relationships and drift off from or be extruded by the group. Such pairs might be described as having a totally permeable membrane. The sole avoidant pair (across the three camps) showed a marked exclusivity and guardedness. They played only together, seldom participating in groups as individuals or as a pair. Their play often took place in private areas at a distance from the others or behind some sort of barrier. They were jealous of the advances of any other child and did not invite others to play with them. When one or another partner was absent from camp, the other appeared "lost," unable to join in with the others. The membrane surrounding this pair was totally impermeable. Thus, in stark contrast to secure pairs, the friendship of these two took them out of commerce with the group, leaving them isolated together.

Finally, we studied in some detail one manifestation of middle childhood peer competence, namely, adherence to peer-group norms with regard to the maintenance of sex boundaries (Sroufe, Bennett, Englund, Urban, & Shulman, in press). Sex cleavage in middle childhood is pronounced, and contact between the sexes is governed by "rules" that may easily be inferred through behavioral regularities and consequences when rules are broken (Thorne, 1986). Essentially, one may not, as an individual, have contact with members of the other sex without some form of clear "cover" (e.g., it was accidental, a counselor might have insisted on the action, the contact was accompanied by insults or some other form of disavowal, etc.). One may engage in certain forms of contact when accompanied by same-sex partners, but even then boundaries must be maintained through body positions and behavior. We found that ratings of the degree of sex-boundary violation correlated with independent behavioral records of the frequency of violations. In addition, such ratings correlated negatively with social competence and history of secure attachment. In accord with our complex model of continuity, we hypothesized that it is the children who maintain sex boundaries at age 10 who will be successful in establishing cross-sex relationships (and participating in "crowds" that are composed of both sexes) in adolescence.

Adaptation in the Adolescent Years: Preliminary Data

Recently, we had the first of what will be three camp reunions. Fourteen 15-year-olds attended. Even with this small sample, and given that the two members of this camp group not in attendance had previously been highly malfunctioning anxiously attached children, significant results were obtained on major variables (e.g., ratings on emotional health and self-esteem, ego-resiliency, and peer competence), again favoring those with histories of secure attachment. One variable of special interest was a rating of the "capacity to be vulnerable," to be open to one's feelings and to engage the range of camp experiences despite feelings aroused. As predicted, this was significantly discriminating of attachment groups and was related to measures of competence in the earlier summer camps. In addition, observational data and counselor judgments confirmed the presence of a "crowd" composed of 2 couples and 1 other boy and 3 other girls. Seven of these 8 teenagers had been securely attached, including those in both couples. The one member of this group who had been anxiously attached was viewed by all judges (unaware of the child's history) as being the most peripheral member of the group. Detailed study of individual functioning, dyadic relationships, and group processes will follow data collection from the other two reunions.

Mechanisms and Processes of Continuity

Following Bowlby (1969/1982), our model of continuity is a process model. We do not believe that early attachment experiences are associated with later quality of personality and social relationships because of some permanent scarring or protection that occurs in the first 18 months (a critical period hypothesis). Rather, we believe that patterns of adaptation show coherence and heterotypic continuity over time because of a trans- active process, wherein expectations concerning self and relationships and patterns of arousal modulation lead to particular forms of engagement with the social and nonsocial worlds. Others commonly react in a com- plementary way to these styles of behavior, with the result being a per- petuation of the pattern (in new forms and in new contexts) in the next developmental period. Thus, a child who has positive expectations con- cerning others, feelings of worth and confidence, and a conception of relationships as responsive and mutually enhancing engages and responds to peers in positive ways, expects and elicits positive and age-appropriate support from adults, and stretches his or her abilities in setting goals and meeting challenges. In so doing, the child creates the opportunities and elicits reactions that ensure experiences that increase the likelihood of being able to profitably face subsequent developmental issues.

Change likewise is conceptualized in terms of disruption of expec- tations or environmental reactions counter to those expectations, espe- cially in the form of alternative relationship experiences. The empirical work discussed earlier implicitly supports this process view. It would be difficult indeed to explain this body of findings without recourse to some such idea. Static trait concepts such as "sociability" or boldness–inhibi- tion are far too simplistic to capture the array of findings and complex linkages (as in effective attachment leading to self-reliance and sex-bound- ary maintenance predicting participation in the heterosexual adolescent peer group). Ad hoc interpretations of each association would lead to a cumbersome explanation. In addition, both continuity and change are too coherent to rely solely on current environmental support. Something is internalized and carried forward by the child from prior experience.

We also have obtained some explicit data on linkages between early relationship experiences and attitudes and expectations concerning self and others (what Bowlby (1973) called "internal working models"). We used a variety of techniques, including analyses of the content of fantasy play in preschool, family drawings at age 8, and Thematic Apperception Test (TAT)-type stories and sentence completion associations at age

12. Although the relationships were usually modest, they were often significant.

In preschool, children who were securely attached at 18 months showed a higher quality of fantasy play than children classified as anxious in infancy (Rosenberg, 1984). Secure children were highly invested in fantasy play, more socially flexible with play partners, and more advanced in play behavior and verbalizations. Children with avoidant histories were rated the lowest on all qualitative variables. Fantasy play themes were also related to experience in early relationships. Play themes of securely attached children were people oriented and balanced, including positive resolutions to negative themes of conflict and sadness. Children with avoidant histories incorporated themes that were less positive and less frequently concerned with interpersonal relationships. For these children, aggression was a prevalent theme in play, and emotions were rarely attributed to characters or action. Children with resistant attachment histories incorporated both relationship themes and negative themes related to environmental danger.

In middle childhood, children's early attachment histories (secure vs. insecure) were related to their drawings of family members in third grade (Fury, 1992). In blind codings, based on the work of Main (Kaplan & Main, 1989), children with secure histories and children with anxious histories were strongly discriminated, both on the basis of ratings and on the basis of combinations of specific signs. Secure children drew figures that were grounded or centered on the page, individuated, and complete. Drawings were distinguished by a natural proximity among family members and the presence of real-world elements such as bicycles, pets, and trees. By contrast, the family drawings of children with avoidant histories were characterized by stiff figures with rigid postures and missing arms or feet and a lack of individuation of and distance between family members. An overall impression of vulnerability characterized the drawings of children classified as resistant in infancy. Figures were either tiny or huge with exaggerated facial features or body parts, were depicted in extreme proximity or separated by barriers, and were drawn randomly on the page (not in the center or grounded). In addition, some drawings reflected elements of both the avoidant and resistant criteria.

On sentence completion (Ramirez, Carlson, Gest, & Egeland, 1991) and story-telling (McCrone, Carlson, & Loewen, 1991) projective tasks collected in middle childhood, ratings were related across measures to concurrent behavior and early history. Across measures, ratings of positive expectations of adult support were related significantly and associated with overall emotional health. Also, "positive expectations concerning mother" expressed in sentence completion responses were associated with positive tone, positive resolutions to conflicts, concern for others, and a view of the self as competent in relationships in projective stories.

Children's expectations of relationships and the self and related affective tone derived from projective measures were associated with counselor rankings of behavior in summer camp and teacher ratings of behavior in school (see Table 3). Differences in children's expectations of peer relationships, views of self in relationships, affective tone, and emotional health on both sentence completion and story-telling measures were related to counselor rankings of social competence and overall emotional health in camp. Given the robustness of the camp variables,

TABLE 3

Correlations Between Projective Assessments and Competence Ratings by Camp Counselors (Composited) and Sixth-Grade Teachers

Measure	Social competence camp[a]		Emotional health camp		Peer competence teacher[b]		Emotional health teacher	
	r	p	r	p	r	p	r	p
SC peer scale	.54	.000	.41	.003	.24	.001	.15	.023
SC global rating	.49	.000	.37	.006	.27	.000	.19	.005
TAT peer scale	.54	.000	.48	.000	.11	.068	.02	.383
TAT global rating	.51	.000	.40	.003	.15	.023	.06	.219
Combined peer scale	.65	.000	.54	.000	.23	.001	.08	.142
Combined global rating	.66	.000	.55	.000	.24	.001	.10	.091

Note. SC = sentence completion and TAT = Thematic Apperception Test. All correlations are Pearson product–moment. All probability statistics are one-tailed.
[a]Sample size for camp data ranged from 44 to 45.
[b]Sample size for teacher data ranged from 173 to 174.

for which we were able to use ratings composited across four well-trained counselors, these relationships were relatively strong. Positive affective tone on both measures and sentence completion ratings of expectations of relationships with mother and peers, expectations of self, emotional health, and worldview were related modestly but significantly to individual sixth-grade teacher ratings of peer competence.

Children's projective responses were also modestly but significantly related to measures of early experience in attachment relationships. Story themes of children with secure attachment histories were balanced with negative and positive aspects. Secure children responded adaptively to a range of emotionally laden stimuli. They expressed openly and resolved in a positive way feelings of vulnerability, conflict, or sadness elicited by the task. These children received low ratings of dependency in relationships. By contrast, children with avoidant histories revealed highly negative story themes and less positive expectations of adult and peer relationships. Avoidance in early relationships was related to low ratings of overall emotional health on both tasks.

Variables related to early attachment and experience with mother at 24 months of age were correlated significantly with projective measures of peer relationships. For example, an avoidant attachment variable (e.g., the number of times classified as avoidant across the 12- to 18-month assessments) correlated significantly with all "peer attitudes" and global ratings from the sentence completions and TAT, with correlations ranging from .13 to .26. The molar rating of the child's overall experience in our 2-year tool-problem setting likewise correlated modestly with the combined TAT and sentence completion measures. When infancy and 2-year measures, and TAT and sentence completion outcomes, were entered into a canonical correlation, the resulting correlation was .32 ($p < .01$).

This set of variables was found to predict socioemotional competence in a series of regression analyses. In separate, simple regression equations, early relationship variables ($R^2 = .21$, $F(2,40)5.29$, $p<.01$) and current projective assessments of expectations of peer relationships ($R^2 = .41$, $F(1,41)28.80$, $p<.001$) predicted later social competence at summer camp independently. Entered in the same equation (current projective ratings entered first followed by early history variables), the two sets of variables produced a multiple R^2 of .44 ($F(3,39)10.08$, $p<.001$). In this model, however, early history variables failed to account for a significant proportion of the variance in social competence (R^2 Change = .02, F Change $(3,39)$ = .83, $p<.44$). This set of findings suggests that the influence of early history on current behavior in peer relationships may be mediated by an internal organization of relationships as measured by projective techniques. Since alternative regression equations were not always consistent, we present these findings as tentative. Nonetheless, we would retain as an active hypothesis for future research that continuity between early experience and later adaptation is mediated by early emerging expectations and self-representations, which are carried forward.

Conclusion

By focusing on age-salient issues, centering on key social relationships, and by aggregating data and emphasizing patterning among variables, we have been able to show a remarkable degree of coherence in individual adaptation over time. For example, numerous aspects of social competence in early and middle childhood were predictable from assessments of the quality of attachment in infancy.

Such prediction of individual adaptation through childhood from assessments in infancy is essentially unprecedented. We believe that one reason for the power of these predictions was our focus on the caregiving matrix, out of which the personality arises. Individual behavior is notably unstable in early infancy and rarely has been shown to have broad predictive significance across such a span of time. Our contention, which we feel has been borne out, is that there is greater stability and predictive significance of the dyadic relationship system. This would seem to be especially true with regard to later aspects of interpersonal life.

We would also argue that these results derive from our focus on age-salient issues. Competence with peers has proved to be one of the most consistently robust outcomes, despite the fact that assessments over time involve diverse social partners and diverse arenas. This strategy is congruent with J. Block's (1991) emphasis on seeking coherence, not homotypic continuity, in adaptation over time and his emphasis on allowing considerable complexity in the linkages sought.

A great deal of research is still required to understand the processes and mechanisms underlying continuity in individual adaptation. Given the complexity of linkages in adaptation described in this chapter—secure attachment predicting later self-reliance, sex boundaries predicting later cross-sex associations, and so forth—explanatory processes will also likely be complex. Coherence of individual adaptation is probably not best viewed as lying solely in static child traits or in continuously present environmental support. Rather, it should be conceived of as a transactive process in which child experience, and expectations and self-representations arising from that experience, lead to styles of environmental engagement and social behavior that encourage perpetuating feedback from the environment. The relative roles of cognitive appraisals and experienced-based patterns of affect modulation are far from clear at this point. However, some such mechanism, internalized through repeated, salient social experiences, must be invoked to account for the complex, cross-time relationships reported here and in other studies.

References

Ainsworth, M., Blehar, M., Waters, E., & Wall, S. (1978). *Patterns of attachment*. Hillsdale, NJ: Erlbaum.

Arend, R., Gove, F., & Sroufe, L. A. (1979). Continuity of individual adaptation from infancy to kindergarten: A predictive study of ego-resiliency and curiosity in preschoolers. *Child Development, 50*, 950–959.

Block, J. (1991, August). *Studying personality the long way*. G. Stanley Hall Award Lecture presented at the 99th Annual Convention of the American Psychological Association, San Francisco.

Block, J. H., & Block, J. (1980). The role of ego-control and ego-resiliency in the organization of behavior. In W. A. Collins (Ed.), *Minnesota Symposia on Child Psychology* (Vol. 13, pp. 39–101). Hillsdale, NJ: Erlbaum.

Bowlby, J. (1973). *Separation*. New York: Basic Books.

Bowlby, J. (1982). *Attachment and loss* (2nd ed.). New York: Basic Books. (Original work published 1969)

Clarke-Stewart, K. A., & Fein, G. (1983). Early childhood programs. In M. M. Haith & J. J. Campos (Eds.), P. H. Mussen (Series Ed.), *Handbook of child psychology: Infancy and developmental psychology* (pp. 917–1000). New York: Wiley.

Egeland, B., & Brunnquell, D. (1979). An at-risk approach to the study of child abuse: Some preliminary findings. *Journal of the American Academy of Child Psychiatry, 18*, 219–225.

Egeland, B., Kalkoske, M., Gottesman, N., & Erickson, M. (1990). Preschool behavior problems: Stability and factors accounting for change. *Journal of Child Psychology and Psychiatry, 31,* 891–909.

Elicker, J., Englund, M., & Sroufe, L. A. (1992). Predicting peer competence and peer relationships in childhood from early parent-child relationships. In R. Parke & G. Ladd (Eds.), *Family-peer relationships: Modes of linkage* (pp. 77–103). Hillsdale, NJ: Erlbaum.

Epstein, S. (1979). The stability of behavior: On predicting most of the people much of the time. *Journal of Personality and Social Psychology, 37,* 1097–1126.

Erickson, M., Sroufe, L. A., & Egeland, B. (1985). The relationship of quality of attachment and behavior problems in preschool in a high risk sample. *Monographs of the Society for Research in Child Development, 50*(1–2, Serial No. 209).

Erikson, E. H. (1963). *Childhood and society* (2nd ed.). New York: Norton.

Fury, G. (1992). *An exploratory study of representational models of attachment as revealed in family drawings in middle childhood.* Unpublished doctoral dissertation, University of Minnesota, Minneapolis.

Gewirtz, J. (1972). *Attachment and dependency.* New York: Holt, Rinehart & Winston.

Hartup, W. W. (1983). Peer relations. In P. Mussen & E. M. Hetherington (Eds.), *Manual of child psychology* (4th ed., pp. 103–196). New York: Wiley.

Havighurst, R. (1948). *Developmental tasks and education.* Chicago: University of Chicago Press.

Kagan, J. (1982). *Psychological research on the human infant: An evaluative summary.* New York: W. T. Grant Foundation.

Kagan, J. (1984). *The nature of the child.* New York: Basic Books.

Kaplan, N., & Main, M. (1989). *A system for the analysis of family drawings.* Unpublished manuscript, Department of Psychology, University of California, Berkeley.

Kestenbaum, R., Farber, E., & Sroufe, L. A. (1989). Individual differences in empathy among preschoolers: Concurrent and predictive validity. In N. Eisenberg (Ed.), *Empathy and related emotional responses: No. 44. New directions for child development* (pp. 51–56). San Francisco: Jossey-Bass.

Lamb, M. (1984). Fathers, mothers, and child care in the 1980's: Family influences on child development. In K. Borman, D. Quarm, & S. Gideonse (Eds.), *Women in the workplace* (pp. 61–88). Norwood, NJ: Ablex.

Magnusson, D., & Bergman, L. (1990). A pattern approach to the study of pathways from childhood to adulthood. In L. Robins & M. Rutter (Eds.), *Straight and devious pathways from childhood to adulthood* (pp. 101–115). Cambridge, England: Cambridge University Press.

Matas, L., Arend, R., & Sroufe, L. A. (1978). Continuity of adaptation in the second year: The relationship between quality of attachment and later competence. *Child Development, 49,* 547–556.

Mathieu, P. (1990). *Developmental antecedents of school achievement: The influence of developmental history.* Unpublished doctoral dissertation, University of Minnesota, Minneapolis.

McCrone, E., Carlson, E., & Loewen, G. (1991, April). *Thematic analysis of friendship motivation related to attachment history: Constructive replication of McAdams and Losoff (1984).* Poster presented at the 1991 biennial meeting of the Society for Research in Child Development, Seattle, WA.

Pancake, V. R. (1988). *Quality of attachment in infancy as a predictor of hostility and emotional distance in preschool peer relationships.* Unpublished doctoral dissertation, University of Minnesota, Minneapolis.

Ramirez, M., Carlson, E., Gest, S., & Egeland, B. (1991, July). *The relationship between children's behavior at school and internal representations of their relationships as measured by the sentence completion method.* Paper presented at the 11th Biennial Meeting of the International Society for the Study of Behavioral Development, Minneapolis, MN.

Rosenberg, D. M. (1984). *The quality and content of preschool fantasy play: Correlates in concurrent social-personality function and early mother-child attachment relationships.* Unpublished doctoral dissertation, University of Minnesota, Minneapolis.

Sander, L. W. (1975). Infant and caretaking environment. In E. J. Anthony (Ed.), *Explorations in child psychiatry* (pp. 129–166). New York: Plenum Press.

Savin-Williams, R. (1979). Dominance hierarchies in groups of early adolescents. *Child Development, 50,* 923–945.

Shapiro, T., & Perry, R. (1976). Latency revisited: The age 7 plus or minus 1. *Psychoanalytic Study of the Child, 31,* 79–105.

Sroufe, L. A. (1979). The coherence of individual development. *American Psychologist, 34,* 834–841.

Sroufe, L. A. (1983). Infant-caregiver attachment and patterns of adaptation in preschool: The roots of maladaptation and competence. In M. Perlmutter (Ed.), *Minnesota Symposium in Child Psychology* (Vol. 16, pp. 41–81). Hillsdale, NJ: Erlbaum.

Sroufe, L. A. (1985). Attachment classification from the perspective of infant-caregiver relationships and infant temperament. *Child Development, 56,* 1–14.

Sroufe, L. A. (1988). The role of infant-caregiver attachment in development. In J. Belsky & T. Nezworski (Eds.), *Clinical implications of attachment* (pp. 18–38). Hillsdale, NJ: Erlbaum.

Sroufe, L. A. (1990). An organizational perspective on the self. In D. Cicchetti & M. Beeghly (Eds.), *The self in transition: Infancy to childhood* (pp. 281–307). Chicago: University of Chicago Press.

Sroufe, L. A., Bennett, C., Englund, M., Urban, J., & Shulman, S. (in press). The significance of gender boundaries in preadolescence. *Child Development.*

Sroufe, L. A., & Egeland, B. (1991). Illustration of person and environment interaction from a longitudinal study. In T. Wachs & R. Plomin (Eds.), *Conceptualization and measurement of organism–environment interaction* (pp. 68–84). Washington, DC: American Psychological Association.

Sroufe, L. A., Egeland, B., & Kreutzer, T. (1990). The fate of early experience following developmental change: Longitudinal approaches to individual adaptation in childhood. *Child Development, 61,* 1363–1373.

Sroufe, L. A., & Fleeson, J. (1988). The coherence of family relationships. In R. A. Hinde & J. Stevenson-Hinde (Eds.), *Relationships within families: Mutual influences* (pp. 27–47). Oxford, England: Oxford University Press.

Sroufe, L. A., Fox, N., & Pancake, V. (1983). Attachment and dependency in developmental perspective. *Child Development, 54,* 1615–1627.

Sroufe, L. A., Schork, E., Motti, E., Lawroski, N., & LaFreniere, P. (1984). The role of affect in social competence. In C. Izard, J. Kagan & R. Zajonc (Eds.), *Emotion, cognition and behavior* (pp. 289–319). New York: Plenum Press.

Sullivan, H. S. (1953). *The interpersonal theory of psychiatry.* New York: Norton.

Thorne, B. (1986). Girls and boys together . . . but mostly apart: Gender arrangements in elementary schools. In W. Hartup & Z. Rubin (Eds.), *Relationships and development* (pp. 167–184). Hillsdale, NJ: Erlbaum.

Troy, M., & Sroufe, L. A. (1987). Victimization among preschoolers: The role of attachment relationship history. *Journal of the American Academy of Child and Adolescent Psychiatry, 26,* 166–172.

Urban, J., Carlson, E., Egeland, B., & Sroufe, L. A. (1991). Patterns of individual adaptation across childhood. *Development and Psychopathology, 3,* 445–460.

Ward, M. J., Vaughn, V., & Robb, M. (1988). Socio-emotional adaptation and infant-mother attachment in siblings: Role of mother in cross-sibling consistency. *Child Development, 59,* 643–651.

Waters, E., Wippman, J., & Sroufe, L. A. (1979). Attachment, positive affect, and competence in the peer group: Two studies in construct validation. *Child Development, 40,* 821–829.

CHAPTER 15

Why Maladaptive Behaviors Persist: Sources of Continuity and Change Across the Life Course

Avshalom Caspi

A dual research agenda defines the study of personality development across the life course: How is continuity possible? How does change occur? My aim in this chapter is to explore those two questions; to consider genetic, environmental, and interactional contributions to behavioral continuity; and to argue that the processes that promote change are unique and not simply the opposite of processes that promote continuity. I do this with reference to antisocial behavior, but I suggest that the framework proposed here offers insights more generally for understanding continuity *and* change in maladaptive behaviors across the life course.

How Is Continuity Possible?

An extensive database describes the continuity of antisocial behavior across the life course. First, children with behavioral disorders in the preschool years continue to show conduct disorders in late childhood (Richman, Stevenson, & Graham, 1982). Second, disorders of conduct in late childhood are associated with a host of social, emotional, and relational difficulties in adolescence and young adulthood (Kazdin, 1987). Third, a history of antisocial behavior in childhood and adolescence has been linked to continued antisocial behavior later in life (Farrington, Loeber, & van Kammen, 1990; Huesman, Eron, Lefkowitz, & Walder, 1984; Magnusson, 1988; McCord, 1983). These robust continuities have been revealed over the past 50 years in different nations and with multiple methods of assessment.

Efforts to go beyond description to the more difficult task of explanation are, however, less developed. What sources of influence contribute to the impressive coherence of antisocial behavior across time and circumstance? The explanation for behavioral continuities may be found in genetic sources, environmental sources, as well as interactional processes of personality functioning.[1]

Genetic Contributions to Behavioral Continuity

If genetic factors influence individual differences in social behavior, it is possible—*but not necessary*—that genetic factors may also influence the continuity of those individual differences (Plomin, 1986; Plomin & Nesselroade, 1990; Rowe, 1987). Three lines of research may shed light on this possibility. (a) If cross-sectional studies show heritability effects on antisocial behavior among adults, adolescents, and children, one may conclude that genes help to control the expression of antisocial behavior at different points in the life course. (b) Of course, antisocial *behavior* per se is not inherited; a variety of biological traits may underlie heritability coefficients for antisocial behavior by predisposing individuals to develop an antisocial phenotype. These traits may be studied to determine whether any are stable across development and whether the processes by which they initiate antisocial behavior might also serve to maintain such behavior. (c) In combination, these two lines of research are suggestive. The critical test of a genetic effect on the continuity of antisocial behavior will be revealed in longitudinal studies that estimate genetic contributions to cross-age correlations.

---

[1]This chapter relies heavily on two previous articles that developed these themes in greater detail (Caspi & Moffitt, in press; Caspi, Moffitt, Sampson, & Laub, 1993).

The genetic contribution to antisocial behavior has been studied using adoption and twin methods. The evidence from studies of adults provides strong support for a detectable genetic contribution to antisocial behavior (Mednick, Gabrielli, & Hutchings, 1984; Rushton, Fulker, Neale, Nias, & Eysenck, 1986; Tellegen et al., 1988). The evidence from studies of adolescents is more equivocal, suggesting a genetic contribution to some forms of antisocial behavior (DiLalla & Gottesman, 1989). The evidence from behavioral–genetic studies of aggressiveness earlier in life is inconsistent (Plomin, Nitz, & Rowe, 1990), but these inconsistencies likely reflect wide differences in measurement procedures (see, e.g., Ghodsian-Carpey & Baker, 1987). In addition, genetic factors may influence temperament characteristics in childhood (e.g., anger, fear, activity) that are linked with later externalizing behavior problems (Buss & Plomin, 1984).

Collectively, the cross-sectional data suggest that genetic factors help to control the expression of antisocial behavior at different points in development and that these factors may possibly influence the continuity of antisocial behavior across the life course as well. However, these studies do not address the mechanisms by which they do so.

There have been numerous efforts to identify some of the biological mechanisms and factors involved in antisocial behavior (see Mednick, Moffitt, & Stack, 1987; Moffitt & Mednick, 1988). Perhaps the best candidate to help account for the *continuity* of antisocial behavior across the life course is compromised cognitive ability: The partial heritability of cognitive abilities is well-documented (Plomin, 1990); the stability of cognitive functions from childhood to adulthood is similarly convincing (Wohlwill, 1980); and the link between cognitive impairment and antisocial behavior has been revealed in studies of children's aggression, adolescents' delinquency, and adults' criminality (e.g., Lynam, Moffitt, & Stouthamer-Loeber, in press). Moffitt's (1990) neuropsychological research pointed to two areas of cognitive functioning that are especially pertinent to the question of antisocial behavior. Findings about *verbal functions* and *executive functions* provide intriguing theoretical implications for understanding sources of continuity in antisocial behavior.

Deficits in verbal functions might contribute to the development of antisocial behavior because language is essential to prosocial processes such as delaying gratification, anticipating consequences, and linking delayed punishments with earlier transgressions. In particular, deficits in verbal skills may contribute to a present-oriented cognitive style that fosters irresponsible and exploitative behavior across the life course (Wilson & Herrnstein, 1985).

Deficits in executive functions (e.g., sustaining attention, abstract reasoning, self-monitoring, and self-awareness) might also contribute to the development of antisocial behavior because these interfere with a child's ability to control his or her own behavior, producing an inattentive, impulsive child who is impaired in considering the future implications of his or her acts. Such a child may have difficulty understanding the negative impact his or her behavior has on others, fail to hold in mind abstract ideas of ethical values and future rewards, and fail to inhibit inappropriate behavior or adapt his or her behavior to changing social circumstances. Executive deficits may thus give rise to early childhood behavior problems that in turn set the stage for emerging delinquent behavior as the child grows physically older but not necessarily more cognitively mature.

Although these neuropsychological correlates of antisocial behavior are consistent and robust, researchers still need to determine whether the genetic factors that produce individual differences in these functions during childhood and adolescence correlate with the genetic factors that produce these individual differences in adulthood. The chances are good that they do. Recent studies suggest that much of the phenotypic stability for cognitive abilities is mediated genetically; that is, genetic factors that produce individual differences in cognitive functions in childhood correlate significantly with genetic factors that produce individual differences in adulthood (DeFries, Plomin, & Labuda, 1987). Longitudinal studies that assess age-to-age genetic continuity and change are clearly needed to further establish such links (Plomin, 1986).

Environmental Contributions to Behavioral Continuity

A second continuity-promoting mechanism is so mundane that it is often overlooked: Behavioral patterns may show stability across the life course because the environment remains stable. In particular, individuals' behavioral patterns may show stability because the interpersonal environments in which individuals reside remain stable. To the extent that parental demands, peer influences, and teacher expectancies remain stable over time, one could expect such environmental stability to promote behavioral continuities. Social–behavior theorists have been saying this for years, of course, but few longitudinal studies have actually assessed the stability and change of interpersonal environments alongside the stability and change of individual behavior patterns.

The studies that have charted characteristics of the child-rearing environment over time have shown that many parenting behaviors remain remarkably stable. For example, Roberts, Block, and Block (1984) found that 73% of the 91 items contained in the Child-Rearing Practices Report showed significant continuities from early childhood through early adolescence. Similar stability has been found in observations of maternal sensitivity from infancy through the preschool years (Pianta, Sroufe, & Egeland, 1989) and in parenting practices that were correlated with children's aggressive acts (Patterson & Bank, 1990). In fact, Patterson and Bank (1990) suggested that there are "parallel continuities" between children's aggressive behaviors and their parents' parenting skills. If the interpersonal environments of most children are as stable as all of these data suggest, then the continuities observed in children's behavior over time may simply reflect the cumulative and continuing continuities of those environments.

The direct corollary of the assertion that behavioral continuities may reflect environmental constancies is, of course, that environmental change will produce behavioral change. Here, the evidence is abundant. For example, Rutter (1987) has noted that residential treatments had a marked influence on current behavior but that these influences did not persist when youngsters returned home to an environment that maintained its delinquency-promoting characteristics. Changes in the prosocial direction were shown by boys in England whose delinquent behavior diminished when their families moved out of London, a result that could not be attributed to selective migration (West, 1982). Also, Elliott and Voss (1974) reported that for many delinquents, the rate of self-reported delinquency declined following drop out from schools, suggesting that a shift from environments associated with failure experiences may serve to reduce delinquency. Finally, a longitudinal study of adolescent mothers showed that the sequelae of unplanned teen parenthood strongly depended on subsequent environmental changes, such as further education, marriage, and independence from the family of origin (Furstenberg, Brooks-Gunn, & Morgan, 1987).

It is important to note, however, that such environmental changes are not random; they may themselves be a function of the individual's personality. Which women choose to return to school? Who are able to enter stable marriages? In short, the behavioral changes reported in many studies may derive from changes in environments that are themselves brought about by stable personality attributes. Indeed, it is possible that features of the environment may reflect the enduring features of individuals who make up the environment. It is even possible that features of the environment may reflect heritable characteristics of individuals.

Plomin and Bergeman (1991) have shown that a variety of measures typically used to study children's environments (e.g., the Home Observation for Measurement of the Environment scales, the Family Environment Scale) are subject to substantial genetic influence. Measures of the person and measures of the environment are *not* pure and distinct from each other: They are confounded. Although the mechanisms that produce genetic correlations between the two remain elusive, it is likely that genetic influences on measures of the environment reflect interactional processes wherein individuals "create" situations that are compatible with their dispositions (Scarr & McCartney, 1983). Clearly, researchers are dealing here with person–environment interactions.

Person–Environment Interactions

There are many kinds of interactions, but there are three that play particularly important roles both in promoting the continuity of personality across the life course and in controlling the trajectory of the life course itself (Caspi & Bem, 1990). *Reactive interaction* occurs when different individuals exposed to the same environment experience it, interpret it, and react to it differently. *Evocative interaction* occurs when an individual's personality evokes distinctive responses from others. *Proactive interaction* occurs when individuals select or create environments of their own. How do these interactional processes promote continuity in antisocial behavior?

Reactive Person–Environment Interaction

Different individuals exposed to the same environment experience it, interpret it, and react to it differently. Each individual extracts a subjective psychological environment from the objective surroundings, and it is that subjective environment that shapes both personality and subsequent interaction.

That is, of course, the basic tenet of the phenomenological approach embodied in the famous dictum that if people "define situations as real, they are real in their consequences" (Thomas & Thomas, 1928). It is also the assumption that connects S. Epstein's (1990) writings on the development of personal theories of reality, Tomkins's (1986) description of scripts about the self and interpersonal interactions, and Bowlby's (1973) analysis of working models that develop in the context of interactional experiences.

All three theories suggest that early experiences can set up anticipatory attitudes that lead the individual to project particular interpretations onto new social relationships and ambiguous situations. This is accomplished through a variety of informational and behavioral processes in which the person interprets new events in a manner that is consistent with his or her experientially established understanding of the self and others.

All three theories also assert that people continually revise their "personal theories," "scripts," and "working models" as a function of experience. However, if these function as filters for social information, the question is raised as to how much revision actually occurs. In fact, social psychologists, who tend to focus on the cognitive rather than the motivational features of internal organizational structures, argue that self-schemata—psychological constructs of the self—screen and select from experience to maintain structural equilibrium (Greenwald, 1980). Once a schema becomes well organized, it filters experience and makes individuals selectively responsive to information that matches their expectations and views of themselves (Markus, 1977). The course of personality development is thus likely to be conservative because features of the cognitive system may impair people's ability to change in response to new events that challenge their beliefs and self-conceptions.

According to contemporary theorists who view the self as "an arrangement of schemas that represent one's past experiences and personal characteristics," the self-concept is dynamic; it activates representations of particular situations and "carries" a person's responses to the interpersonal world (Markus & Cross, 1990, p. 594). If so, the self-concept of antisocial people should differ greatly from that of their non-anti-social counterparts. Indeed, research shows that antisocial people appear to have different cognitive standards regarding the use of aggressive behavior. For example, they believe that aggression will yield tangible rewards and desirable results (Boldizar, Perry, & Perry, 1989; Perry, Perry, & Rasmussen, 1986). They are also more likely to believe that aggression is a legitimate response to solving problems (e.g., "It's OK to hit someone if you just go crazy with anger"); that behaving aggressively helps to avoid a negative image (e.g., "If you back down from a fight, everyone will think you are a coward"); that aggressive acts improve one's social reputation and increase self-esteem (e.g., "It's important to show everyone how tough you are"); and that victims do not suffer (Slaby & Guerra, 1988).

Collectively, then, this arrangement of beliefs and self-conceptions may support the use of aggression in many social encounters. And, of course, these beliefs are not fictions. The social environment contains a rich reinforcement schedule for these aggressive acts and thus confirms the antisocial person's belief system (Perry, Kusel, & Perry, 1988).

It is not clear, however, whether these beliefs guide behavioral action independent of information-processing biases, or whether—as is more likely—beliefs and self-conceptions influence the type of social information that is attended to and processed by antisocial people (Slaby & Guerra, 1988).

Numerous studies have focused on the social information-processing strategies of aggressive children. Most notable is the social–cognitive model proposed by Dodge (1986), who posited individual differences in five distinct social information-processing steps.

1. When *encoding information* about a social event, aggressive children seek out less information about the event (Dodge & Newman, 1981; Slaby & Guerra, 1988).

2. When *interpreting the cues* in new social situations, aggressive children are prone to attribute hostile intention to ambiguous events (e.g., Dodge, 1980; Nasby, Hayden, & DePaulo, 1979) and to expect hostility from others in the social environment (e.g., Dodge & Frame, 1982).

3. When *searching for possible responses* to the situation, aggressive children are more likely to generate aggressive responses (Dodge, 1986), and they also possess significantly less knowledge about interpersonal problem solving (e.g., Hains & Ryan, 1983; Slaby & Guerra, 1988).

4. When *considering the consequences* of generated alternative responses, aggressive people may truncate the process of weighing alternatives as a result of their rapidly escalating emotional reactions (Katz, 1989).

5. When *carrying out selected responses*, aggressive people may be impaired in their ability to monitor the consequences of their actions because their verbal and self-control deficits place them at a disadvantage in interpersonal exchanges.

Of course, the social world is not passive. As I discuss shortly, aggressive behavior is likely to evoke responses from the surrounding environment that confirm and sustain aggressive children's subjective interpretations of that environment as hostile. Thus begins a feedback process that militates more adaptive options and strengthens the chain of continuity.

Evocative Person–Environment Interactions

Each individual evokes distinctive responses from others: One person acts, the other reacts, and the person reacts back in mutually interlocking evocative interaction. Such interactions continue throughout the life course and may promote the continuity of antisocial behavior patterns.

Already very early in life children evoke consistent responses from their social environments (Chess & Thomas, 1987). Indeed, numerous studies have shown that an infant's temperament may affect disciplinary strategies and subsequent interactions with adults and peers (Bell & Chapman, 1986). For example, Maccoby and Jacklin (1983) showed that over time, mothers of children with a "difficult" temperament reduced their efforts to actively guide and direct their children's behavior and became increasingly less involved in the socialization process. In their ongoing longitudinal study, Block and Block (1980) found that parents of highly active children were impatient and hostile with their children and frequently got into power struggles with them (Buss, 1981). Moreover, when the children were 7 years old, they were described by their teachers as aggressive, manipulative, noncompliant, and more likely to push limits and stretch the rules in many social encounters (Buss, Block, & Block, 1980). These findings suggest that early developing temperament differences are linked to a matrix of aversive interpersonal interactions with peers, parents, and teachers. Indeed, it is possible that antisocial children evoke reactions from the social environment that then help to maintain and escalate a behavioral trajectory characterized by increasingly more serious problems.

Research at the Oregon Social Learning Center has shown just how such evocative person–environment interactions can sustain aversive patterns of behavior (Patterson, 1982, 1986; Patterson & Bank, 1990). It appears that children's coercive behaviors often provoke adult family members to counter with highly punitive and angry responses, often escalating to an ever-widening gulf of irritation until the parents of such children eventually withdraw from aversive interactions with their children. One outcome of such negative reinforcements is that children who coerce others into providing short-term payoffs in the immediate situation may thereby learn an interactional style that continues to "work" in similar ways in later social encounters and with different interaction partners. The immediate reinforcement not only short-circuits the learning of more controlled interactional styles that might have greater adaptability in the long run, but it also increases the likelihood that coercive behaviors will recur whenever similar interactional conditions arise again.

However, the long-term costs associated with these short-term rewards are severe. Early coercive family interactions portend deteriorated family management practices when antisocial children reach adolescence. At this point, parents of antisocial children are less likely to supervise and monitor their pubescent boys; their inept disciplinary strategies, in turn, predict persistent and progressively more serious delinquency among their offspring (e.g., Laub & Sampson, 1988; Loeber & Stouthamer-Loeber, 1986).

The social learning interpretation of coercive family systems is that "family members and antisocial children alternate in the roles of aggressors and victims, each inadvertently reinforcing the coercive behavior of the other" (Patterson & Bank, 1990). Parents and children thus maintain and escalate "coercive cycles" by evoking predictable reactions and counterreactions from each other. There is, however, an additional interpretation: Parents and children possess similar aggressive traits as determined by their shared genes. Rowe (1987) observed that shared heredity may render the social learning interpretation incomplete and suggested that social–interactional analyses of biological and adoptive parent–child dyads are needed to estimate the contribution of social learning mechanisms to behavioral continuity independent of shared heredity.

Although no such studies have been conducted to my knowledge, experimental research has clearly shown that children evoke predictable responses from adults independent of shared heredity (e.g., Anderson, Lytton, & Romney, 1986). It appears that adults respond to the behaviors of children rather than create differences between children. Indeed, it may well be that early temperament differences contribute to the development of conduct disorders by evoking responses from the interpersonal social environment that exacerbate the child's tendencies (Lytton, 1990).

It is also through evocative interaction that phenomenological interpretations of situations—the products of reactive interaction—are transformed into situations that are "real in their consequences." In particular, early experiences can set up expectations that lead an individual to project particular interpretations onto new situations and relationships and hence to behave in ways that corroborate those expectations.

For example, because aggressive children expect others to be hostile, they may behave in ways that elicit hostility from others, thereby confirming their initial suspicion and sustaining their aggression. Individuals also elicit and selectively attend to information that confirms rather than disconfirms their self-concepts (Darley & Fazio, 1980; Snyder, 1984; Swann, 1983, 1987). This promotes stability of the self-concept, which, in turn, promotes the continuity of behavioral patterns that are congruent with that self-concept (Andrews, 1988; Backman, 1985, 1988; Secord & Backman, 1965; also see Carson, 1969; Snyder & Ickes, 1985).

In these several ways, then, reactive and evocative person–environment interactions enable an ensemble of behaviors, expectations, and self-concepts to evoke maintaining responses from others—thereby promoting continuity of antisocial styles across time and circumstance.

Proactive Person–Environment Interactions

Individuals often seek out situations that are compatible with their dispositions, and recent analyses have suggested that individuals' dispositions can lead them to select situations that, in turn, reinforce and sustain those same dispositions (Ickes, Snyder, & Garcia, in press; Snyder & Ickes, 1985). It has been proposed that this dispositionally guided selection and creation of environments becomes increasingly important and influential as the individual gains increased autonomy from the imposed settings of early childhood (Scarr & McCartney, 1983). In fact, this developmental phenomenon may account for the oft-noted age-related increase in the magnitude of stability coefficients across the life span (Caspi & Bem, 1990). As self-regulatory competencies increase with age, individuals begin to make choices and display preferences that may reinforce and sustain their salient characteristics.

The environments that are most consequential for personality are probably interpersonal environments, and it is in friendship formation and mate selection that the personality-sustaining effects of proactive interaction are the most intriguing. Friends tend to be similar with respect to values, attitudes, and behaviors (e.g., Kandel, 1978). Even aggressive children succeed in forming ties to particular subgroups of children. In particular, boys and girls tend to affiliate selectively with friends who match their antisocial behavior (Cairns, Cairns, Neckerman, Gest, & Gariepy, 1988; Giordano, Cernkovich, & Pugh, 1986; Rowe & Osgood, 1984).

Billy and Udry (1985; Billy, Rodgers, & Udry, 1984) examined the contribution of three mechanisms to similarities between friends: *selection*, in which individuals acquire friends on the basis of behavioral similarity; *influence*, in which peers influence their friends to behave in certain ways; and *deselection*, in which individuals deselect friends whose behavior is different from their own. In general, it appears that social selection is the most important factor contributing to similarities in attitudes, behaviors, and, more generally, deviant life styles. Children and adolescents do not congregate randomly; they choose activities that are compatible with their own dispositions and select companions who are similar to themselves.

Once social selection effects take place, they set in motion important social influence effects. This reciprocal dynamic of social selection and social influence is especially interesting with respect to problem behaviors. For example, Dishion (1990) and Patterson and Bank (1990) have suggested that each individual "shops" for settings and people that maximize his or her positive payoffs. The trial-and-error process of shopping and being rejected inevitably leads the problem child to find a group of peers that will reinforce his or her behaviors. In turn, membership in a delinquent peer group is a key determinant of drift into subsequent and more severe delinquency (Elliott & Menard, in press).

Indeed, in their social–ecological analysis of the development of aggression, Cairns and his colleagues have found that aggressive children's social networks are quite stable over periods of at least 1 year (Cairns et al., 1989; Cairns, Perrin, & Cairns, 1985). Even when specific peer associations change, the change must be evaluated with caution. Adolescents may switch alliances and cliques, but the new affiliations resemble the old ones in terms of deviance. Cairns and Cairns (1993) suggested that these affiliations serve as guides for norm formation and the consolidation of behavior patterns over time. Continuities in social networks may thus contribute to behavioral stability because the demands of the social environment remain relatively similar over time. Moreover, consistency in how members of the social network relate to the individual may contribute to behavioral stability because this affects how individuals view and define themselves.

Just as people tend to befriend similar others, they tend to marry partners who are similar to themselves (E. Epstein & Guttman, 1984). Moreover, it appears that similarities between spouses reflect active personal preferences, not simply the outcome of social homogamy (Mascie-Taylor & Vandenberg, 1988). Although only a few studies have directly examined assortative mating for aggressive reaction patterns, there is a good deal of evidence of congruence for traits related to antisocial behavior (e.g., Baker, Mack, Moffitt, & Mednick, 1989; Buss, 1984a; Zuckerman, 1979).

Assortative mating has important genetic and social consequences (Buss, 1984b) and may also have important psychological implications. From the perspective of personality development, marriage to a similar partner serves to create an environment that reinforces initial tendencies; through assortative mating people may set in motion processes of social interchange that help to sustain their dispositions across time and circumstance. Caspi and Herbener (1990) have documented this effect by showing that marriage to a similar other promotes consistency in the intraindividual organization of personality attributes across adulthood. In addition, marital assortment may promote family transmission effects to the extent that marital assortment gives rise to shared experiences that create similarities between family members (Caspi, Herbener, & Ozer, 1992).

In combination, studies of friendship formation and mate selection suggest that continuities may emerge not in spite of changing relationships and situations but because individuals often select environments that are correlated with their dispositions. A more complete account of continuity and change thus requires that researchers examine the sustaining role of environmental conditions and how individuals in various settings and relationships are successively drawn in as "accomplices" in the maintenance of behavior patterns across the life course (Wachtel, 1977). One does not have to embrace the most radical proposition contained in Sullivan's (1953) conception of personality as the "relatively enduring pattern of recurrent interpersonal situations which characterize a human life" (p. 111) to appreciate its more subtle implication: Inquiries about sources of individual continuity and change may benefit from examining not only the individual but also those significant others in his or her life that contribute to the continuity and change of personality.

Life-Course Consequences of Person–Environment Interactions

I have noted that the processes of reactive, evocative, and proactive interaction enable an individual's personality both to shape itself and to promote its own continuity throughout the life course. These same processes also enable an individual's personality to influence the life course itself. In particular, person–environment interactions can produce two kinds of consequences in the life course: cumulative consequences and contemporary consequences (Caspi & Bem, 1990).

Consider the case of a boy who, in late childhood, responds to frustration with explosive temper tantrums. His ill-temperedness may provoke school authorities to expel him (evocative interaction) or cause him to experience school failure so negatively (reactive interaction) that he chooses to quit as soon as he is legally permitted to do so (proactive interaction). In either case, leaving school might limit his future career opportunities, forcing him into frustrating low-level jobs. This low occupational status might then lead to an erratic work life characterized by frequent job changes and bouts of unemployment, possibly disrupting his marriage and leading to divorce. In this hypothetical scenario, the occupational and marital outcomes are *cumulative* consequences of his childhood personality. Once set in motion by childhood temper tantrums, the chain of events takes over and culminates in the adult outcomes— even if he is no longer ill-tempered as an adult.

On the other hand, if he does carry his ill-temperedness into adulthood, then *contemporary* consequences are also likely to arise. He is likely to explode when frustrations arise on the job or when conflicts arise in his marriage. This can lead to an erratic work life, low-level occupational status, and divorce. In this scenario, the same occupational and marital outcomes are contemporary consequences of his current personality rather than consequences of earlier events such as quitting school.

Caspi, Bem, and Elder (1989; Caspi, Elder, & Bem, 1987) explored these two hypothetical scenarios in their work using data from the longitudinal Berkeley Guidance Study. They identified men who had a history of temper tantrums during late childhood and then traced the continuities and consequences of this personality style across the subsequent 30 years of the subjects' lives.

They began their research with the following continuity question: Do ill-tempered boys become ill-tempered men? Apparently so. Correlations between the temper tantrum scores in late childhood and independent personality ratings 20 years later revealed that ill-tempered boys were later described as being significantly more undercontrolled, irritable, and moody than their even-tempered peers.

They then examined the subjects' work histories. The major finding was that ill-tempered boys who came from middle-class homes suffered a progressive deterioration of socioeconomic status (SES) as they moved through the life course. They were somewhat more likely than their even-tempered peers to terminate their formal education earlier; the occupational status of their first jobs was significantly lower; and, by midlife (age 40), their occupational status was indistinguishable from that of men born into the working class. A majority of them held jobs of lower occupational status than those held by their fathers at a comparable age. They also had more erratic work lives, changing jobs more frequently and experiencing unemployment between 18 and 40 years of age.

Did these men become occupationally disadvantaged because their earlier ill-temperedness started them down a particular path (cumulative consequences) or because their current ill-temperedness impaired them in the world of work (contemporary consequences)? The path analysis displayed in Figure 1 reveals evidence—albeit indirect—for both kinds of consequences.

Cumulative consequences were implied by the effect of childhood ill-temperedness on occupational status at midlife: Tantrums predicted lower educational attainment ($\beta = -.34, p < .05$), and educational attainment, in turn, predicted occupational status ($\beta = .59, p < .001$). However, there was no direct effect of ill-temperedness on occupational status ($\beta = -.10$). In other words, middle-class boys with a history of childhood ill-temperedness arrived at lower occupational status at midlife because they truncated their formal education, not because they continued to be ill-tempered.

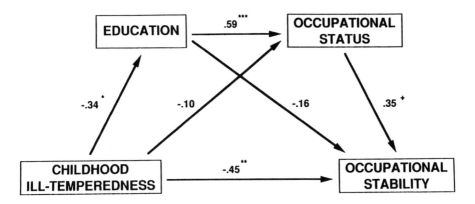

FIGURE 1. Midlife occupational status and stability of men with middle-class origins as a function of childhood ill-temperedness. (Adolescent IQ is included as an exogenous variable in this model; its correlation with temper tantrums is $-.09$, ns [$N = 45$]. $*p < .05$. $**p < .01$. $***p < .001$. $^+p < .10$. Adapted from Caspi, Elder, & Bem (1987). Reprinted with permission.

Contemporary consequences were implied by the strong direct link between ill-temperedness and occupational stability ($\beta = -.45, p < .01$). Men with a childhood history of ill-temperedness continued to be ill-tempered in adulthood, where it got them into trouble in the work world.

As noted earlier, the processes of reactive, evocative, and proactive interaction not only shape personality and mediate its continuity over time but they also enable the personality to influence the trajectory of the life course itself.

It follows from all that has been said that early individual differences have lawful implications for the course of later behavior and development. I have contended, following Block (1981), that

> how experience registers, how environments are selected or modified, and how the stages of life are negotiated depend, importantly and coherently, on what the individual brings to these new encounters—the resources, the premises, the intentions, the awareness, the fears and the hopes, the forethoughts and the afterthoughts that are subsumed by what we call personality. (pp. 40–41)

I have also tried to elucidate some of the processes through which this might be accomplished. It is now time to consider the possibility of change (Sampson & Laub, in press-a).

How Does Change Occur?

More often than not, unpromising origins set in motion a cumulative sequence of life disadvantage. However, as Rutter (1988, p. 3) argued, researchers know little about "escape from the risk process" and about whether processes that promote change are unique or simply the opposite of processes that promote continuity (Sampson & Laub, in press-a).

Hints about the process of change may be gleaned from recent studies that have focused on those salient life events that appear to modify life-course trajectories. In particular, three vastly different prospective studies converge in identifying life events that may serve to modify problem trajectories. These life events include military service, marriage, and work, and the study of these "turning points" offer important clues about how change may occur in the life course.

Military Service

The first study, an investigation of children who grew up in the Great Depression, illustrates how the assumption of new social roles may induce change in life opportunities. In exploring how the large number of children growing up in families on public aid rose above their misfortune, Elder (1986, 1987) found that men who grew up in deprived circumstances could break the cycle of disadvantage by entering the service, especially if they did so at a relatively young age.

Three features of military life appeared to have promoted change in the life course (Elder, 1986, 1987; Elder & Caspi, 1990). The first feature was the "knifing-off" of past experience; the military separated recruits from their past and made their prior identities irrelevant. The second feature was the "time-out," or "psychosocial moratorium," offered by military service; the military gave youths a chance to take a break from the conventional expectations and pressures of the age-graded life course and to consider where they were going. The third feature was the broadened range of perspectives, social knowledge, and basic skills instilled by the military; the military offered youths a source of self-esteem and new skills that they could apply on reentry into civilian life.

These are not the exhaustive features of the transition to military life, but together they defined a developmental pathway that might have offered a promising route to life change. These features were also identifiable in a study of men who were paroled from prison to military service during World War II (Glaser, 1988; cited in Ohlin & Blumstein, 1988). Most of the men received honorable discharges, and although no "untreated" group of prisoners was available for comparison on outcome, job skills learned in the army were associated with low rates of criminal recidivism after discharge. Glaser noted that interposing the military between the move from prisoner to civilian roles made the transition smoother; levels of regimentation and supervision were decreased gradually rather than abruptly. Military service also broke up old friendship networks and created new, less criminogenic ones. The parolees gained a new role label, *military veteran*, that avoided the stigmatic label of *ex-convict*, and they obtained an alibi for their sparse employment histories so that their criminal pasts were not suspected by employers.

Marriage

A second study of change in the life course focused on two groups of youths (Quinton & Rutter, 1988; Rutter, Quinton, & Hill, 1990). One was a sample of inner-London youths institutionalized in group homes because of family dysfunctions (e.g., parental criminality, abuse, desertion). The other was a sample of noninstitutionalized individuals of the same age living in the same inner-London borough. The results showed that the high-risk group experienced more troublesome outcomes in adulthood than the relatively low-risk group. However, there was also considerable heterogeneity in the adult outcomes. What accounted for these wide variations among youth at risk for later difficulties?

It appears that marital support in early adult life provided an important protective mechanism that inhibited persisting psychosocial difficulties. For example, the women at risk for poor psychosocial outcomes in adult life were able to avert later problems if they were married to supportive spouses. Positive school experiences among girls was another factor that promoted change in the life course, especially indirectly through its effect on stable marriage choices. Moreover, these results were not an artifact of selection effects; they were maintained even when controls for numerous measures of childhood deviance were introduced to the analysis. In sum, the findings indicated "substantial heterogeneity in outcomes, indicating the need to account for major discontinuities, as well as continuities in development. In that connection, marital support from a nondeviant spouse stood out as a factor associated with a powerful protective effect" (Rutter et al., 1990, p. 152).

In their dual concern with continuity and change, Rutter and his colleagues also offered a useful metaphor: chain links. Continuity from childhood adversity to adult difficulties involves multiple links in a chain, with each link dependent on the presence of other links. However, there are also many opportunities for change, for each link in the chain can be unfastened. Thus, much like Elder's (1986, 1987) study of military experience, Quinton and Rutter's (1988) study suggested that adult transitions in the life course can "modify the effect of adversities experienced in childhood" (Rutter et al., 1990, p. 152).

Work

In a third study along similar lines, Sampson and Laub (1990, in press-b) theorized that social ties to adult institutions of informal social control (e.g., family, community, work) may modify the persistence of antisocial behavior from childhood through adulthood. Their research has focused on the transition to adulthood and, in turn, the new role demands from full-time employment, military service, and marriage. Unlike much life-course research, however, Sampson and Laub (1990, in press-b) emphasized the quality or strength of social ties more than the occurrence or timing of discrete life events. Thus, Sampson and Laub (in-press-a) argued that "marriage per se may not increase social control, but close emotional ties increase the social bonds between individuals and, all else equal, should lead to a reduction in criminal behavior." Similarly, "employment alone may not increase social control. It is employment coupled with job stability, job commitment, and ties to work that should increase social control, and, with all else being equal, lead to a reduction in criminal behavior" (Sampson & Laub, in press-a). According to their theory of informal social control, it is the "social capital" inherent in particular institutional relationships that may serve to modify risk trajectories.

To test these hypotheses, Sampson and Laub (1990, in press-b) analyzed the natural histories of two groups of boys who differed dramatically in childhood antisocial behavior; one was a group of 500 delinquents and the other a group of 500 control subjects matched on age, IQ, SES, and ethnicity. The results showed marked adult differences between the two groups of boys. For example, as adults, the former delinquents were more likely than the control subjects to be arrested, to drink excessively, and to experience erratic employment careers. There was, however, also considerable heterogeneity in adult outcomes that could be accounted for by the quality and strength of social ties in the transition to adulthood.

Consistent with their theory of adult development and informal social control, Sampson and Laub (1990, in press-b) found that job stability and marital attachment in young adulthood were significantly related to changes in adult crime: The stronger the adult ties to work and family, the less crime and deviance among *both* delinquents and controls. These results maintained even with controls for measures of childhood deviance, thus ruling out important selection effects. Hence, much like Quinton and Rutter (1988), the Sampson and Laub (1990, in press-b) study suggested that social ties embedded in the transition to adulthood (e.g., marital attachment, job stability) may help to explain wide variations in adult outcomes among youths at risk for persistent difficulties.

Change in the Life Course: Developmental Experiences and Situational Imperatives

Change is clearly possible, but researchers still have to identify the processes that enable people to alter the course of their lives (Anthony & Cohler, 1987; Masten & Garmezy, 1985). As Rutter (1987) noted, researchers must unravel the processes that operate at key turning points when a risk trajectory is recast to a more adaptive path.

From the studies summarized earlier, it is possible to derive several general propositions about the developmental and situational mechanisms that might promote change in the life course (Rutter, 1987). Other research and theory supports some of these observations, but here these observations are offered more in the spirit of generative hypotheses than as fully confirmed principles (Caspi, Moffitt, Sampson, & Laub, 1993).

1. Life-course events such as military service, marriage, and work can cause radical changes in the organization of the self, but receptivity to such events is the most pronounced during the transition to adulthood.

It may be no coincidence that studies grappling with the puzzle of life-course change have pointed to experiences in late adolescence and young adulthood that appear to deflect life trajectories. The period of late adolescence and young adulthood may be salient because it is characterized by a convergence of changes in multiple domains: cognitive, psychosocial, and institutional.

Cognitively, the maturation of formal operations in adolescence means that youths have become reliably capable of thinking in terms of life span possibilities and alternatives; possibilities and alternatives are now considered in reference to the past and to the future, and youths are increasingly aware of the contrast between ideals and reality (Inhelder & Piaget, 1958).

Psychosocially, the period of late adolescence and young adulthood offers new challenges in achieving personal identity (Erikson, 1959). Youths must now assume full responsibility in new domains, in personal partnerships, and in work accomplishments; success in these domains may retrack developmental trajectories onto more adaptive paths.

The transition from late adolescence to young adulthood is not, of course, the only period of development that brings with it cognitive and psychosocial transitions. The transitional experience of this period is, however, unique in that it coincides with institutionalized events characterized by a high degree of salience, such as graduations, initiations, and marriages. These institutionalized transitions increase the likelihood of a reorientation in life structure, direction, and purpose, in part because they may increase self-awareness and because they make life planning a conscious act (Rutter, 1987).

However, simply changing environments is not sufficient. The situational imperatives involved in redirecting life-course trajectories are stringent, a point that is made collectively apparent by the three aforementioned studies of "turning points" in the life course. Those three studies revealed that to produce change, new situations must accomplish several aims.

2. To affect change, new situations should alter people's exposure to environments that perpetuate risk.

I have already shown that in the usual course of development, people evoke experiences and select environments that are positively correlated with their characteristics and backgrounds. It is possible, however, to alter or diminish such person–environment congruence by providing new environments that are negatively correlated with people's characteristics and backgrounds (Scarr & McCartney, 1983). Indeed, select contexts in late adolescence and young adulthood may most effectively promote change when they alter people's exposure to the environmental conditions that perpetuate continuity (Quinton & Rutter, 1988).

For example, military service may acquire special developmental significance in the life course because it releases youths from the limitations imposed by earlier conditions of life, removes them from discordant environments, and alters their networks of social relationships. Similarly, marriage may serve to alter life-course trajectories because it is associated with a reduction of activity in those social networks that lead youths to trouble.

However, even this may not be enough for the production of long-term change. Unless old options are challenged or eliminated, and unless new opportunities are provided, individuals will often resort to familiar techniques of self-verification rather than engage in the more arduous efforts aimed at changing themselves (Caspi & Moffitt, in press). As Rutter (1987) noted, removing people from a "risky" environment that perpetuates continuity is useful only insofar as new opportunities and life chances are simultaneously made available.

3. New situations should reconstruct pathways and connections between available social opportunities.

As noted earlier, the continuity of maladaptive behavior across the life course is partly maintained by its *cumulative* consequences. This implies that early behavior (e.g., delinquency) influences later behavior (e.g., adult crime) because social reactions to early behavior generate negative consequences that further diminish life chances. Official labeling, incarceration, school failure, and other negative life events associated with delinquency close down the doors of opportunity and interfere with successful adult development through the cumulative continuity of lost opportunity, above and beyond that generated by an early propensity toward antisocial behavior (Sampson & Laub, in press-a).

If the chain of continuity involves such multiple links (Rutter et al., 1990), severing one link may break the chain of continuity. However, to be effective, life-course events must be able to influence the direction that lives can take. For example, educational settings not only socialize students for a culture; education is also a fixed capital asset, in that it provides the credentials that can open up occupational opportunities and social positions (Meyer, 1978). Similarly, military service, and the legitimation it confers on discharged recruits, provides an entrance ticket to new social opportunities and serves as a springboard for upward mobility (Gal, 1986). Both events may trigger life-course change because they sever a link in the chain of continuity and reconstruct pathways between social opportunities.

4. New situations should provide opportunities to perform tasks that help people acquire new skills and that may enhance a personal sense of efficacy.

Doing well is rewarding, and performance accomplishments are likely to increase a person's sense of self-efficacy and appraisal of internal control. It is thus possible that positive experiences in military service, marriage, and work may provide sources of self-esteem during this transitional phase of the life course. In particular, structured settings that give youth a sense of being needed and that provide them with productive roles to perform may contribute to the development of a more generalized perception of control over life paths. As Elder (1986) observed,

> being needed they had the chance and responsibility to make a real contribution to the welfare of others. Being needed gives rise to a sense of being committed to something larger than the self. However onerous the task may be, there is gratification and even personal growth to be gained in being challenged by a real undertaking if it is not excessive or exploitative. (p. 242)

Of course, doing well at new tasks also implies that new skills have been acquired and honed, and it is possible that salutary effects may be more properly attributable to the learning of new skills in new settings than to generalized feelings of control and self-esteem. Unfortunately, the available evidence does not allow researchers to discriminate between these two accounts, but there is no reason to rule out their complementary effects (Rutter, 1987).

5. New situations should compel individuals to engage in social comparisons with a new and wider range of people and thereby provide an opportunity for change through the setting of new achievement goals.

When people change situations, they change reference groups; in turn, new reference groups usually bring about new social comparisons. It is thus possible that the resocialization functions associated with military service and stable work may derive from social comparisons with a wider range of people, some superior, others equal, and still others inferior. This compositional effect of new situations can be understood in relation to social comparison theory (Festinger, 1954).

In general, people wish to compare themselves with others who are relatively similar to themselves in order to understand their world. However, people are also motivated to enhance their self-evaluation (Tesser, 1984), and to do this they may seek out comparisons with dissimilar others. For example, when group members discover discrepancies among themselves, each member may be motivated to improve performance. This may be accomplished through upward comparisons with more successful group members (Wood, 1989). It is also possible that downward comparisons, with less fortunate others, may enhance self-evaluations, albeit as a defensive strategy (Wills, 1981).

Although comparisons with dissimilar others may be unfavorable, they may also provide fodder for change and encourage efforts aimed at self-improvement. Elder (1987) cited one recorded account of such social comparisons among war veterans:

> When I was in the service ... I picked up a lot of ideas ... about how to live my own life and get more out of it ... You know, you talk with one fellow and he's planning to be a doctor, you talk with another and he's

planning to be a carpenter, and somebody else wants to be an aviator. Well, when you talk these things over with them and get their slant on things, it sort of opens up horizons ... you start thinking in broader terms than you did before. (p. 461)

In the service of self-enhancement, the social comparison process may be complemented by a reflection process (Tesser, 1984). In addition to comparing themselves with others, people may raise their own self-evaluations by pointing out the accomplishments of others with whom they are associated in some way, even if they themselves are not directly responsible for those accomplishments. "Basking in reflected glory" (Cialdini et al., 1976) may be facilitated by the compositional structure of military and work settings that promote psychological closeness between individuals and reward entire groups for the quality of others' performance.

Conclusions

The historian C. Vann Woodward sought to diffuse the controversy over continuity and change by reminding his audience that "however passionate the advocates of the one or the other, they would end (if they lacked the wisdom to begin) with the admission that there would be no history at all without some of both" (1989, p. 43). Longitudinal studies of human development may offer the same tonic for psychology by addressing the dual research agenda: How is continuity possible? How does change occur?

Longitudinal research has taught investigators to treat the continuity of individual differences as a problematic phenomenon requiring both confirmation and explanation. No longer can it be assumed that continuity is guided by inertia. Instead, researchers have learned that there are vigorous processes that promote continuity across the life course. No longer can they assume implicitly that continuities in maladaptive behaviors are simply manifestations of intrapersonal dispositions. Instead, they have learned to seek the explanation for continuity in the interaction between the person and the environment.

My aim in this chapter has been to elucidate some of these processes, with special reference to the problem of antisocial behavior. I have argued that early experiences can set up anticipatory attitudes that lead the individual to project particular interpretations onto new social relationships and ambiguous situations. In particular, antisocial persons *react* to the world in distinct ways; they extract unique subjective psychological environments from their objective surroundings, and it is these subjective environments that shape both their personality and subsequent social interactions. In addition, antisocial people are likely to *evoke* responses from the surrounding environment that confirm and sustain their subjective interpretation of that environment as hostile. And, finally, as self-regulatory capacities increase with age, antisocial people begin to make choices and seek out situations that are compatible with their dispositions. The situations that are most consequential are one's interpersonal environments, and it is in friendship formation and mate selection that the personality-sustaining effects of *proactive* interaction are most apparent in the lives of antisocial individuals. These interactional mechanisms thus set in motion feedback processes that curtail opportunities for change and strengthen the chain of continuity across time and circumstance.

Of course, none of this eliminates the possibility of change. Researchers are gaining instead a finer appreciation of the special conditions under which *systematic* change may be promoted and produced, and they are learning that the situational requisites that define turning points in behavioral development are more specialized than previously thought. The processes promoting continuity are aggressive foes. Those in the mental health professions must now recognize that in order to promote salutary outcomes, they have to do more than provide people with opportunities for change. They also have to eliminate the opportunities that allow active processes of continuity to flourish and to guide the trajectory of the life course.

References

Anderson, K. E., Lytton, H., & Romney, D. M. (1986). Mothers' interactions with normal and conduct-disordered boys: Who affects whom? *Developmental Psychology, 22,* 604–609.

Andrews, J. D. W. (1988). *The active self in psychotherapy: An integration of therapeutic styles.* New York: Gardner Press.

Anthony, E. J., & Cohler, B. J. (1987). *The invulnerable child.* New York: Guilford Press.

Backman, C. W. (1985). Interpersonal congruency theory revisited: A revision and extension. *Journal of Social and Personal Relationships, 2,* 489–505.

Backman, C. W. (1988). The self: A dialectical approach. In L. Berkowitz (Ed.), *Advances in experimental social psychology* (Vol. 21, pp. 229–260). San Diego, CA: Academic Press.

Baker, L. A., Mack, W., Moffitt, T. E., & Mednick, S. A. (1989). Etiology of sex differences in criminal convictions in a Danish adoption cohort. *Behavior Genetics, 19,* 355–370.

Bell, R. Q., & Chapman, M. (1986). Child effects in studies using experimental or brief longitudinal approaches to socialization. *Developmental Psychology, 22,* 595–603.

Billy, J. O. G., Rodgers, J. L., & Udry, R. (1984). Adolescent sexual behavior and friendship choice. *Social Forces, 62,* 653–678.

Billy, J. O. G., & Udry, R. (1985). Patterns of adolescent friendship and effects on sexual behavior. *Social Psychology Quarterly, 48,* 27–41.

Block, J. (1981). Some enduring and consequential structures of personality. In A. I. Rabin, J. Aronoff, A. Barclay, & R. Zucker (Eds.), *Further explorations in personality* (pp. 27–43). New York: Wiley.

Block, J., & Block, J. H. (1980). The role of ego-control and ego-resilience in the organization of behavior. In W. A. Collins (Ed.), *Minnesota Symposia on Child Psychology* (Vol. 13, pp. 39–101). Hillsdale, NJ: Erlbaum.

Boldizar, J. P., Perry, D. G., & Perry, L. C. (1989). Outcome values and aggression. *Child Development, 60,* 571–579.

Bowlby, J. (1973). *Attachment and loss: Vol. 2. Separation.* New York: Basic Books.

Buss, A. H., & Plomin, R. (1984). *Temperament: Early developing personality traits.* Hillsdale, NJ: Erlbaum.

Buss, D. M. (1981). Predicting parent–child interactions from children's activity level. *Developmental Psychology, 17,* 59–65.

Buss, D. M. (1984a). Marital assortment for personality dispositions: Assessment with three different data sources. *Behavior Genetics, 14,* 111–123.

Buss, D. M. (1984b). Toward a psychology of person–environment correspondence: The role of spouse selection. *Journal of Personality and Social Psychology, 47,* 361–377.

Buss, D. M., Block, J. H., & Block, J. (1980). Preschool activity level: Personality correlates and developmental implications. *Child Development, 51,* 401–408.

Cairns, R. B., & Cairns, B. D. (1993). *Adolescence in our time: Lifelines and risks.* Manuscript in preparation.

Cairns, R. B., Cairns, B. D., Neckerman, H. J., Gest, S. D., & Gariepy, J-L. (1988). Social networks and aggressive behavior: Peer support or peer rejection? *Developmental Psychology, 24*, 815–823.

Cairns, R. B., Perrin, J. E., & Cairns, B. D. (1985). Social structure and social cognition in early adolescence: Affiliative patterns. *Journal of Early Adolescence, 5*, 339–355.

Carson, R. C. (1969). *Interaction concepts of personality.* Chicago: Aldine.

Caspi, A., & Bem, D. J. (1990). Personality continuity and change across the life course. In L. Pervin (Ed.), *Handbook of personality theory and research* (pp. 549–575). New York: Guilford Press.

Caspi, A., Bem, D. J., & Elder, G. H., Jr. (1989). Continuities and consequences of interactional styles across the life course. *Journal of Personality, 57*, 375–406.

Caspi, A., Elder, G. H., & Bem, D. J. (1987). Moving against the world: Life-course patterns of explosive children. *Developmental Psychology, 23*, 308–313.

Caspi, A., & Herbener, E. S. (1990). Continuity and change: Assortative marriage and the consistency of personality in adulthood. *Journal of Personality and Social Psychology, 58*, 250–258.

Caspi, A., Herbener, E. S., & Ozer, D. J. (1992). Shared experiences and the similarity of personalities: A longitudinal study of married couples. *Journal of Personality and Social Psychology, 62*, 281–291.

Caspi, A., & Moffitt, T. E. (in press). The continuity of maladaptive behavior: From description to understanding in the study of antisocial behavior. In D. Cicchetti & D. Cohen (Eds.), *Manual of developmental psychopathology.* New York: Wiley.

Caspi, A., & Moffitt, T. E. (in press). When does personality matter? A paradoxical theory of personality coherence. *Psychological Inquiry.*

Caspi, A., Moffitt, T. E., Sampson, R. J., & Laub, J. H. (1993). *The natural history of antisocial behavior: Individual, ecological, and interactional contributions to continuity and change across the life course.* Manuscript in preparation.

Chess, S., & Thomas, A. (1987). *Origins and evolution of behavior disorders: From infancy to early adult life.* Cambridge, MA: Harvard University Press.

Cialdini, R. B., Borden, R. J., Thorne, A., Walker, M. R., Freeman, S., & Sloan, L. R. (1976). Basking in reflected glory: Three (football) field studies. *Journal of Personality and Social Psychology, 34*, 366–375.

Darley, J., & Fazio, R. H. (1980). Expectancy confirmation processes arising in the social interaction sequence. *American Psychologist, 35*, 867–881.

DeFries, J. C., Plomin, R., & Labuda, M. C. (1987). Genetic stability of cognitive development from childhood to adulthood. *Developmental Psychology, 23*, 4–12.

DiLalla, L. F., & Gottesman, I. I. (1989). Heterogeneity of causes for delinquency and criminality: Lifespan perspectives. *Development and Psychopathology, 1*, 339–349.

Dishion, T. J. (1990). The peer context of troublesome child and adolescent behavior. In P. Leone (Ed.), *Understanding troubled and troubling youth* (pp. 128–153). Newbury Park, CA: Sage.

Dodge, K. A. (1980). Social cognition and children's aggressive behavior. *Child Development, 51*, 162–270.

Dodge, K. A. (1986). A social information processing model of social competence in children. In M. Perlmutter (Ed.), *Minnesota Symposia on Child Psychology* (Vol. 18, pp. 77–125). Hillsdale, NJ: Erlbaum.

Dodge, K. A., & Frame, C. L. (1982). Social cognitive biases and deficits in aggressive boys. *Child Development, 53*, 629–635.

Dodge, K. A., & Newman, J. P. (1981). Biased decision-making processes in aggressive boys. *Journal of Abnormal Psychology, 90*, 375–379.

Elder, G. H., Jr. (1986). Military times and turning points in men's lives. *Developmental Psychology, 22*, 233–245.

Elder, G. H., Jr. (1987). War mobilization and the life course. *Sociological Forum, 2*, 449–472.

Elder, G. H., Jr., & Caspi, A. (1990). Studying lives in a changing society: Sociological and personological explorations. In A. Rabin, R. Zucker, R. Emmons, & S. Frank (Eds.), *Studying persons and lives* (pp. 201–247). New York: Springer-Verlag.

Elliott, D. S., & Menard, S. (in press). Delinquent friends and delinquent behavior: Temporal and developmental patterns. In D. Hawkins (Ed.), *Some current theories of deviance and crime.* New York: Springer-Verlag.

Elliott, D. S., & Voss, H. L. (1974). *Delinquency and dropout.* Lexington, MA: Lexington Books.

Epstein, E., & Guttman, R. (1984). Mate selection in man: Evidence, theory, and outcome. *Social Biology, 31*, 243–278.

Epstein, S. (1990). Cognitive-experiential self-theory. In L. Pervin (Ed.), *Handbook of personality: Theory and research* (pp. 165–192). New York: Guilford Press.

Erikson, E. (1959). Identity and the life cycle. *Psychological Issues, 1*, 1–171.

Farrington, D. P., Loeber, R., & van Kammen, W. B. (1990). Long-term criminal outcomes of hyperactivity-impulsivity-attention deficit and conduct problems in childhood. In L. N. Robins & M. R. Rutter (Eds.), *Straight and devious pathways to adulthood* (pp. 62–81). New York: Cambridge University Press.

Festinger, L. (1954). A theory of social comparison processes. *Human Relations, 7*, 117–140.

Furstenberg, Jr., F. F., Brooks-Gunn, J., & Morgan, S. P. (1987). *Adolescent mothers in later life.* New York: Cambridge University Press.

Gal, R. (1986). *A portrait of the Israeli soldier.* Greenwood, CT: Greenwood Press.

Ghodsian-Carpey, J., & Baker, L. A. (1987). Genetic and environmental influences on aggression in 4- to 7-year-old twins. *Aggressive Behavior, 13*, 173–186.

Giordano, P. C., Cernkovich, S. A., & Pugh, M. D. (1986). Friendship and delinquency. *American Journal of Sociology, 91*, 1170–1202.

Greenwald, A. G. (1980). The totalitarian ego: Fabrication and revision of personal history. *American Psychologist, 35*, 603–618.

Hains, A. A., & Ryan, E. B. (1983). The development of social cognitive processes among juvenile delinquents and nondelinquent peers. *Child Development, 54,* 1536–1544.

Huesman, L. R., Eron, L. D., Lefkowitz, M. M., & Walder, L. O. (1984). Stability of aggression over time and generations. *Developmental Psychology, 20,* 1120–1134.

Ickes, W., Snyder, M., & Garcia, S. (in press). Personality influences on the choice of situations. In S. Briggs, R. Hogan, & W. Jones (Eds.), *Handbook of personality psychology.* San Diego, CA: Academic Press.

Inhelder, B., & Piaget, J. (1958). *The growth of logical thinking from childhood to adolescence.* New York: Basic Books.

Kandel, D. (1978). Homophily, selection, and socialization in adolescent friendships. *American Journal of Sociology, 84,* 427–436.

Katz, J. (1989). *Seductions of crime.* New York: Basic Books.

Kazdin, A. E. (1987). *Conduct disorders in childhood and adolescence.* Newbury Park, CA: Sage.

Laub, J. H., & Sampson, R. J. (1988). Unraveling families and delinquency: A reanalysis of the Glueck's data. *Criminology, 26,* 355–380.

Loeber, R., & Stouthamer-Loeber, M. (1986). Family factors as correlates and predictors of juvenile conduct problems and delinquency. In M. Tonry & N. Morris (Eds.), *Crime and justice* (Vol. 7, pp. 29–149). Chicago: University of Chicago Press.

Lynam, D., Moffitt, T. E., & Stouthamer-Loeber, M. (in press). Explaining the relations between IQ and delinquency: Class, race, test motivation, school failure, or self-control. *Journal of Abnormal Psychology.*

Lytton, H. (1990). Child and parent effects in boys' conduct disorder: A reinterpretation. *Developmental Psychology, 26,* 683–697.

Maccoby, E. E., & Jacklin, C. N. (1983). The "person" characteristics of children and the family as environment. In D. Magnusson & V. L. Allen (Eds.), *Human development: An interactional perspective* (pp. 75–92). San Diego, CA: Academic Press.

Magnusson, D. (1988). *Individual development from an interactional perspective.* Hillsdale, NJ: Erlbaum.

Markus, H. (1977). Self-schemata and processing information about the self. *Journal of Personality and Social Psychology, 35,* 63–78.

Markus, H., & Cross, S. (1990). The interpersonal self. In L. Pervin (Ed.), *Handbook of personality: Theory and research* (pp. 576–608). New York: Guilford Press.

Mascie-Taylor, C. G. N., & Vandenberg, S. G. (1988). Assortative mating for IQ and personality due to propinquity and personal preference. *Behavior Genetics, 18,* 339–345.

Masten, A., & Garmezy, N. (1985). Risk, vulnerability, and protective factors in developmental psychopathology. In B. B. Lahey & A. E. Kazdin (Eds.), *Advances in clinical child psychology* (Vol. 8, pp. 1–52). New York: Plenum Press.

McCord, J. (1983). A longitudinal study of aggression and antisocial behavior. In K. T. Van Dusen & S. A. Mednick (Eds.), *Prospective studies of crime and delinquency* (pp. 269–276). Boston: Kluwer-Nijhoff.

Mednick, S. A., Gabrielli, W. F., & Hutchings, B. (1984). Genetic factors in criminal behavior: Evidence from an adoption cohort. *Science, 224,* 891–893.

Mednick, S. A., Moffitt, T. E., & Stack, S. A. (Eds.). (1987). *The causes of crime: New biological approaches.* New York: Cambridge University Press.

Meyer, J. W. (1978). The effects of education as an institution. *American Journal of Sociology, 83,* 55–77.

Moffitt, T. E. (1990). The neuropsychology of delinquency: A critical review of theory and research. In N. Morris & M. Tonry (Eds.), *Crime and justice* (Vol. 12, pp. 99–169). Chicago: University of Chicago Press.

Moffitt, T. E., & Mednick, S. (Eds.). (1988). *Biological contributions to crime causation.* Dordrecht, The Netherlands: Martinus Nijhoff.

Nasby, W., Hayden, B., & DePaulo, B. M. (1979). Attributional bias among aggressive boys to interpret unambiguous social stimuli as displays of hostility. *Journal of Abnormal Psychology, 89,* 459–468.

Ohlin, L., & Blumstein, A. (1988). *Final report of the desistence-persistence working group.* Castine, ME: Castine Research, Program on Human Development and Criminal Behavior.

Patterson, G. R. (1982). *Coercive family process.* Eugene, OR: Castalia.

Patterson, G. R. (1986). Performance models for antisocial boys. *American Psychologist, 41,* 432–444.

Patterson, G. R., & Bank, L. (1990). Some amplifying mechanisms for pathologic processes in families. In M. Gunnar (Eds.), *Minnesota Symposium on Child Psychology* (Vol. 22, pp. 167–209). Hillsdale, NJ: Erlbaum.

Perry, D. G., Kusel, S. J., & Perry, L. C. (1988). Victims of peer aggression. *Developmental Psychology, 24,* 807–814.

Perry, D. G., Perry, L. C., & Rasmussen, P. (1986). Cognitive social learning mediators of aggression. *Child Development, 57,* 700–711.

Pianta, R. C., Sroufe, L. A., & Egeland, B. (1989). Continuity and discontinuity in maternal sensitivity at 6, 24, and 42 months in a high risk sample. *Child Development, 60,* 481–487.

Plomin, R. (1986). *Development, genetics, and psychology.* Hillsdale, NJ: Erlbaum.

Plomin, R. (1990). The role of inheritance in behavior. *Science, 248,* 183–188.

Plomin, R., & Bergeman, C. S. (1991). The nature of nurture: Genetic influence on "environmental" measures. *Behavioral and Brain Sciences, 14,* 373–386.

Plomin, R., & Nesselroade, J. R. (1990). Behavioral genetics and personality change. *Journal of Personality, 58,* 191–220.

Plomin, R., Nitz, K., & Rowe, D. C. (1990). Behavioral genetics and aggressive behavior in childhood. In M. Lewis & S. M. Miller (Eds.), *Handbook of developmental psychopathology* (pp. 119–133). New York: Plenum Press.

Quinton, D., & Rutter, M. (1988). *Parenting breakdown: The making and breaking of intergenerational links.* Aldershot, England: Avebury.

Richman, N., Stevenson, J., & Graham, P. J. (1982). *Pre-school to school: A behavioural study.* San Diego, CA: Academic Press.

Roberts, G. C., Block, J. H., & Block, J. (1984). Continuity and change in parents' child rearing practices. *Child Development, 55,* 587–597.

Rowe, D. C. (1987). Resolving the person–situation debate: Invitation to an interdisciplinary dialogue. *American Psychologist, 42,* 218–227.

Rowe, D. C., & Osgood, D. W. (1984). Heredity and sociological theories of delinquency: A reconsideration. *American Sociological Review, 49,* 526–540.

Rushton, J. P., Fulker, D. W., Neale, M. C., Nias, D. K. B., & Eysenck, H. J. (1986). Altruism and aggression: The heritability of individual differences. *Journal of Personality and Social Psychology, 50,* 1192–1198.

Rutter, M. (1987). Psychosocial resilience and protective mechanisms. *American Journal of Orthopsychiatry, 57,* 316–331.

Rutter, M. (1988). *Studies of psychosocial risk: The power of longitudinal data.* Cambridge, England: Cambridge University Press.

Rutter, M., Quinton, D., & Hill, J. (1990). Adult outcome of institution-reared children: Males and females compared. In L. N. Robins & M. R. Rutter (Eds.), *Straight and devious pathways to adulthood* (pp. 134–157). New York: Cambridge University Press.

Sampson, R. J., & Laub, J. H. (1990). Crime and deviance over the life course: The salience of adult social bonds. *American Sociological Review, 55,* 609–627.

Sampson, R. J., & Laub, J. H. (in press-a). Crime in the life course. *Annual Review of Sociology.*

Sampson, R. J., & Laub, J. H. (in press-b). *Unraveling crime and deviance: Informal social control and the life course.* Cambridge, MA: Harvard University Press.

Scarr, S., & McCartney, K. (1983). How people make their own environments: A theory of genotype → environment effects. *Child Development, 54,* 424–435.

Secord, P. F., & Backman, C. W. (1965). Interpersonal approach to personality. In B. H. Maher (Ed.), *Progress in experimental personality research* (Vol. 2, pp. 91–125). San Diego, CA: Academic Press.

Slaby, R. G., & Guerra, N. G. (1988). Cognitive mediators of aggression in adolescent offenders: 1. Assessment. *Developmental Psychology, 24,* 580–588.

Snyder, M. (1984). When beliefs create reality. In L. Berkowitz (Ed.), *Advances in experimental social psychology* (Vol. 18, pp. 248–305). San Diego, CA: Academic Press.

Snyder, M., & Ickes, W. (1985). Personality and social behavior. In E. Aronson & G. Lindzey (Eds.), *Handbook of social psychology* (Vol. 2, pp. 883–947) New York: Random House.

Sullivan, S. (1953). *The interpersonal theory of psychiatry.* New York: Norton.

Swann, W. B., Jr. (1983). Self-verification: Bringing social reality into harmony with the self. In J. Suls & A. B. Greenwald (Eds.), *Psychological perspectives on the self* (Vol. 2, pp. 33–66). Hillsdale, NJ: Erlbaum.

Swann, W. B., Jr. (1987). Identity negotiation: Where two roads meet. *Journal of Personality and Social Psychology, 53,* 1035–1051.

Tellegen, A., Lykken, D. T., Bouchard, T. J., Wilcox, K. J., Segal, N. L., & Rich, S. (1988). Personality similarity in twins reared apart and together. *Journal of Personality and Social Psychology, 6,* 1031–1039.

Tesser, A. (1984). Self-evaluation maintenance processes: Implications for relationships and for development. In J. C. Masters & K. Yarkin-Levin (Eds.), *Boundary areas in social and developmental psychology* (pp. 271–299). San Diego, CA: Academic Press.

Thomas, W. I., & Thomas, D. (1928). *The child in America.* New York: Knopf.

Tomkins, S. (1986). Script theory. In J. Aronoff, A. I. Rabin, & R. A. Zucker (Eds.), *The emergence of personality* (pp. 147–216). New York: Springer.

Wachtel, P. L. (1977). *Psychoanalysis and behavior therapy.* New York: Basic Books.

West, D. J. (1982). *Delinquency.* Cambridge, MA: Harvard University Press.

Wilson, J. Q., & Herrnstein, R. J. (1985). *Crime and human nature.* New York: Simon & Schuster.

Wills, T. A. (1981). Downward comparison principles in social psychology. *Psychological Bulletin, 90,* 245–270.

Wohlwill, J. (1980). Cognitive development in childhood. In O. G. Brim, Jr., & J. Kagan (Eds.), *Continuity and change in human development* (pp. 359–444). Cambridge, MA: Harvard University Press.

Wood, J. (1989). Theory and research concerning social comparisons of personal attributes. *Psychological Bulletin, 106,* 231–248.

Woodward, C. V. (1989, February 20). That noble dream: The "objectivity question" and the American historical profession. *The New Republic,* p. 40.

Zuckerman, M. (1979). *Sensation seeking: Beyond the optimal level of arousal.* Hillsdale, NJ: Erlbaum.

CHAPTER 16

Vulnerability and Resilience

Norman Garmezy

I t was a privilege to be invited to write a chapter in a book honoring a dear friend, Jack Block, one that also honors, via attachment and collaborative as well as singular achievements, the research of Jack's lifetime research partner and wife, Jeanne Block. In paying tribute to Jack's contributions to psychological science, I also feel it necessary to recognize the seminal influences generated by one of the most productive and honored research and marital partnerships in the history of contemporary psychology.

Jack and Jeanne deserve the honorifics reflected in the writings of those who have contributed to this volume. However, most of all, I prefer the tribute rendered to Jeanne by her lifelong companion in his foreword

Appreciation is expressed to the William T. Grant Foundation and the John D. and Catherine T. MacArthur Foundation for support for this research.

to her book, *Sex Role Identity and Ego Development* (J. H. Block, 1984). Jack wrote,

> The achievements in thinking and writing reflected in this work Jeanne accomplished over a period spanning less than a decade—while her scientific and professional life was extremely active, while she was the prime mover of a monumental longitudinal study of personality and cognitive development, while she was engaged with large family responsibilities and pleasures, and while she was buffeted by a chronic illness early understood to be ominous. My partner in life and in science for thirty-two years, Jeanne died of cancer after a long and gallant struggle. If hers was a life fatefully, unfairly, cut short, it was also a life extraordinarily full, lived with zest and wisdom. She was a woman of valor, grace, intelligence, verve, warmth and love. I miss and our children miss her heartening presence. But for us and for all who knew her, the meaning and usefulness of her life extend beyond us through her work to a better understanding of how our society shapes its children into the women and men they become. (J. Block, 1984, pp. xii–xiii)

In honoring Jack and Jeanne, this book makes overt the appreciation of researchers for their unerring longitudinal study of personality development, begun initially with young boys and girls who are now in young adulthood. For 30 years the Blocks developed the personality constructs of ego-control and ego-resiliency. If there is an awakening in the United States today as to the nature and content of resilience, it would appear to be a function of two elements: (a) a growing appreciation of a latent construct that can be termed *adaptability* and (b) an awareness of the omnipresent qualities of various types of competencies that appear to serve as protective factors despite the presence of risk reflected in deviant families, distorted rearing practices, family poverty, and the stress of disadvantaged ecologies. This shift from the hitherto dominant emphasis on psychopathology under these deviant conditions might well have occurred earlier if sufficient attention had been paid to the Blocks' research on ego-control and ego-resiliency. These twin constructs were formulated some 40 years ago in Jack's (1950) doctoral dissertation on the construct of ego-control and in Jeanne's (1951) dissertation a year later on the topological representation of ego structure. This early research provided the seed ground for the current excitement about resiliency. Today, it elicits for many an image of drama, whereas for the Blocks four decades earlier it was cast in the rightful image of science.

In the content that follows I will examine the nature of vulnerability indicators and the contributions to the construct derived from studies of children of schizophrenic and of affectively disordered parentage. Attention to the current emergence of a growing interest in resilience follows accompanied by the Blocks' contributions via their constructs of ego-control and ego-resilience.

Vulnerability and Resilience

I have chosen as my contribution to this book a discussion of the twin constructs of vulnerability and resilience. Vulnerability represents, on the one hand, a heightened probability for maldevelopment ostensibly because of the presence of a single or of multiple risk factors. Whereas vulnerability provides a singular emphasis on risk elements, resilience is defined by the presence of any or many of these self-same risk factors, but the accompanying adaptive outcomes are now presumed to be a function of evident, or unidentified, positive elements within the individual and external environments that serve a protective function.

Epidemiology has fostered the extensive knowledge of risk factors. In the most basic definitional sense, "epidemiology is concerned with the patterns of disease occurrence in human populations and of the factors that influence these patterns" (Lilienfeld & Lilienfeld, 1980). These factors are diverse and can include genetic, biological, behavioral, sociocultural, economic, and demographic variables. These often form the base for etiological studies of diseases and their processes of activation and sustainment.

Clinical epidemiology is the application of epidemiological principles and methods to problems in clinical medicine. In many ways, the epidemiologist is similar in orientation to the behavioral scientist in the emphasis on hypothesis generation accompanied by tests of these hypotheses with groups of individuals. Because the emphasis, however, is on pathogenesis, potential causative agents with a disease-oriented goal, the epidemiologist does differ from the behavioral scientist, whose orientation in stress research, as an example, is not solely on the disordered or the maladroit but on those who, despite exposure to risk factors, continue along a path of positive adaptation.

Furthermore, both groups are interested in repeated observations, often in varying circumstances, in order to test the power or efficacy of a given risk factor. It is under such multiple conditions of exposure to risk that differentiation is sought between victim and survivor. Once identified, the questions that are central reflect *how* and *what* inquiries rather than *why*. It is at this point that the study of resilience loses its newspaper or magazine heraldry and gets down to the hard bedrock of scientific search. And here one finds the danger of disappointment for those who embrace the construct as inherently valid. At the International Society for the Study of Behavioral Development's (ISSBD) meetings in 1991, I participated in a conversation hour devoted to resilience. I began my presentation with the statement that resilience has for each of us a personal validation—we know resilient people or we confirm the construct with stories reported in newspapers or via television that give personal testimony to the triumph of the individual capable of "overcoming the odds" (Werner & Smith, 1992). Often, these are seen as the heroes of society, yet the very drama of their achievements is to be resisted lest it confound the scientific challenge. That is the warning, and it is accompanied by the critical question: Where do researchers stand in their studies of vulnerability and resilience, and what are the contexts for such studies?

Genetic Vulnerabilities

First, there is vulnerability with particular reference to potential genetic factors. Increasingly, studies of the major psychiatric disorders appear to provide a partial but sturdy image of the role of genetics. Most striking is bipolar disorder; schizophrenia, too, earns a secondary but significant place in terms of underlying genetic elements. Genetic studies of high-risk families, concordance rates for monozygotic (MZ) versus dizygotic (DZ) pairs and MZ pairs reared apart provide stimulating evidence that there is a gene or genes that heighten the probability of developing one of these serious mental disorders if the disorder is markedly present in the family genealogy. Gershon (1988) made this evident in his research devoted to the discovery of specific risk factors and genetic linkage markers in the affective disorders.

Referring to the distinction drawn from family study data in which symptoms were evaluated in depressed relatives of bipolar and unipolar patients, Gershon (1988) noted the following:

> The underlying assumption was that the depressed relatives of normal controls were more likely to represent sporadic cases, whereas depressed relatives of affective patients were, by definition, familial cases. The two types of depression did differ clinically in the sense that the presence of severe impairment or incapacitation occurred more often in the familial cases, the duration was longer, and there were more frequent multiple episodes. (p. 128)

Furthermore, the incidence rates in biological relatives of adoptive patients is higher than for adoptive relatives. The predisposition, however, is separate for chronic schizophrenia, suggesting that the two disorders, although manifestly genetic in transmission, are distinctly different forms of mental disorder.

Thus, there is evidence for a genetic bifurcation between affective disorders and schizophrenia. On the other hand, other studies have shown evidence that in MZ twins concordant for affective disorders, there are indications of discordance for polarity in which one twin has the bipolar disease and the other suffers from a unipolar disorder (i.e., depression only). The same findings hold for first-degree relatives with bipolar patients having more unipolar first-degree relatives than bipolar ones. This type of genetic overlap has suggested the operation of the same genetic diathesis. At this point no genetic marker has been found that would both identify and specify the genetic risk, but the future is brightened by fundamental advances in neurogenetics.

Reider and Gershon (1978) have suggested certain criteria in identifying a genetic marker. Such criteria are significant because it is evident from MZ studies that concordance rates as such suggest that there are those with a biological vulnerability to the disorder who do not manifest illness. These are the discordant pairs of MZ twins, and the reasons for the discordance have not been truly explored. For these investigators, just as environmental and heterogeneous genetic factors can coexist in the etiology of mental retardation, so, too, may they exist in psychiatric disorders. Reider and Gershon recognized that there are likely to coexist primary factors that can be represented in a single gene or by interactions with other genes that may affect neurophysiological or psychological attributes. Contributing factors could play a role in potentiating the disorder. In consequence, stated Reider and Gershon, having a primary genetic factor for schizophrenia would not necessarily eventuate in disorder. However, they added, those who have the primary factor should contribute more to the schizophrenia pool than would those drawn from a random sample serving as controls who lack that factor. In sum, a genetic marker must (a) heighten the probability of a psychiatric illness; (b) not be the result of the disorder but a heritable factor in developing the illness; and (c) be observable in the well state and able to be independently determined in both wellness and illness.

Environmental Vulnerabilities

What, then, about the play of environmental variables? Discordant twin pairs suggest the potential operation of such factors, but twin studies do not appear to be the optimum roadway into the problem. Gottesman and Shields (1972), in a definitive study and evaluation of twins using hospital data, mental status interviews, neuropsychological tests, personality inventories, and so forth, reached several tentative conclusions accompanied by some pessimism about the dilemma of resolving the potential role of environmental factors. They reported that very little distinguishes the sick from the healthy other than the illness. Personality factors such as submissiveness reflect more the nature of twin pairing rather than disorder-heightening potential. The environmental range for twins tends not to be highly differentiated.

The "high-risk" paradigm so much in vogue more than a decade ago (Watt, Anthony, Wynne, & Rolf, 1984) has not provided a powerful set for differentiation. Gottesman and Shields (1972) made clear an obvious reality: Most schizophrenic adults are not twins, and few are reared by schizophrenic parents. They concluded that environmental stressors have proved to be too idiosyncratic and that "there are limitations to the resolving power of the twin method for highlighting environmental factors of general importance and specificity even with identical twins discordant for schizophrenia" (p. 314).

However, environmental influences may yet appear. There are two major long-term studies that have tracked the children of schizophrenic parents into adulthood. One is the study conducted in Denmark by Mednick and Schulsinger (1968; Mednick, Parnas, & Schulsinger, 1987; Mednick & Silverton, 1988; Schulsinger, 1976) and their colleagues; the second is the research conducted by Erlenmeyer-Kimling et al. (1990) and Erlenmeyer-Kimling, Golden, and Cornblatt (1989) in New York City. This investigative team has reported their earlier results (1984) with cohorts now grown to adulthood. Although these studies will not shed light on the twin data, they may in time report differentiators among more adaptive and ill adults who were the children of schizophrenic parents (Watt et al., 1984).

Linking Vulnerabilities

The issue of risk status, however, has brought forth a research movement that combines psychobiological and psychological inquiry presumed to have been imposed on the genetic substrate. This took the form of a research consortium focused on children at risk for schizophrenia that was composed of laboratories primarily located in the United States but also represented by programs in Denmark, Finland, Norway, Canada, Israel, and Switzerland. A partial culmination of this consortium was an extensive volume *(Children at Risk for Schizophrenia: A Longitudinal Perspective)* edited by Norman Watt, E. J. Anthony, L. C. Wynne, and J. Rolf (1984) in which all research groups presented their basic findings. Basically, the consortium sought to add to the database in the search for etiological or, more appropriately, predisposing factors in children of schizophrenic parents. The target was the discovery of vulnerabilities, those hypothesized risk factors that antedated the disorder, via cues selected in considerable part from psychology's armamentarium of measures. None were far-fetched and all were built on either reasonable rationales or, in some cases, the use of demonstrably relevant factors in adult schizophrenia to study child and adolescent vulnerabilities. In other cases there were factors that might have conduced to disabilities in functional competence and were possible precursors to more severe psychiatric disorders.

In an earlier book, *Child Personality and Psychopathology: Current Topics*, I provided a chapter on the children who were vulnerable to psychopathology (Garmezy, 1975). Reports of deviant early neurological development and visual motor impairment, plus obstetrical complications in infants at risk, were among the contents that marked the studies of children at risk for schizophrenia. The tabulation of dependent variables covered 6 pages of central variables that ranged across neurological assessments; Piagetian tasks; psychophysiology; attentional studies; psychological assessments; school observations; social behavior; electrophysiology; motor tasks; developmental tasks of arousal, autonomic functioning, and vestibular functioning; mother–child interaction; cognitive styles; competence measures; birth and obstetrical data; infant temperament; maternal attitudes toward pregnancy; neurological assessments; school records; peer sociometric ratings; biochemical measures reflecting catecholamine metabolism; word association tasks; pediatric assessments; court records; social competence; family process variables; and so forth. The list evokes a laundry-list quality, yet virtually all of these dependent variables presented a reasonable justification for their inclusion. This plentitude of riches, in part, stemmed from ignorance based on the lack of longitudinal studies of the life course of individuals who became schizophrenic. That is a general statement regarding the absence of a longitudinal skein for at-risk people. Furthermore, virtually all early studies were retrospective, and content from the great psychiatric leaders were in short supply.

With the developmental tradition so aptly represented in this volume, I pause to present a bit of Emil Kraepelin. In 1919 in a volume titled *Dementia Praecox and Paraphrenia*, Kraepelin wrote a masterly 250-

page description of the phenomenology of schizophrenia that I cited at the Second Rochester International Conference on Schizophrenia (Wynne, Cromwell, & Matthysse, 1978). A final chapter, of only 4-½ pages titled "How to Combat Schizophrenia," contained Kraepelin's longitudinal backward extension of the factors influencing the development of schizophrenia. Here in 199 words is the commentary based on retrospective evidence of one of the true giants in the history of psychiatry:

> In children of such characteristics as we so very frequently find in the previous history of dementia praecox one might think of an attempt at prophylaxis especially if the malady had been already observed in the parents or brothers or sisters. Whether it is possible in such circumstances to ward off the outbreak of the threatening disease, we do not know. But in any case it will be advisable to promote to the utmost of one's power general bodily development and to avoid one-sided training in brain work; as it may well be assumed that a vigorous body grown up under natural conditions will be in a better position to overcome the danger than a child exposed to the influences of effeminacy, or poverty, of exact routine, and especially of city education. Childhood spent in the country with plenty of open air, bodily exercise, escalation beginning late without ambitious aim, [and] simple food would be the principal points to keep in view. (Kraepelin, 1919, p. 279)

Then, with reference to another psychiatric great, Adolf Meyer (Lief, 1948), Kraepelin concluded that "Meyer, who regards dementia praecox essentially as the effect of unfavorable influences of life and education on personalities with abnormal dispositions, hopes by all these measures to be able to prevent the development of the malady" (p. 279).

Quite old-fashioned in wording, Kraepelin (1919), as I pointed out 15 years ago, had provided a first pass at implicating factors that are now assumed to be related to children vulnerable to schizophrenia. First, there is the genetic emphasis—"the malady observed in parent, brothers, and sisters." Second, the genetic hypothesis is joined by specific environmental stressors: the lack of participation in a world of activity; excessive rumination and reflection ("brain work" as "a retreat from participation"); a failure to engage in social and sexual activities that reflect the normative developmental phase of adolescence; compulsive routines; problems of sexual identity; overideational reflectiveness sans activity; compulsivity; and the great stressor in America from the 1970s and into the 1990s of the correlates that accompany lower social class and poverty status.

The important element in these contents is the evidence of the early seed ground for the life span developmental view that would later become evident in the children-at-risk research programs. The point is that these multiple and variable tasks had a thread that linked them to the disorder, one it was hoped would provide clues via the longitudinal study of the antecedents to schizophrenia. Although some served to differentiate across comparison groups, many did not. It was a round-robin of potential risk factors but not a determinate resolution of the isolation of specific vulnerabilities.

Affective Disorders and Vulnerability Indicators

An interesting comparison is afforded by more recent studies of children at risk for affective disorders (Downey & Coyne, 1990; Hammen et al., 1991; Orvaschel, 1983). The contrast is striking, for unlike the outpouring of variables appropriated to children seen in the schizophrenia-at-risk domain, the study of precursors to affective disorders seems to focus on the validation of the disorder in children. Because this linkage has now gained validity, researchers can turn to the major task that lies ahead. However, the uncertainty in previous years of the appropriateness of attaching depression to children has left its mark in the form of a significant delay in studying the attributes of these children (Garmezy & Masten, in press).

The elements in this disparity between research on children at risk for schizophrenia versus the depressive disorders are interesting in terms of differential precedents in the two disorders: (a) The literature of adult schizophrenia for at least a half century reveals a strong psychological laboratory orientation influenced by the presence of pioneering psychopathologists that has been lacking in studies of early influencing factors in the affective disorders; (b) the issue of both a theoretical and empirical challenge, at least until recently, as to whether childhood depression exists has provided a more turbulent history of early disbelief prior to the emergence of the children-at-risk studies; and (c) there have been comparatively few clinical and experimental psychologists in the 1960s and 1970s who focused on affective disorder in contrast to many who were clearly identified with and influenced the experimental laboratory study of schizophrenia in the search for the roots of behavioral deficits in the disorder.

Now having affirmed the reality of childhood depression, one can see the emergence of studies of adaptive and maladaptive children at risk for affective disorders (Downey & Coyne, 1990; Hammen et al., 1987; Hammen, Burge, & Adrian, 1991; Hammen, Burge, & Stansbury, 1990; Orvaschel, 1983). What will undoubtedly follow will be the amassing of laboratory-oriented studies of the performance of these at-risk children.

However, the question that will remain will be, "What should be studied?" A likely beginning point could be drawn by an age-downward assessment of precursors of diagnostic signs and symptoms that are associated with the affective disorders of adult life. For example, one might begin with the affectively laden emergent behavioral and feeling-state indicators that are characteristic of the disorder and look for early signs of their presence in at-risk children. This at-risk group would be compared with a substantial normative comparison group to provide basal differentiators (were these to exist) drawn from such at-risk pioneering studies.

As genetic studies of affective disorders broaden to include more readily acquired family genealogies, it seems evident that investigations are likely to incorporate a continuum of risk factors based on incidence and prevalence data for affective disorder not only in parents and grandparents but in other first-degree relatives as well. Using the focus of children at risk for depressive disorders, a beginning point likely would lie in the study of diagnostic signs and symptoms (Wetzel, 1984).

One might look into *affectively laden emergent behavioral and feeling-state indicators* in at-risk children such as dysphoric mood, anxiety and apprehension, a sense of inadequacy, fearfulness, anger, guilt, hopelessness, and fatigue (cognitive and physical). Another arena may be *cognitive thought processes* such as negative views of the world, fear and discouragement of the future, recurrent thoughts of death and suicide, low self-esteem, fear of failure, slowed thinking, disinterest in activities and people, anhedonic qualities, inability to concentrate, self-reproach, and so on.

At the behavioral level, Wetzel (1984) noted dependency, submissiveness, poor communication skills, marked inhibition, control by others, withdrawal under frustration, inactivity, slowed motor responsiveness, and agitation under threat of failure. Physical functioning can be manifested by appetite disturbances, low energy level, excessive fatigue not commensurate with age, tension, sex drive disturbance, sleep disturbance, and the like.

What these evident behaviors now require is a downward extension into childhood that embraces age-appropriate tasks presented via age-appropriate methods. Just as behavioral and laboratory observations became the pattern of research of the children-at-risk-for-schizophrenia groups, so, too, can a new set of laboratory and behavioral studies be generated and initially tested for their reliability and validity via studies performed across laboratories.

A major problem looms—the lack of normative data on these potentially useful variables across different age groups of children. This lack reduces the investigator to between-groups comparisons. However, just as researchers have available distributions of intelligence test and achievement test data across ages, they also need other sets of data central to at-risk studies. These data are often lacking in nonrisk children, and their absence is another containing factor in advancing knowledge of the performance of children at risk for depressive disorders.

Poverty: The Correlate of Vulnerability

I end this brief discussion of psychopathology now to give attention to a far more pressing issue of vulnerabilities than is provided by the major mental disorders. It is the issue of poverty and its consequences for America. Here, indeed, is the seed ground for cumulative chronic adversities that are the precursors to psychiatric vulnerability. I illustrate the problem with Figure 1, which represents the transgenerational effects of poverty across successive generations. It is taken from a book pub-

DISADVANTAGED CHILDREN

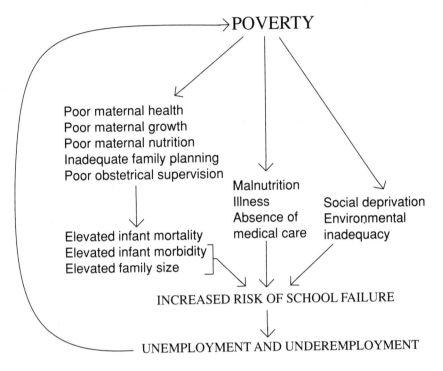

FIGURE 1. A transgenerational model of poverty and its consequences and correlates. From Birch and Gussow (1970). Reprinted with permission.

lished more than two decades ago written by Birch, a distinguished pe-
diatrician–researcher, and Gussow (1970). They titled the book *Disadvantaged children: Health, nutrition, and school failure.* The content
and viewpoint set forth in this volume has equivalent or perhaps even
greater significance today.

Birch provided an illustrative generational model of the consequences and correlates of poverty. From the knowledge base available
today, it may well be called a transgenerational model of poverty (Garmezy, 1991).

The most significant element in the figure is the additive pattern of
chronic adversities (Garmezy & Masten, in press) that accompany pov-

erty. The significance of the Birch and Gussow (1970) diagram lies in the cumulating life stressors of children born into poverty and their consequences for development. These multiple stressors exceed similar cumulative counts of children at risk for mental disorder evident in research conducted by Rutter (1979), Kolvin, Miller, Fleeting, and Kolvin (1988), and Sameroff, Seifer, and Zax (1982).

Birch and Gussow (1970) pointed to the cyclical nature of poverty, its locus in impoverished environments, including the fetal environment, poor health, school dropout, inadequate employment or unemployment, and so on. Poverty today is a cancer that is eating at the very spirit of America, and its correlates are near universal: poor maternal health and nutrition; infant mortality (the United States is now ranked 24th in the world, a slippage that accelerated during the past decade); poor health status; school dropout; shortened life span development; inadequate medical care (reflected, in part, by the hospital closings that are taking place in inner cities); the deterioration of the neighborhoods; the rise of drugs and violence, and so forth.

When Rutter and Madge wrote *Cycles of Disadvantage* (1976) 6 years later, their British statistical data paralleled Birch and Gussow's (1970) findings. Their study also implicated intergenerational continuity that emphasized the situational, sociological, geographical, and familial continuities of poverty with a frequency of outcome in *some* families, reviewed across two generations, that included crime and psychiatric disorder.

However, here is the hopeful sign, and it brings this chapter to the nature of resilience, the second portion of its title. Rutter and Madge (1976) reported that half of the children living under conditions of disadvantage did not repeat that pattern in their own adult lives. On the other hand, there were others who moved downward from more provident life circumstances. When the consequences of disadvantage were examined over *three* generations, the case for intergenerational continuity was further weakened—a hopeful augury.

The Nature of Resilience

Investigators have arrived at the most significant of questions: Among the disadvantaged, what factors influence upward mobility? What factors influence decline? Long and Vaillant's (1984) follow-up study of the Glueck and Glueck (1950) investigations of delinquency sheds some light on these two questions. They traced the midlife outcomes of 456 inner-city men who had been reared as children in families marked by extreme poverty and a chaotic family life. Initially, the investigators created four categories of families: (a) chronically dependent; (b) multiproblem; (c) nondependent, nonproblem; and (d) Social Class V group—the lowest in the social stratum but neither dependent nor multiproblem in the familial pattern.

The delinquent multiproblem group on follow-up was clearly on a downgrade and located in the lower category. A control group in childhood had not been known to the police. On review, the family lives of the controls were stable, as was their employment. Many of the children reared in poverty had escaped their parents' social class confines. In sum, even the transmission of a parental chaotic life-style was neither a necessary nor a sufficient condition for predicting status outcome in later life.

Why this more hopeful augury from the past? For Long and Vaillant (1984), there was a specific set of protective factors (which one cannot liken to America's present economic crisis). In the late 1940s, employment levels were high, America's wealth was on the rise, midlevel jobs were plentiful, and millions of soldiers returning from World War II had been offered and accepted occupational training under the GI Bill. Contrast this with the Gulf war with Iraq, after which many American soldiers faced forced dismissal from the service and entry into a stagnant economy marked by high unemployment and minimum-wage jobs.

Yet, despite the presence of these factors, the Long and Vaillant (1984) findings may yet be replicable. A review of the literature on resilience (Garmezy, 1985; Werner & Smith, 1982, 1992) suggests the presence of three core factors (there are others as yet unexplored) that may operate as protective factors for individuals in stressful life situations. One set implicates temperament and personality attributes such as activity level, reflectiveness when confronted with new situations, cognitive skills, and positive responsiveness to others. Another core of variables is to be found in families, including those in poverty: warmth, cohesion, and the presence of some caring adult, such as a grandparent who assumes a parental role in the absence of responsive parents or if there is marital discord or dissolution between the parents.

A third factor is the availability of social support. This can come in the form of a strong mother substitute, a concerned teacher, a caring agency, institution, or a church that fosters a child's tie to the larger nondelinquent community.

The study of resilience has been advanced by Werner and Smith, whose longitudinal study of the children of Kauai, Hawaii (Werner, Bierman, & French, 1971; Werner & Smith, 1977) is the most significant long-term longitudinal study (30-plus years) in this area. Werner and her colleagues' developmental observations, which have been noted and described over a span of four books that stretched from the prenatal period to adulthood, are supportive of the three broad factors outlined earlier. They wrote of the rewards that can accompany a beleaguered child of competence and determination as well as a belief system whereby a child grown to adulthood can meet a stressful external world.

With regard to families, I point to this source as the critical element for the development of sustaining competencies in the child. Families, by appropriate modeling and support, provide the base for social competence and the demands for needed academic competence. Their involvement implicates building within the child familial responsibilities and values that carry over into the school situation. Clark (1983), in his book titled *Family Life and School Achievement: Why Poor Black Children Succeed or Fail,* wrote of 17 patterns in the homes of high- and low-achieving children that differentiated the groups. I suggest that only a few of these elements provide an image of nurturance and support that is likely to be basic for the development in children, including those in poverty, of a sense of personal power and achievement motivation. Here are some of the factors that Clark perceived as characteristic in home or in school of successful poor Black children:

1. Frequent school contact is initiated by parents.

2. The school's teachers are stimulating and supportive.

3. Parents expect to play a major role in the child's schooling and expect the child to do likewise.

4. Parents establish clear, specific role boundaries and status structures while serving as the dominant authority.

5. Conflict between family members is infrequent.

6. Parents frequently engage in deliberate achievement-training activities.

7. Parents exercise firm, consistent mentoring and rule enforcement.

8. Parents provide liberal nurturance and support.

9. Parents are able to defer to the child's knowledge on intellectual matters.

Clark's (1983) observations add to the consistency of those factors now evident in the literature on resilience. They parallel the seminal work of Comer (1980). Researchers can more firmly establish the correlates of the adaptive child in poverty by a systematic investigation of such children and their families. Although the influencing factors are even now becoming evident, the nature of the underlying processes is still unknown. Furthermore, researchers have not yet looked to the biological attributes of these children, to their social environments, or to the external contexts that relate to their survivorship.

The Construct of Ego-Resiliency: Its Relatedness to Vulnerability and Adaptation

The research agenda that links to survivorship owes a great deal to the decades-long research of Jack and Jeanne Block (J. H. Block & Block, 1980) and their concepts of ego structure, ego-resilience, and ego-control. Their long-term longitudinal study has provided strong evidence of the resiliency construct, and I seek in closing to make evident the pioneering nature of their research contributions to the current interest in vulnerability and to resistance to stress.

In a major review article, J. H. Block and Block (1980) set forth the meaning they had assigned to the construct of ego-resilience and its relatedness to other concepts such as mobility, cognitive controls, competence, and coping and coping strategies. A critical paragraph provides the salience of their construct to the properties currently assigned to *resiliency, vulnerability,* and *risk and protective factors.*

> Ego-resiliency, when dimensionalized, is defined at one extreme by re-sourceful adaptation to changing circumstances and environmental con-tingencies, analysis of the "goodness of fit" between situational demands and environmental contingencies, and flexible invocation of the available repertoire of problem-solving strategies ("problem-solving" being defined to include the social and personal domains as well as the cognitive). The opposite end of the ego-resilience continuum (ego-brittleness) implies lit-tle adaptive flexibility, an inability to respond to the dynamic require-ments of the situation, a tendency to perseverate or to become disorgan-ized when encountering changed circumstances or when under stress, and a difficulty in recouping after traumatic experiences. (p. 48)

The Blocks surrounded ego-resilience with behavioral elements reflecting the adaptiveness inherent in defining the construct: "resourceful," "in-tegrated performance under stress," multiple "solutions when confronted by a barrier," the ability "to process two or more competing stimuli," "engaged with the world but not subservient to it," and "adaptively organized under environmental presses" (J. H. Block & Block, 1980, pp. 48–49).

By contrast, they perceived the ego-unresilient (brittle) person to be "fixed in his/her established pattern of adaptation," to have "only a small adaptive margin," to be "stereotyped in responding to new situations," "to become immobilized, rigidly repetitive, or behaviorally diffuse under stress," "anxious when confronted by competing demands," "slow to re-cover after stress," and "is disquieted by changes in either the personal psychological environment or the larger world, and cannot modify his/her preferred personal tempo in accordance with reality considerations" (J. H. Block & Block, 1980, p. 48).

Of equal importance in defining their construct was their search for the correlates of resiliency. Here, too, they anticipated the efforts of those who have followed in their path. They wrote the following:

> Experimental influences on ego-resiliency also appear to be substantial. Referencing the longitudinal data collected over many years at the Insti-

tute of Human Development, we found that individuals we would call ego-resilient tended to come from families earlier and independently characterized as having loving, patient, competent, and integrated mothers, free interchange of problems and feelings, sexual compatibility of parents, agreement on values and concern with philosophical and moral issues, among other qualities. (J. H. Block & Block, 1980, p. 51)

In comparing the home life of ego-brittle individuals, the Blocks again provided content now recognized as valid in other contexts: homes that were "conflictful, discordant, with neurotic and anxious mothers ambivalent about their maternal role, and without intellectual or philosophical emphasis, among other qualities" (J. H. Block & Block, 1980, p. 51).

If I have any hesitancy with these descriptive realities, it lies in descriptive leanings that one often associates with middle-class patterns (e.g., "intellectual or philosophical emphasis"). In fact, these very virtues in varied forms have also been reported for families who, despite living under highly disadvantaged economic and social circumstances, strive to set goals and aspirations for their children.

Jack Block and Jeanne Block have been the true pioneers of the emergent area of resilience research. The ongoing longitudinal research program conducted by Jack Block at the University of California, Berkeley, will provide investigators with contents relevant to children's survivorship in an increasingly stressful world, findings that have a demonstrable significance not only for families and communities but also for the nation at large.

References

Birch, H. G., & Gussow, J. D. (1970). *Disadvantaged children: Health, nutrition and school failure.* New York: Grune & Stratton.

Block, J. (1950). *An experimental investigation of the construct of ego-control.* Unpublished doctoral dissertation, Stanford University, Stanford, CA.

Block, J. H. (1951). *An experimental study of a topological representation of ego structure.* Unpublished doctoral dissertation, Stanford University, Stanford, CA.

Block, J. H. (1984). *Sex role identity and ego development.* San Francisco: Jossey-Bass.

Block, J. H., & Block, J. (1980). The role of ego-control and ego-resiliency in the organization of behavior. In W. A. Collins (Eds.), *Development of cognition, affect, and social relations* (Vol. 13, pp. 39–101). Hillsdale, NJ: Erlbaum.

Clark, R. M. (1983). *Family life and school achievement: Why poor black children succeed or fail.* Chicago: Chicago University Press.

Comer, J. P. (1980). *School power.* New York: Free Press.

Downey, G., & Coyne, J. C. (1990). Children of depressed parents: An integrative review. *Psychological Bulletin, 108,* 50–76.

Erlenmeyer-Kimling, L., Cornblatt, B. A., Bassett, A. S., Moldin, S. O., Hilldoff-Adamo, U., & Roberts, S. (1990). High risk children in adolescence and young adulthood: Course of global adjustment. In L. Robins & M. Rutter (Eds.), *Straight and devious pathways from childhood to adulthood* (pp. 351–364). Cambridge, New York: Cambridge University Press.

Erlenmeyer-Kimling, L., Golden, R. R., & Cornblatt, B. A. (1989). A taxometric analysis of cognitive and neuromotor variables in children at risk for schizophrenia. *Journal of Abnormal Psychology, 98,* 201–208.

Garmezy, N. (1975). The experimental study of children vulnerable to psychopathology. In A. Davids (Ed.), *Child personality and psychopathology: Current topics* (Vol. 2, pp. 171–216). New York: Wiley.

Garmezy, N. (1985). Stress-resistant children: The search for protective factors. In J. E. Stevenson (Ed.), *Recent research in developmental psychopathology* (pp. 213–233). Elmsford, NY: Pergamon Press.

Garmezy, N. (1991). Resilience and vulnerability to adverse developmental outcomes associated with poverty. *American Behavioral Scientist, 34,* 416–430.

Garmezy, N., & Masten, A. S. (in press). Chronic adversities. In M. Rutter, L. Hersov, & E. Taylor (Eds.), *Child and adolescent psychiatry: Modern approaches* (3rd ed.). Oxford, England: Blackwell Scientific.

Gershon, E. S. (1988). Discovering biologically specific risk factors and genetic linkage markers in affective disorders. In D. L. Dunner, E. S. Gershon, & J. E. Barrett (Eds.), *Relatives at risk for mental disorder* (pp. 127–141). New York: Raven Press.

Glueck, S., & Glueck, E. (1950). *Unraveling juvenile delinquency.* New York: Commonwealth Fund.

Gottesman, I. I., & Shields, J. (1972). *Schizophrenia and genetics: A twin study vantage point.* San Diego, CA: Academic Press.

Hammen, C., Adrian, C., Gordon, D., Burge, D., Jaenicke, C., & Hiroto, D. (1987). Children of depressed mothers: Maternal strain and symptom predictors of dysfunction. *Journal of Abnormal Psychology, 96,* 190–198.

Hammen, C., Burge, D., & Adrian, C. (1991). Timing of mother and child depression in a longitudinal study of children at risk. *Journal of Consulting and Clinical Psychology, 59,* 341–345.

Hammen, C., Burge, D., & Stansbury, K. (1990). Relationship of mother and child variables to child outcomes in a high-risk sample: A causal modeling analysis. *Developmental Psychology, 26,* 24–30.

Kolvin, I., Miller, F. J. W., Fleeting, M., & Kolvin, P. A. (1988). Risk and protective factors for offending with particular reference to deprivation. In M. Rutter (Ed.), *Studies of psychosocial risk: The power of longitudinal data* (pp. 77–95). Cambridge, England: Cambridge University Press.

Kraepelin, E. (1919). *Dementia praecox and paraphrenia.* Edinburgh, Scotland: Livingston.

Lief, A. (1948). *The commonsense psychiatry of Dr. Adolf Meyer (1945).* New York: McGraw-Hill.

Lilienfeld, A. M., & Lilienfeld, D. E. (1980). *Foundations of epidemiology* (2nd ed.). New York: Oxford University Press.

Long, J. V. F., & Vaillant, G. E. (1984). Natural history of male psychological health: XI. Escape from the underclass. *American Journal of Psychiatry, 141,* 341–346.

Mednick, S. A., Parnas, J., & Schulsinger, F. (1987). The Copenhagen high risk project, 1962–1986. *Schizophrenia Bulletin, 13,* 485–495.

Mednick, S. A., & Schulsinger, F. (1968). Some premorbid characteristics related to breakdown in children with schizophrenic mothers. *Journal of Psychiatric Research, 6,* 267–291.

Mednick, S. A., & Silverton, L. (1988). High-risk studies of the etiology of schizophrenia. In M. T. Tsuang & J. C. Simpson (Eds.), *Handbook of schizophrenia: Nosology, epidemiology and genetics* (Vol. 3, pp. 543–562). New York: Elsevier Science.

Orvaschel, H. (1983). Maternal depression and child dysfunction: Children at risk. In B. B. Lahey & A. E. Kazdin (Eds.), *Advances in clinical psychology* (Vol. 6, pp. 169–197). New York: Plenum Press.

Reider, R. O., & Gershon, E. S. (1978). Genetic strategies in biological psychiatry. *Archives of General Psychiatry, 35,* 866–873.

Rutter, M. (1979). Protective factors in children's responses to stress and disadvantage. In M. W. Kent & J. E. Rolf (Eds.), *Primary prevention of psychopathology: Social competence in children* (Vol. 3, pp. 49–74). Hanover, NH: University Press of New England.

Rutter, M., & Madge, N. (1976). *Cycles of disadvantage: A review of research.* London: Heinemann Educational Books.

Sameroff, A. J., Seifer, R., & Zax, M. (1982). Early development of children at risk for emotional disorder. *Monographs of the Society for Research in Child Development, 47* (7, Serial No. 199).

Schulsinger, H. (1976). A ten-year follow-up of children of schizophrenic mothers. *Acta Psychiatric Scandinavica, 53,* 371–386.

Watt, N., Anthony, E. J., Wynne, L., & Rolf, J. (Eds.). (1984). *Children at risk for schizophrenia: A longitudinal perspective.* Cambridge, England: Cambridge University Press.

Werner, E. E., Bierman, J. M., & French, F. E. (1971). *The children of Kauai.* Honolulu: University of Hawaii Press.

Werner, E. E., & Smith, R. S. (1977). *Kauai's children come of age.* Honolulu: University of Hawaii Press.

Werner, E. E., & Smith, R. S. (1982). *Vulnerable but invincible: A longitudinal study of resilient children and youth.* New York: McGraw-Hill.

Werner, E. E., & Smith, R. S. (1992). *Overcoming the odds: High-risk children from birth to adulthood.* Ithaca, NY: Cornell University Press.

Wetzel, J. W. (1984). *Clinical handbook of depression.* New York: Gardner Press.

Wynne, L. C., Cromwell, R. L., & Matthysse, S. (Eds.). (1978). *The nature of schizophrenia: New approaches to research and treatment.* New York: Wiley.

CHAPTER 17

Implications of Cognitive–Experiential Self-Theory for Personality and Developmental Psychology

Seymour Epstein

C ognitive–experiential self-theory (CEST) is a broadly integrative theory of personality that is compatible with psychodynamic theories of personality, learning theories, phenomenological theories, and modern cognitive views about information processing. It achieves its integrative power through two major assumptions: First, in addition to accepting the Freudian unconscious, it introduces a subconscious system—the experiential system—that is intimately associated with emotional experience and that automatically organizes experience and directs behavior. Second, it integrates the conflicting views on basic sources of motivation of other schools of psychology by assuming the existence of four basic sources of human motivation.

Preparation of this chapter and the research reported in it were supported by National Institute of Mental Health (NIMH) Grant MH 01293 and NIMH Research Scientist Award 5 K05 MH00363 to Seymour Epstein.

In this chapter, I review some of the assumptions of CEST, explore how the experiential system acquires and encodes the constructs in its system at two levels of complexity, and consider the implications of CEST for new directions in research, particularly in personality and developmental psychology.

Basic Assumptions

I begin with a brief summary of the most relevant aspects of CEST. The interested reader can find more detailed accounts elsewhere (e.g., Epstein, 1973, 1980, 1983a, 1991a; Epstein & Erskine, 1983).[1]

According to CEST, people automatically construct an implicit theory of reality that contains a self-theory, a world theory, and connecting propositions. An implicit theory of reality consists of a hierarchical organization of schemata and networks of schemata. Toward the apex of the theoretical structure are highly general, abstract schemata, such as that the self is worthy, people are trustworthy, and the world is basically predictable, controllable, and good. Because of their central role, invalidation of these basic schemata can destabilize the entire personality. Evidence of this is provided by the precursors of personality disorganization in acute schizophrenic reactions (Epstein, 1979a) and in posttraumatic stress disorder (Epstein, 1991b; Horowitz, 1976; McCann & Pearlman, 1990). At the other end of the hierarchy are narrow, situation-specific schemata. Unlike the broader schemata, the narrower ones are readily changed without jeopardizing the stability of the personality structure. Thus, the hierarchical structure of schemata provides a way for the psychic structure to be simultaneously flexible and stable.

There are three major systems for processing information, each operating according to its own inferential rules: the rational system, the experiential system, and the primary-process system. The rational system operates according to socially prescribed rules of inference and evidence that are linear, analytical, and abstract. The experiential system operates according to principles that are holistic, concretive, and associationistic. Behavior is a joint function of the rational and experiential systems. The

---

[1] All Epstein citations refer to S. Epstein unless otherwise noted.

experiential system, unlike the rational system, is intimately related to emotions. The greater the emotional arousal, the more the balance of influence shifts in the direction of the experiential system. Although acquisition of constructs in the experiential system is related to emotional consequences, once a certain way of behaving has become sufficiently practiced, it becomes automated and is thereafter carried out routinely, with minimal emotional arousal (Smith, 1984).

The primary-process system is the system that Freud (1900/1953) inferred from his analysis of dreams. It operates by loose association, symbolic representation, condensation, and displacement. In this chapter, my concern is primarily with the experiential system because this is the system that contains a person's implicit theory of reality that automatically organizes experience, directs behavior, and influences conscious thought.

There are two kinds of schemata in an implicit theory of reality: descriptive schemata and motivational schemata. Descriptive schemata refer to beliefs about what the self and the world are like (e.g., "Authority figures are dangerous"). Motivational schemata refer to beliefs about means–ends relations, (e.g., "If I placate authority figures, they will not harm me"). Schemata of both kinds represent, to a considerable extent, generalizations from emotionally significant past experiences.

Attributes of the Experiential System

The experiential system is a conceptual system that humans share with other higher order animals. It has evolved over millions of years and, accordingly, has highly adaptive properties. It operates in relatively simple as well as in more complex ways. At the simple level, it fosters fast and crude processing of information; at more complex levels, it is a source of intuitive wisdom and creativity.

The experiential system is neither inferior nor superior to the rational system. It is simply a different way of understanding reality. Each system has its advantages and disadvantages, and they can best be used in a supplementary fashion. The experiential system is more rapid, less effortful, and therefore more efficient in many circumstances. The rational system is better suited for abstraction and delay of action. Table 1 shows

TABLE 1

Comparison of the Experiential and Rational Systems

Experiential system	Rational system
1. Holistic	1. Analytic
2. Emotional: pleasure–pain oriented (what feels good)	2. Logical: reason oriented (what is sensible)
3. Associationistic connections	3. Cause–effect connections
4. Behavior mediated by "vibes" from past experiences	4. Behavior mediated by conscious appraisal of events
5. Encodes reality in concrete images, metaphors, and narratives	5. Encodes reality in abstract symbols, words, and numbers
6. More rapid processing: oriented toward immediate action	6. Slower processing: oriented toward delayed action
7. Slower to change: changes with repetitive or intense experience	7. Changes more rapidly: changes with speed of thought
8. More crudely differentiated: broad generalization gradient; categorical thinking	8. More highly differentiated; dimensional thinking
9. More crudely integrated: dissociative, organized in part by emotional complexes (cognitive–affective modules)	9. More highly integrated
10. Experienced passively and preconsciously: we are seized by our emotions	10. Experienced actively and consciously: we are in control of our thoughts
11. Self-evidently valid: "experiencing is believing"	11. Requires justification via logic and evidence

Adapted from Epstein, Lipson, Holstein, and Huh (1992). Reprinted by permission.

a comparison of the characteristics of the two systems. An additional way that the experiential system differs from the rational system can be inferred from its holistic and concretive properties. Namely, the experiential system is relatively context specific compared with the rational system, which is more context general. These two approaches are equally adaptive but in different ways. The experiential system achieves specificity in judgment by restricting its holistically derived schemata to contexts judged to be relevant on the basis of past experience. By contrast, the rational system achieves specificity in judgment by bringing to bear a confluence of contextually general abstract principles.

Emotions and the Experiential System

A personal theory of reality is not developed for its own sake but for its affective advantages. Initially, individuals acquire schemata because of their consequences with respect to maximizing pleasure and minimizing pain. However, once an organized schema system is formed, cognitions influence emotions as much as the reverse.

The operation of the experiential system is assumed to be intimately associated with the experience of affect, including "vibes," which refer to diffuse feelings, such as agitation, irritability, and disquietude, of which people may or may not be aware. When a person responds to a significant event, the sequence of reactions is assumed to be as follows: The experiential system automatically searches its memory banks for related events, including affective components. The recalled feelings influence the course of further reactions, which are actions in subhuman animals and conscious and unconscious thoughts as well as actions in humans. If the feelings that are stirred up are pleasant, the person is motivated to act and think in ways to reproduce the feelings. If the feelings are unpleasant, the person automatically acts and think in ways to avoid recapitulating the feelings. All of this occurs instantaneously and normally outside of conscious awareness. The result is that people are generally unaware of intervening interpretative and affective reactions and assume that they react directly to external events. It follows that the influence of subtle feelings (vibes) on conscious thought is a pervasive source of biased thinking, which has implications for people's ability to think rationally. To the extent that this sequencing of reactions, as proposed by CEST, is correct, and I later indicate that there is strong evidence to support it, conscious thought is more under the influence of unconscious processes than even Freud had imagined.

Because of the intimate relation between feelings and the experiential system, emotions can be used to infer the basic schemata in a person's implicit theory of reality. It can be assumed that whenever an event elicits an emotional response, a significant schema in a person's implicit theory of reality has been implicated. In other words, the degree of emotional arousal can serve as a barometer of the significance of events in a person's experiential system. Accordingly, by noting the events that elicit emotional responses, some of the more important schemata in a person's theory of reality can be inferred.

A second way that emotions can be used to infer schemata is through knowledge of the relation between specific thoughts and specific emotions. According to cognitively oriented students of emotion (e.g., Averill, 1980; Beck, 1976; Ellis, 1973; Epstein, 1984; Lazarus, 1991), specific emotions are instigated by specific preconscious thoughts. This position has been supported by clinical observation and, more formally, by research that has examined the relation of thoughts and emotions in everyday life (e.g., Epstein, 1976, 1983b). It follows from this view that people who characteristically have certain emotions characteristically think in certain ways. For example, it can be inferred that angry people have central schemata that people behave badly and deserve to be punished; frightened people have central schemata of the world as a dangerous place and that they should therefore be constantly prepared for flight; and sad people have central schemata about having sustained significant losses or of being personally inadequate and that, in either case, there is nothing that can be done to rectify the situation. As a result of the intimate association between the experiential system and emotions and vibes, the functioning of the experiential system has important implications for physical as well as mental well-being.

Four Basic Needs and Four Basic Belief Dimensions

Which Need Is the Most Fundamental?

Nearly every major theory of personality proposes a single need that it regards as being more fundamental than any other. For Freud and most learning theorists, it was the pleasure principle, or the need to maximize pleasure and minimize pain. For Bowlby and the object-relations theorists, it was the need for relatedness. For Rogers and other phenomenological psychologists, it was the need to maintain the coherence of the conceptual system. For Allport and Kohut, it was the need to enhance self-esteem. (For a more thorough discussion of these positions, see Epstein, in press-a.) Who is right? From the perspective of CEST, all are right and all are wrong. They are all right because each of these needs is fundamental, and they are all wrong because of their failure to recognize the importance of the other needs. According to CEST, these four needs are equally basic because each can dominate the others and because there are equally serious consequences, including disorganization of the entire personality, when the fulfillment of any of these needs is seriously threatened.

There are two additional developments in CEST that are based on the assumption that there are four equally important needs. One is that maintaining a balance among them is important. The other is that the four basic needs give rise to four basic belief dimensions, and a person's locations on these dimensions are among the most fundamental schemata in a person's implicit theory of reality.

Maintaining a Balance Among the Basic Needs

Given four equally important basic needs, it follows that behavior must represent a compromise among them and, relatedly, that they serve as checks and balances against each other, which helps to keep behavior within adaptive limits.

It has been widely observed that well-adjusted people, rather than being highly realistic, exhibit self-esteem- and optimism-enhancing biases in their evaluations of self and world (Taylor & Brown, 1988). These findings have been interpreted by some as indicating that reality orientation is not an important criterion of mental health. From the perspective of CEST, a different interpretation is in order: Although reality orientation is extremely important, there are other equally important considerations. For example, given the needs to assimilate the data of reality into a coherent conceptual system and to enhance self-esteem, behavior can be expected to represent a compromise between these two needs, thereby resulting in a limited bias toward self-esteem enhancement. That is, the need for assimilating the data of reality constrains the need for self-esteem enhancement and vice versa. The net result is a moderate self-enhancing tendency in normal individuals. Similarly, a modest degree of optimism enhancement that is characteristic of most normal individuals can be attributed to a compromise between the need to assimilate the data of reality and the need to maximize pleasure by viewing the world in positive terms.

One of the hallmarks of maladaptive behavior is a failure to maintain a balance among the basic needs. This can account for why depressed individuals, under many circumstances, are more realistic than nondepressed individuals. It is not that they are more motivated to assimilate the data of reality in a realistic manner but that they are less motivated to enhance self-esteem. This interpretation is supported by the observation that depressed individuals have low self-esteem and appear motivated to maintain negative self-views. (For a more thorough discussion of this issue, see Epstein, 1992a.)

What are the conditions that promote an imbalance among the basic needs? Imbalances arise when individuals sacrifice other needs in order to fulfill threatened needs. For example, if a person's need to maintain the stability and coherence of his or her conceptual system is severely threatened, the fulfillment of the need for relatedness, self-enhancement, or maximizing the favorability of his or her pleasure–pain balance may be sacrificed. The individual will do so because of a desperate desire to keep the person's conceptual system from disorganizing. From this perspective, the attempts by some social psychologists to establish which of several basic needs (e.g., the need to maintain familiar cognitions, the need for self-enhancement) is more important is misguided. Any of the basic needs can become prepotent if it is sufficiently threatened. Individuals with delusions of grandeur have sacrificed their need to realistically assimilate the data of reality for their need to enhance self-esteem; depressed people have sacrificed their need to enhance their self-esteem for their need to maintain the stability and coherence of their conceptual systems; and disorganized schizophrenics have sacrificed their need to maintain the stability and coherence of their conceptual systems for their need to minimize psychological pain (Epstein, 1979a).

Competition among the basic needs can account for what otherwise appears to be self-defeating behavior, such as maintaining negative views about the self despite disconfirming evidence. How can such behavior, which seems to accomplish nothing but contribute to misery, be explained? It is noteworthy that it was just this phenomenon that led Freud

(1900/1953) to replace his original theory of personality, which emphasized the pleasure principle, with a new theory that attributed equal importance to a presumed "repetition compulsion" in the service of a "death instinct." Such behavior also led Allport (1961) to introduce the concept of functional autonomy, according to which certain behavior maintains itself in the absence of reinforcement. Allport acknowledged that although he considered this phenomenon to be of paramount importance, he was at a complete loss as to how to explain it. According to CEST, the place to seek a solution is not in a death instinct or in behavior that is self-maintaining in the absence of reinforcement but in the influence of competing needs, such as the need to maintain the coherence and stability of a person's conceptual system. In order to maintain coherence it may be necessary to confirm beliefs, even negative ones that are a source of misery. Thus, people are motivated to maintain significant negative beliefs in their conceptual system because to do otherwise would destabilize their conceptual system (Swann, 1984, 1987). I discuss this further in the next section.

It is important to recognize that there are different ways of achieving a balance among needs, some of which are more adaptive than others. Ultimately, what is important is the degree to which a person's basic needs are all fulfilled. A balance that is achieved among equally unfulfilled competing needs is a prescription for chronic tension, not good adjustment. Well-adjusted people fulfill their basic needs in a harmonious, even synergistic, manner, with the fulfillment of one need contributing to, rather than competing with, the fulfillment of other needs. They construct an implicit theory of reality that is stable yet flexible and that facilitates deriving joy from living, establishing rewarding relationships, and maintaining favorable levels of self-esteem in a mutually facilitative manner.

The Basic Beliefs

The four basic needs give rise to four basic beliefs, which become central schemata in a personal theory of reality. As a result, these beliefs are highly influential in determining how people view themselves and the world and, accordingly, in how they interpret events and behave in the world. Moreover, as previously noted, should any of them be invalidated, it will destabilize the entire conceptual system.

How do the four basic needs shape the acquisition of four corresponding basic beliefs? Needs are motivational constructs that have an affective component and that determine what is important to a person and what the person is attempting to accomplish. When a need is fulfilled, positive affect is experienced, and when a need is frustrated, negative affect is experienced. It follows that needs will determine what a person attends to and what the person experiences as positively and negatively reinforcing. Accordingly, basic needs influence the acquisition of descriptive schemata about what the self and world are like and motivational schemata about what one has to do to achieve need fulfillment and to avoid need frustration.

Before examining the relation of specific needs to specific beliefs, it is important to recall that it is the perception, not the objective occurrence of events, that is important with respect to the influence of events on beliefs. Schemata influence, as well as are influenced by, the perception of events. Accordingly, the influence of significant life events on whether a person develops an optimistic or a pessimistic outlook must be understood in terms of how the person experienced those events, not on how someone from an "objective" perspective might judge them. This assumption accounts for why some people who have been exposed to highly aversive environments nevertheless develop optimistic orientations, whereas others who have been exposed to objectively favorable environments develop pessimistic outlooks.

Corresponding to the need to maximize pleasure and minimize pain is a person's basic belief about the world along a dimension varying from benignity to malevolence. If a person's need to maximize pleasure and minimize pain has been well served in his or her perceived environment, the person will internalize this experience and tend to view the world in favorable terms. Dimensions of personality attributes corresponding to this dimension are optimism versus pessimism and security versus insecurity.

Corresponding to the need to represent the data of reality in a stable and coherent conceptual system is a view of the world along a dimension of meaningfulness (including commitment, predictability, and controllability) versus meaninglessness (including alienation, chaos, and uncontrollability). Depending on their emotionally significant past experiences, people's schemata will fall at different points along this dimension. Personality attributes that correspond to this dimension are commitment versus alienation (Kobasa, Maddi, & Kahn, 1982) and a belief in internal versus external control (Rotter, 1966).

Corresponding to the need for relatedness is a view of people on a dimension ranging from trustworthy, accepting, comforting, and supportive to untrustworthy, rejecting, and threatening. Personality attributes related to this dimension are trusting (Erikson, 1963), warm-hearted, and sociable versus suspicious, rejecting, and hostile.

Corresponding to the need for self-enhancement is a view of the self along a dimension varying from loveworthy, moral, competent, and strong to immoral, unloveworthy, incompetent, and weak. Personality attributes related to this dimension are high versus low self-esteem, self-accepting versus self-rejecting, confident versus nonconfident, competent versus incompetent, and morally self-accepting versus guilt ridden.

The Lower and Higher Reaches of the Experiential System

As previously noted, the experiential system copes with a range of complexity. The same fundamental attributes that allow it to solve simple problems rapidly and effortlessly are also involved in more complex levels of information processing.

The Lower Reaches of the Experiential System

The functioning of the experiential system as a quick and crude way of processing information represents the lower levels of the system. By *lower*, I do not mean inadequate or maladaptive. The system, although it has its limitations, is adaptive even in its lower reaches. In fact, the more effortful, slower processing procedure of the rational system is much less adaptive in many real-life situations.

Research Evidence

Classical conditioning provides an example of the operation of the experiential system at its lowest level of functioning. In classical conditioning, an animal (subhuman or human) is presented with a conditioned stimulus, such as a tone, that precedes an unconditioned stimulus, such as food. Over several trials, a connection is formed between the conditioned and unconditioned stimulus, such that the conditioned stimulus evokes a conditioned response (e.g., salivation) that originally occurred only in response to the unconditioned stimulus. This process illustrates several of the attributes of the experiential system, as outlined in Table 1: associationistic processing, automatic processing, concretive representation, gradual development over repeated trials, absence of conscious effort, affective influence, and arbitrary outcome orientation. The response is generally holistic because the animal reacts not only to the tone but to the entire laboratory context in which the tone is presented.

A level of processing that is somewhat more complicated than conditioning is exhibited in heuristic processing. In an article that has had a great influence on social–cognitive theorizing and research, Tversky and Kahneman (1974) introduced the construct of "heuristics," which they defined as cognitive shortcuts that people use naturally in decisional processes. They and other cognitive psychologists have found that such processing is a prevalent source of irrational reactions in many real-life situations. For example, people typically report that protagonists in vignettes become more upset following arbitrary unfortunate outcomes that were preceded by acts of commission than by acts of omission, by near than by far misses, by free than by constrained behavior, and by unusual than by usual acts. Because they react as if the behavior were responsible for the arbitrary outcomes, their thinking is clearly associationistic and in the mode of the experiential system.

A vast amount of research on heuristics (see the review in Fiske & Taylor, 1991) has produced results that are highly consistent with the principles of the experiential system as proposed by CEST. Although the data-driven views on heuristics derived from social–cognitive research and the theory-driven views of CEST are generally highly compatible, the two approaches differ in two important respects. One is that CEST attributes heuristics to the normal mode of operation of an organized conceptual system—the experiential system—that is different from a rational conceptual system. The other is that heuristic processing, according to CEST, having withstood the test of time over millions of years of evolution, is assumed to be primarily adaptive.

In contrast to the views of CEST, cognitive psychologists, such as Kahneman and Tversky (1973) and Nisbett and Ross (1980), regard heuristics as individual "cognitive tools" that are used within a single, general conceptual system that also includes rational, analytical processing. These theorists further regard heuristics as quirks in thinking that although sometimes adaptive are common sources of error in everyday life and therefore would be desirable to eliminate. From this perspective, it has been surprising how resistant some of these blatantly irrational ways of responding have been to elimination through training. From the perspective of CEST, given their general adaptivity in the broader scheme of things, such resilience is to be expected.

My associates and I have conducted a series of experiments to demonstrate that heuristic processing is the normal, adaptive mode of operation of an organized conceptual system that differs from a rational system according to certain principles. Depending on conditions, we assume that the heuristic way of responding can be either adaptive or maladaptive. One aim of the research was to explore what these conditions are.

In our first series of studies, we demonstrated that people are well aware that they and others operate by implicit inferential rules that differ from rational principles (Epstein, Lipson, Holstein, & Huh, 1992). When subjects responded to vignettes by indicating how foolish they thought the protagonists would feel about behavior that was arbitrarily followed by unfortunate outcomes (e.g., loss of money, car accidents), they reported that the protagonists would consider their behavior to be significantly more foolish when the behavior was arbitrarily associated with near than with far misses, with unusual than with usual acts, and so forth, thereby verifying previous findings. When asked to indicate how they themselves would react in the same situations, the results were the same. However, when asked to judge how a rational person would respond, the phenomenon all but disappeared. It did not completely disappear because some subjects believed that their associationistic way of reacting was reasonable and appropriate.

We further demonstrated in the same series of studies that priming the experiential system interfered with people's ability to subsequently think rationally. That is, they tended to rationalize their experiential thinking and therefore to maintain it on a presumably rational basis. This latter finding has important implications because it suggests that conscious, rational thinking is unknowingly influenced by preconscious automatic processing according to the principles of the experiential system.

In another series of studies (Kirkpatrick & Epstein, 1992), we demonstrated that by creating conditions that bypassed people's desire to present themselves as rational or that strongly engaged their experiential system, we could obtain much stronger evidence in support of the principles of the experiential system than under conditions that had previously been investigated (e.g., Miller, Turnbull, & McFarland, 1989). In one of the studies, subjects were asked to imagine a situation in which they could win by drawing a winning ticket from a bowl that contained 10% winning tickets. They were asked to indicate whether, if given the choice, they would choose to draw from a "small bowl" that contained 1 in 10 winning tickets or a "large bowl" that contained 10 in 100 winning tickets and if they would be willing to pay (from 1¢ up to $1) for the privilege of drawing from the bowl of their choice rather than having it done randomly for them. They reported no preference between the bowls, with 49% selecting the large one and 51% the small one, and almost all said they would not pay 1¢ for the privilege of drawing from one rather than the other. Many spontaneously commented that the choice was of no consequence given the identical probabilities. These results were disappointing because we had hypothesized that they would prefer the large bowl because the experiential system is a relatively primitive concretive system that should be more responsive to absolute numbers than to ratios. It occurred to us that subjects might have engaged in some impression management in their desire to appear rational. We therefore repeated the experiment, but this time asked them to indicate how they thought most people (not themselves) would react. A significant majority (64%) said that most people would prefer to draw from the large bowl, thereby confirming the original hypothesis. Moreover, a majority (60%) believed that most people would pay for the opportunity to choose from their preferred bowl.

Because we suspected that a real situation would engage the experiential more than an imaginary one, we conducted a third study in which subjects received real money if they drew a red jelly bean from among a greater number of white jelly beans. This time, 77% expressed a preference for drawing from the large bowl, and 50% paid dimes (which we had given them at the beginning of the experiment) for the privilege of drawing from their preferred bowl. After having participated in the experiment, 94% estimated that others would choose the large bowl, and 75% estimated that others would pay for the privilege.

Our series of experiments demonstrated that people operate by two different sets of rules that correspond to those of the rational and experiential systems. The results further demonstrated that the operation of the experiential system can most clearly be observed when people are confronted with emotionally significant real experiences and when conditions are established that circumvent their need to present themselves as rational.

We have found that the perspective of CEST can resolve some of the anomalies in research on heuristic processing undertaken from other viewpoints. Recall that the experiential system is assumed to operate in a context-specific manner. Accordingly, the responses it fosters are apt to be appropriate when problems are presented in natural contexts and inappropriate when they are presented in unnatural contexts.

The importance of considering whether the correct response to a problem is natural (defined as the customary, expected kind of response for the situation in question) is well demonstrated in research on conjoint probability. Tversky and Kahneman (1982) introduced the famous "Linda vignette," which is undoubtedly the most researched vignette of all time, to investigate people's understanding of conjoint probability. The Linda problem, which seems so easy to solve, has been the source of endless controversy and speculation because it evokes so many conjunction errors (defined as judging a joint occurrence of two events as being more likely than of one of its components). Linda is described as a 31-year-old woman who is single, outspoken, and highly intelligent. In college she was a philosophy major who participated in antinuclear demonstrations and was concerned with issues of social justice. Subjects are asked to rank order the likelihood that among other possibilities, Linda is a bank teller, an activist in the feminist movement, and a bank teller who is also an activist in the feminist movement. Tversky and Kahneman reported that 85% of their subjects rated the joint probability as higher than one of its components, thereby violating the conjunction rule. Most often, subjects said it was more likely that Linda is a bank teller and a feminist than that she is a bank teller. This finding has been replicated repeatedly under varied circumstances. It has also been found that the ability to solve the problem is highly resistant (but not impervious) to improvement with training. How is one to explain why the Linda problem is so difficult to solve and why training has been so ineffective?

In our own investigation of conjoint probability, Denes-Raj and I presented subjects with the Linda problem and two conceptually similar but contextually different problems: a "Lottery" problem and a formal statistical problem (Epstein & Denes-Raj, 1992). With respect to context and the kind of response required, the Linda problem can be classified as "concrete, unnatural," the Lottery problem as "concrete, natural," and the formal statistical problem as "abstract, natural." We hypothesized that correct solutions would be facilitated by natural and concrete as opposed to unnatural and abstract representations. Subjects responded to the three problems by rank ordering the likelihood of the following three outcomes: that one event would occur, that the other would occur, and that both would occur. The three events in the Lottery were winning in a firefighter's lottery with odds of 1 in 1,000, winning in a state lottery with odds of 1 in 1 million, and winning in both lotteries. In the formal statistical problem, subjects were asked to estimate the joint probability of two events occurring, one with a probability of one tenth and the other with a probability of one half. Estimates greater than one tenth were counted as conjunction errors. The results were completely in accord with the hypothesis: Sixty-eight percent of the subjects made conjunction errors in the concrete, unnatural Linda problem; 39% in the abstract, natural problem; and 6% in the concrete, natural Lottery problem.

This study demonstrated that almost everyone intuitively understands the conjunction rule and applies it correctly in concrete, natural contexts. They do not apply it in unnatural contexts because they do not perceive it to be relevant. The study further demonstrated that there is a clear difference between abstract, analytical knowledge and intuitive knowledge and that the latter in certain circumstances is superior to the former.

In several studies, my associates and I have observed conflicts between the two ways of processing information that are consistent with the assumption that there are different systems that operate according to the principles enumerated in Table 1. For example, in the "jelly bean" study described previously, subjects frequently commented that although they "knew" the odds were identical, they "felt" the larger bowl offered a better chance of a favorable outcome because it contained more red beans. Many looked sheepish and made self-conscious comments about their irrationality when they paid 10¢ in order to guarantee a choice between what they recognized were identical probabilities.

In recently completed unpublished studies, my associates and I obtained additional evidence in support of different ways of processing information that correspond to the experiential and rational systems. Several studies have demonstrated that in some circumstances people rely on associationistic, outcome-oriented processing and in others on cause–effect analysis. In a study in which we asked subjects to list the first three thoughts that came to mind in response to outcomes described in vignettes, the first thoughts were often consistent with the principles of the experiential system and the third thoughts with the principles of the rational system. For example, when subjects were presented with a vignette that described a person who had an accident when backing out of a place that his friend had requested him to park in, they frequently reported that their first thought was that the accident was their friend's fault. Their third thought often consisted of identifying the first thought as irrational and accepting the responsibility as their own.

Another study investigated outcome-oriented processing, using a vignette adapted from a study by Miller and Gunasegaram (1990). In the adaptation, three protagonists had to each throw a coin that came up heads in order for each to receive $100. The first two threw heads and the third threw tails. Subjects reported their first three thoughts in response to this question: If you were in the position of the first two protagonists, would you invite the third protagonist to join you in a gambling vacation at Las Vegas? Most subjects reported that their first thought was that they would not. By their third thought, however, most dismissed the poor performance of the third protagonist as a chance occurrence and said they would invite him. Consistent with CEST, the first thought was automatic, associationistic, and arbitrarily outcome-oriented, all attributes of the experiential system, whereas the third thought was reflective and took into account reasonable cause and effect connections, which is characteristic of the rational system.

If there are two fundamental ways of processing information, it is reasonable to consider that there may be important individual differences in the relative degree to which people rely on each. In order to test for the existence of a broad factor of heuristic processing that differs from rational–analytical processing, we (Epstein, Heier, & Denes-Raj, 1992) had subjects respond to 11 vignettes taken from a variety of studies on heuristic processing. The subjects indicated their reactions from three orientations: how they thought most people would react, how they themselves would react, and how they thought a completely rational person would react. The subjects also took a variety of self-report personality scales that we thought might be related to heuristic processing, including the following: the Constructive Thinking Inventory (CTI; Epstein & Meier, 1989); Caccioppo and Petty's (1982) Need for Cognition Scale; a measure of affect intensity patterned after Larsen and Diener's (1987) Affect Intensity Measure; a measure of evaluation of intuition and thinking patterned after scales in the Myers-Briggs Type Indicator; a specially constructed bipolar scale of the degree to which one typically makes decisions based on the heart versus the mind; a specially constructed faith in intuition scale (FAIS) that measures the degree to which a person relies on unmodulated intuitive impressions, such as trusting one's first impressions; and a rational versus experiential scale (RVE) based on a general factor from a factor analysis of the items in the other scales.

The results indicated that each of the orientations produced a general factor of heuristic processing that included responses to almost all of the vignettes in the self- and other orientations and to all of the vignettes in the rational orientation. Given the large number of correlations, a probability value of .01 was set as the criterion for significance. The number of heuristic responses from a self-orientation, from an other orientation, and from a rational orientation produced different, coherent patterns of significant correlations with the personality scales. Heuristic responses from a self-orientation were significantly correlated with the broad RVE scale ($r = -.20$); with the FAIS ($r = .24$); with the CTI scales of Global Constructive Thinking ($r = -.21$), Emotional Coping ($r = -.23$), and Behavioral Coping ($r = -.19$); with two of the subscales of Emotional Coping, Absence of Negative Overgeneralization ($r = -.19$); and Nonsensitivity ($r = -.27$); and with the Action-Oriented scale of the Behavioral Coping scale ($r = -.21$). The overall pattern suggested that high self-acknowledged heuristic processing in response to vignettes from a self-orientation is associated with self-reported excessive reliance on intuitive solutions to everyday problems, with poor general cognitive coping strategies and, relatedly, with being excessively sensitive to psychological assaults.

The score on heuristic responding from the perspective of how others are assumed to react was significantly correlated with the CTI scale of Emotional Coping ($r = -.19$) and its subscales of Absence of Negative Overgeneralization ($r = -.18$) and Nonsensitivity ($-.18$). Thus, people who assume that others are particularly prone to extreme heuristic processing tend to be poor emotional copers and, in particular, to overgeneralize broadly and to be excessively sensitive to psychological assaults. The similarity in the pattern of relationships produced by the self- and other orientations may be a consequence of people, particularly those who are nonreflective, assuming that others respond as they do.

Heuristic responding from a rational orientation indicates the degree to which irrational heuristic reactions are judged to be rational. From the perspective of CEST, high scores reveal a failure to distinguish between the two processing systems by judging what is automatic and natural to be rational. This score correlated significantly with the self-report FAIS scale ($r = .21$) and with the CTI subscales of Polarized Thinking ($r = .21$) and Stereotyped Thinking ($r = .22$). The results suggest that those who view nonrational heuristic responses as rational tend to have excessive faith in their intuition and to think in a more simplistic, undifferentiated manner than others.

Evidence in Everyday Life

In addition to experimental evidence, there is abundant evidence in real life attesting to the existence of parallel processing systems that operate according to the principles of the experiential and rational systems. Psychotherapists, for example, have long been aware of the difference between intellectual knowledge and insight. Self-knowledge related to emotionally significant experiences is widely recognized by psychotherapists to be a more potent source of change than intellectual information.

The widespread occurrence of conflicts between the heart and the mind (between "hot" and "cold" cognitions) provides further support for two fundamentally different ways of processing information. If cognitions were all represented in a single conceptual system, there would be no reason for the conflicting components to divide according to whether they do or do not involve emotions or real-life experience. Sappington (1990), among others, has provided evidence for separate emotional and nonemotional ways of processing information that may either conflict with or supplement each other.

Perhaps the most compelling evidence for the existence of an experiential system that processes information in a fundamentally different manner from an analytical, rational system is the ubiquity of religion throughout recorded history. Analytical, reflective thinking combined with controlled empirical observation are apparently unable to provide as emotionally satisfying an understanding of self and world for many people as is provided for them by the concretive, holistic symbolic thinking characteristic of organized religion.

Religion is well designed to satisfy the four fundamental needs identified by CEST. It satisfies the need for meaning by providing concretive, narrative explanations of the origins of the world and of the emergence of humankind. It provides an illusion of control over and predictability of nature by the use of ritual and magic. It satisfies the need for relatedness by social activities (e.g., group worship, communal chanting, choir singing), by uniting people through a common faith, and by deities with whom people can communicate. It satisfies the need for pleasure by providing attractive visual stimulation (e.g., stained glass windows, Christmas trees, architectural works, festivals), auditory stimulation (e.g., music), and kinesthetic sensations (e.g., dancing, whirling) and by providing techniques for achieving ecstatic and serene states (e.g., meditation, prayer). Relatedly, it satisfies the need to avoid pain by providing magical procedures for ridding people of maladies and evil spirits and by providing procedures and beliefs for reducing the aversiveness of critical life experiences (e.g., the promise of rewarding the just and punishing the wicked in a future life). It satisfies the need for self-esteem by providing people with the belief that their religion confers virtue and superiority on them over those with other religions. It also raises self-esteem by connecting people with powerful deities or ones who will forgive and love them, no matter what their lapses.

The ubiquity of prejudice can also be attributed to the experiential system. According to a song from the musical *South Pacific*, people have to be carefully taught to hate those whose "eyes are ugly made" and whose "skin is of a different shade." According to CEST, it is the absence, not the presence, of prejudice that must be carefully taught, for people are disposed toward developing prejudices because of the propensities of their experiential systems. Its attributes of concretive, holistic, and categorical processing combined with its orientation toward immediate action encourage people to generalize broadly and to seek targets for their frustration.

The widespread prevalence of superstitious thinking also provides evidence of a system that functions by principles that are clearly not rational. Table 2 summarizes some recently acquired data on superstitious and other irrational beliefs as a function of age. At least 40% of grade school and college students and more than 60% of adults reported having at least one superstition.

TABLE 2

Percentages of Superstitious and Esoteric Thinking in Children, Their Parents, and College Students

Item	Children	College	Adult
Some people can project their thoughts into others' minds.	19	18	18
Some people can read others' thoughts.	23	27	15
If I wish hard enough for something, it can make it happen.	15	11	8
The moon or stars can affect people's thinking.	5	13	19
I believe in ghosts.	60	48	60
I believe in flying saucers.	22	15	20
There are people who can see into the future.	20	25	25
I have at least one good-luck charm.	45	56	72
I believe in good and bad magic.	25	13	11
I have at least one superstition.	46	40	63

Note. Children (n = 189) were aged 9–12 years, college students (n = 284) were aged 18–22 years, and adults (n = 159) were aged 27–65 years.

Age was found to be inversely associated with belief in good and bad magic and with the belief that wishing can make things happen, but it was directly associated with the belief that the moon and stars can affect people's thinking, which is probably associated with astrology.

Of greater interest were items not so transparently associated with age-related interests. There were two items that qualified: having at least one superstition of any kind and having at least one good-luck charm. Adults reported a considerably greater incidence on these items than did children. Fully 72% of adults reported that they had a good-luck charm as compared with 45% of children, and 63% of adults reported having at least one superstition as compared with 46% of children. These findings suggest that rather than being displaced by rational processes, as would be expected from Piagetian theory, irrational and rational modes of thinking operate in parallel throughout a lifetime.

The Higher Reaches of the Experiential System

Although the experiential system encodes events concretely and holistically, it is nevertheless able to generalize, integrate, and direct behavior in complex ways. It does this through prototypical, symbolic, and narrative representations, analogy and metaphor. Representations in the experiential system are also connected through their associations with emotions.

Unfortunately, there is not much in the way of research that can be cited with respect to the higher functioning of the experiential system. This is an area that is sorely in need of exploration by psychologists sophisticated in research procedures. To illustrate the nature of the issues that are involved I will cite a case history that first made me aware of the possible significance of such processing for mental and physical well-being.

Case History

The case is that of a middle-aged woman who entered psychotherapy following a diagnosis of terminal cancer. She wrote a book (A. Epstein, 1989) describing in detail the rich fantasies elicited in the course of her therapy. She believed that expressing and working on the fantasies contributed to a rapid reorganization of her personality and an eventual complete recovery from the cancer. Whether this view is correct is not the issue of current concern. However, given recent findings on the relation of emotions to the immune system, it would be unwise to summarily reject her hypothesis. There may be much more to the power of the higher reaches of the experiential system than most researchers suspect. Only future research will tell. In any event, there is much of interest that can be learned from her detailed descriptions of spontaneous fantasies about how the experiential system encodes information and establishes generalizations in the form of images and narratives.

The following is an example of a fantasy reported early in therapy. The session began with the client stating that she wished to explore a mood of isolation and loneliness that had inexplicably descended on her. In the previous session she had been distressed over the hostility she had expressed to her mother. She was instructed by the therapist to adopt a relaxed, meditative state, immerse herself in the feeling of isolation, and wait for a fantasy to occur. After several false starts, the following fantasy emerged:

> I saw some figures with shrouds—very unclear. Then as they took on a more distinct form, I saw that they were witches standing around a fire.

(Name of therapist) told me to ask them to come over to talk to us. They were frightening to me in the light of the fire, but they were more horrible as they came closer. They laughed at me and started to poke at me with their sticks. The visualization was so real and their presence was so chilling to me that I burst into tears over the interaction with them.

(Name of therapist) told me to ask them what I could do to get rid of the awful fear of isolation. Finally they revealed their price: It was that I make a sacrifice so that they could become beautiful and mingle with other people. When I heard their price I began to tremble. In an almost inaudible voice I whispered, "They want my children so they can turn them into witches like them, but I'll never do it. I'll never give them my children!"

(Name of therapist) then told me to destroy them, but I told him that I couldn't possibly do it. He urged me to try to turn my fear to wrath, to try to imagine a creature that could help me. The image that came to me was a white winged horse. He told me to mount the horse and to supply myself with a weapon that would destroy them. I refused to kill them myself, but said that the wings of the horse would fan the flames of their fire, which would turn back on them and destroy them.

There was only one problem with this scenario—the horse and I were one now and I couldn't get airborne. The wings were so heavy that I couldn't flap them hard enough to catch the breeze. The harder I tried, the more I failed and the more the witches laughed at me. (Name of therapist) ... told me that another horse who loved the first horse very much would join her and together they would destroy the witches. The other horse flew above me and made a vacuum into which I could take off. Once in the air, I flew effortlessly and fanned the fire into a huge blaze. The witches ran here and there trying to avoid the flames, but in the end they were consumed by the fire.

I practiced the scene over and over again until it became easy, but I never enjoyed it. I liked to fly, but I felt sorry for the witches, no matter how mean they were to me. (Name of therapist) felt that it was a mistake to feel sympathy for them because they would take advantage of any mercy that I displayed. He felt that they would use any deception and illusion they could to control me. I was not so sure but I did agree with him that I must assume the right to soar into the world and be free of their influence.

After the session, (name of therapist) and I discussed the meaning of the images. Although I had begun with the concept of isolation in mind, I knew that the witches related to my mother, particularly the way she would poke at me and shame me. They probably represented my fear of isolation if I did not acquiesce to her demands. (Name of therapist) added that in destroying the witches I was only destroying the hostile parts of our relationship, the witch part of it, and leaving the loving part intact. This was necessary for me to be free, autonomous, and not en-snared by fear of abandonment.

The concept that I had a great deal of conflict between the need for association and the need for autonomy was not new. I believed I had to buy affection and that no one would love me if I were myself, i.e., if I attended to my own wants. I knew also that I felt that I had to carry the burden of being responsible for my mother's well-being, that she would die at some level if I broke the bond with her. (A. Epstein, 1989, pp. 45–47)

Case Discussion

This fantasy well represents the client's conflict between relatedness and autonomy that is the essence of her overprotective relationship with her mother, and it also suggests what the conditions are for resolving it.

There are several aspects of the fantasy that warrant comment. First, it is noteworthy that the only aspect of the representation that initially reached awareness was an enduring mood, which consisted of a deep feeling of loneliness. Previously, I noted that emotions provide important clues about how people interpret events. There is reason to believe that this also applies to moods but on a much grander scale (Epstein, 1985). Rather than reflecting construals of specific events, moods reflect how people construe their situation in the world (e.g., as being condemned to a life of loneliness). Thus, moods, like emotions, can provide important clues about the fundamental schemata in personal theories of reality.

In which system was the fantasy encoded: the rational conceptual system, the experiential conceptual system, or the primary-process system? Considering that the production is unrealistic rather than realistic, spontaneous rather than deliberative, and intimately associated with affect, it is not likely to be a production of the rational system. Considering further that it is highly coherent, takes into account causal relations and constraints of time and place, and, unlike a dream, is not at all fragmented, it is more likely to be a product of the experiential than of the primary-process system. Accordingly, it may be able to provide interesting insights into the operation of the upper reaches of the experiential system.

The fantasy suggests that the experiential system is capable of making complex, highly abstract generalizations. It can accomplish this by using symbols, such as witches, that represent emotionally significant generalizations from real-life experiences, which it then incorporates into narratives that convey important messages about how to behave in the world to obtain what one wants and to avoid what one fears. In this respect, it is noteworthy that the client's feeling of isolation provided an automatic source of motivation against striving for autonomy. In effect, it reminded her of the price she would have to pay if she succeeded in such efforts, thereby directing her behavior and very likely her conscious thoughts in other directions. Recall that this is exactly the way I said the experiential system operates: by being responsive to feelings (including subtle vibes as well as more articulated emotions and moods) that are automatically triggered by representatives of past experience.

Does the experiential mind, then, have a unique wisdom that knows things that the rational mind does not? Judging from this fantasy, the answer appears to be yes. The client was aware before the fantasy that conflicting needs between relatedness and autonomy posed a serious problem for her. She was also aware that her mother overprotected her, that she felt compelled to please her mother, that this compulsion carried over to other people, and that she resented her need to please others. She was not aware, however, that at a deeper level, she believed her mother had robbed her of her childhood. It took her some time after reporting the fantasy to come to the realization that the children the witch wanted her to sacrifice might represent her own childhood. She also later became aware that the reason she may have displaced the childhood from her own to that of her children was that she could react with indignation to the demand to sacrifice her children, whereas she would feel guilty if she refused to sacrifice herself for her mother. This brings up for consideration the therapeutic implications of fantasies, which further suggests an inherent wisdom of the experiential system. The fantasy, in effect, informed her that there are conditions in which love does not require sacrificing one's autonomy and that autonomy can be a freeing experience that can be enjoyed without guilt or fear. It is true that she knew this before intellectually, but the fantasy taught her to believe it in a way that mattered and that could affect her feelings and behavior. It is noteworthy, in this respect, that she replayed the scene in which she soared freely time and again, savoring every moment of her newly imagined freedom.

This leads to the interesting speculation that it may be possible to reach and influence the experiential system through providing corrective experiences in fantasy in the absence of intellectual insight. This, then, suggests a form of therapy in which there is an attempt to locate through fantasy the major schemata in the experiential system that are the source of a person's problems in living. The next step is to correct these schemata through the use of fantasy, by communicating with the experiential system in a language it understands. This fairly accurately describes the major thrust of the therapy of the client in the case history. The result, as previously noted, was that she effected a major reorganization of her personality in a relatively brief period (3 months). It remains to be seen how generally effective such a procedure is. At the least, it raises important questions about the nature of the upper reaches of the experiential system and of its power to influence mental and physical well-being.

Implications of CEST for Personality and Developmental Psychology

As a global theory of personality, CEST has widespread implications for many different areas of human behavior, including personality psychology (Epstein, 1973, 1980, 1981, 1983a, 1984, 1991c, 1992c), developmental psychology (Epstein, 1973, 1985, 1991a; Epstein & Erskine, 1983), abnormal psychology (Epstein, 1979a, 1981, 1987, in press-b), psychotherapy (Epstein, 1983a, 1984, 1985, 1987), social psychology (Epstein, 1984, 1985,

1989), advertising (Epstein, 1991c), politics (Epstein, 1991c), superstition (Epstein, 1991c), and religion and spirituality (Epstein, 1991c). Because it is impossible to discuss all of these within the confines of a brief article, I concentrate on the implications of CEST for new directions in personality and developmental psychology.

Personality Psychology Research

Recent social–cognitive theories of the self have had two notable deficiencies (Epstein, 1992a, in press-a; Westen, 1992), although, fortunately, this is beginning to change. One is that they have tended to neglect different levels of processing, and the other is that they have neglected the role of emotions and motivation in the self-concept. CEST, on the other hand, has emphasized both of these since its introduction nearly two decades ago (Epstein, 1973). Thus, an important new direction for social–cognitive self-theories is the incorporation of multiple levels of processing and motivational constructs in their self-systems. Although there is a beginning in this direction, there are still important questions to be addressed that have not yet been acknowledged. For example, if there are two different systems of information processing, experiential and rational, then it is not meaningful to refer to "the" self-concept because a person's self-concept in one system may be different from that in the other. As an example, consider self-esteem. People may be high in self-reported self-esteem yet low in self-esteem inferred from behavior (Savin-Williams & Jaquish, 1981). It is therefore important to assess the attributes of a person's self-concept at different levels of awareness and to examine the functional relations of the different levels to other variables because self-reported self-esteem has different correlates than inferred self-esteem (Savin-Williams & Jaquish, 1981). Not only should the different levels be examined individually, but valuable information can be gained from the discrepancies between them. Certainly, it is of interest to consider what it means for a person to have high self-esteem at the self-report level and low esteem at the inferred level.

CEST draws attention to the importance of considering basic needs as broad, central motives. Recently, social and personality psychologists have emphasized midlevel motivational constructs (e.g., Emmons, 1986; Markus & Nurius, 1986). Important as these are, they do not replace the need to examine more central motives. A complete theory of personality should be multitiered, not only at the structural level but also at the motivational level. It would therefore be desirable for researchers to explore the basic motives in human personality as they have already done with respect to basic traits (which mounting evidence suggests are the "Big Five"). Whether the "Big Four" motives postulated by CEST will be verified remains to be seen. In addition to determining what the most central motives are, it is important to investigate their relations to each other and to lower order constructs. It should be possible to establish a hierarchy of motives that includes central motives, midlevel motives, and more situationally specific, lower level motives.

A particularly important consequence of recognizing that there are multiple basic motives is that it draws attention to the importance of their interaction, an area that, with rare exception (e.g., Epstein, 1973, 1980; McCann & Pearlman, 1990), has been neglected. As I have already suggested, a requirement of successful adjustment is the maintenance of a balance among the basic motives. This has widespread implications for understanding motivation and adjustment that are overlooked by theories of personality that emphasize single basic motives. Nevertheless, some research has been conducted on the relative importance of at least two basic needs contrasted with each other: the need to maintain familiar beliefs about the self and the need to enhance the self. Initially, the concern was with which of these is more important. Research has become more sophisticated and has begun to examine the conditions under which each of these is likely to be predominant (e.g., Swann, 1990). Similar research remains to be done with other basic needs to establish under which conditions certain needs tend to become prepotent over others and what the ramifications of this are for the overall personality structure. Such research should also investigate individual differences. It can be expected, for example, that for some individuals maintaining the coherence of their belief system is of paramount importance, whereas for others it is enhancing their self-esteem, and for yet others maintaining relatedness or maximizing pleasure and minimizing pain. A profile of the relative importance of different basic needs would provide important diagnostic information about individuals.

No less important than basic needs are basic beliefs. Researchers need to learn more about the relation between beliefs and needs. This will indicate a great deal about affect regulation. How does the favorability of an individual's basic belief with respect, for example, to self-evaluation or the evaluation of the benevolence of the world (optimism–pessimism) influence people's tonic and phasic levels of positive and negative affect? Does maintaining a low tonic level provide a safeguard against distress produced by unexpected aversive experiences (Epstein, 1992a)? The observation that defensive pessimism provides a protection against disappointment (Norem & Cantor, 1986) suggests that this is indeed the case. Such research should be extended to basic beliefs other than those associated with pessimism. The whole area of affect regulation as related to cognition is an extremely important one that warrants increased research attention. (For further discussion of this issue, see Epstein, 1992a.)

Because basic beliefs are fundamental postulates in a person's implicit theory of reality, they have important implications with respect to the stability of people's personality structure. Research is needed to examine how serious threats to specific basic beliefs are related to defensive operations, to changes in beliefs, and to disorganization and reorganization of personality structure. To conduct such research, it is necessary to have instruments for assessing basic beliefs. At least three such self-report instruments are available (Catlin & Epstein, in press; Epstein, 1990; Janoff-Bulman, 1989; McCann & Pearlman, 1990) and have produced interesting results with respect to the influence of significant life events, including different kinds of trauma, on basic beliefs. McCann and Pearlman (1990) made a compelling case for their conclusion that the effect of a traumatic event cannot be determined by the event itself but only by the interaction of the event with the person's schemata. This can account for why only weak, albeit significant, correlations have been obtained in studies that have examined the relation between specific critical life events and specific basic beliefs (e.g., Catlin & Epstein, 1992; Janoff-Bulman, 1989). Different people have different sensitivities, or areas of vulnerability, derived from previous adverse experiences. Therefore, the same critical event does not have a uniform influence on the changes it induces in people's schemata. As to provoking disorganization, events that impinge on sensitivities are the ones that can be expected to be most likely to produce personality disorganization (Epstein, 1991a, 1991b; Janoff-Bulman, 1989; McCann & Pearlman, 1990). This is an important area of research that can contribute to the understanding of the organization of personality and how new information interacts with a person's implicit conceptual system, both modifying and being modified by it.

CEST has interesting implications for coping with stress. If the experiential system determines how effectively people adjust in their everyday lives, then it suggests that it has a kind of overall intelligence that is analogous to, but different from, intellective intelligence. That is, there must be important individual differences in the efficacy of the experiential system. Evidence in support of this position is provided by research with the CTI, a self-report measure of adaptive and maladaptive automatic thinking (e.g., Epstein, 1990, 1992b; Epstein & Katz, 1992; Epstein & Meier, 1989; Katz & Epstein, 1991). The use of the CTI opens up new ways of investigating coping ability because it is based on a model that emphasizes flexibility of coping rather than specific ways of coping, such as positive thinking or believing that events can or cannot be controlled. Unlike optimism and belief in one's ability to control events, which can be adaptive or maladaptive depending on the circumstances, constructive thinking is always adaptive. In the important respect of emphasizing flexibility, the construct of constructive thinking has much in common with Block and Block's (1980; Funder, Block, & Block, 1983) construct of ego-resiliency. It will be interesting in future research to compare these two constructs.

Research on constructive thinking, as measured by the CTI, may be able to account for certain anomalous findings in stress research, such as contradictory findings about whether behavioral self-blame (unlike characterological self-blame) is generally adaptive (Janoff-Bulman, 1979). I suspect that whether measures of specific coping styles are adaptive depends on whether they are indicative of constructive thinking in the specific kind of situation in question. It is noteworthy, in this respect,

SEYMOUR EPSTEIN

that when constructive thinking was partialed out of relations between various measures of coping style, they were no longer correlated significantly with the criteria to which they had previously been demonstrated to be significantly related (Epstein, 1990; Epstein & Katz, in press; Epstein & Meier, 1989). In other words, their relation with adjustment was completely determined by their degree of overlap with global constructive thinking.

Perhaps the most important implication of CEST for new directions in personality research stems from its assumption of an experiential system that operates by different rules from those of a rational system, as well as from those of the Freudian unconscious. If this is true and, as I have demonstrated earlier, there is considerable evidence that it is, then psychologists must change the way they think about unconscious influences on feeling, behavior, and conscious thinking. It means that heuristic processing of information is the predominant mode for solving problems in everyday living and that rational problem solving is much less prevalent than commonly assumed. It further means that people's ability to be rational is compromised by the influence of their experiential system on their rational system. It follows that the only way to be truly rational is to be in touch with one's experiential system, thereby allowing one to compensate for its biasing effect. Research is needed to determine how people can be trained to reduce the influence of the experiential system on the rational system.

A promising place to begin is to teach people the inferential rules of the experiential system and the conditions that are most likely to strongly engage it. Knowing how and when it operates, people may be able to control its influence when they wish to do so. An additional avenue worth exploring is how to contact the intuitive wisdom of the experiential system and how to promote adaptive interaction between the two systems. The use of fantasy and conventional and private symbols that can communicate with the experiential system in its own medium would seem to provide a promising approach. Researchers need to learn more about how the experiential system generalizes, such as through the use of prototypes, analogies, metaphors, symbols, scripts, and narratives. It is also important to determine to what extent people can produce changes in important schemata in their experiential system through manipulation of their fantasies, as in the example that was cited in which the client practiced soaring freely as a flying horse, which helped convince her, at a deep experiential level, that autonomy was both desirable and attainable. It is noteworthy in this respect that the flying fantasy had to be preceded by a fantasy in which another horse accepted and encouraged her autonomy. It will be interesting to see in future research whether an effective technique for changing experiential schemata is to have people experiment in fantasy with conditions that make certain desirable but feared reactions acceptable.

If the influence of the experiential system on conscious thought is as pervasive as I have suggested, then much of what has been attributed to the Freudian unconscious needs to be reassigned to the experiential system. This would, of course, considerably extend unconscious influences on feeling, behavior, and conscious thought. One reason to suspect that the experiential system will be found to exert a far more widespread influence than the Freudian primary-process system is that the former, unlike the latter, is an adaptive system for adjusting to reality. It is unreasonable to assume that the primary-process system can have the widespread influence on everyday behavior that Freud assigned to it, given its essentially maladaptive attributes of associationistic thinking, wish fulfillment, condensation, and displacement. Rather, the importance of the primary-process system may have to be restricted to its relation to altered states of consciousness, as in dreams and psychotic states.

Other promising areas for exploration include the relative advantages and disadvantages of the experiential and rational systems and how the two systems can best be used in supplementary fashion. Additionally, the implications of disharmony within and between the experiential and rational systems would be worth exploring. I suspect that mental and physical well-being are more strongly influenced by the degree of harmony within the experiential system and the fulfillment of the four basic needs that it intrinsically seeks to accomplish than with the amount of coherence between the rational and experiential systems. This is an important issue because my hypothesis runs counter to the prevailing wisdom that the major task of therapy is to achieve "insight" (i.e., making the unconscious

conscious) so that the higher order intelligence of the rational system can be brought to bear on solving a person's real-life problems. It is noteworthy, in this respect, that CEST offers a framework for integrating diverse psychotherapeutic approaches, including experiential therapies, insight therapies, and cognitive–behavioral therapies.

If the experiential system is more influential than the rational system in determining success in everyday living, as research findings so far suggest, then it is ironic indeed that people require a minimum of 12 years of formal training of the rational system and none at all for the experiential system. One important new direction worth exploring, as I have already noted, is the development of ways to train the experiential system. People need not only to learn how to use their rational minds to detect and compensate for the limitations of their experiential systems but to develop techniques for communicating with and learning from the intuitive wisdom inherent in the upper reaches of their experiential systems.

Developmental Psychology

Much of what I have said about the implications of CEST for new directions in personality can be equally well applied to developmental psychology by considering changes over time. For example, the presence and relative dominance of the basic needs and beliefs can be examined at different age levels. In young children, the need for relatedness can be expected to be more important than the need for self-esteem enhancement. With increasing maturity, the balance should shift to a more equal status between the two, yet this should differ among individuals depending on their experiences.

A particularly important area of research is examination of the influence of stressful events, such as sexual abuse, loss of a parent, and physical abuse at different age levels on basic beliefs. Important information about the structure of personality that could be useful in theory construction and remediation can be obtained by examining the process of assimilation of these episodes over time. There is reason to suspect that negative events are generally reworked over time to have less negative and sometimes even positive consequences (Epstein, 1979b). Clearly, some people develop resiliency from exposure to adversity and others are crushed by it. There needs to be more understanding about this process.

A related important area of research is the investigation of susceptibility to dissociation and disorganization as a function of the invalidation of basic beliefs at different age levels. Are children more or less subject to dissociation and disorganization than adults following the invalidation of basic beliefs? Examination of the development of basic needs and beliefs and how they influence and are influenced by significant life events over time could indicate a great deal about the organization and functions of personal theories of reality. Relatedly, it is important to study how irrational schemata acquired during the early years, when cognitive capacity is limited, are retained versus modified by later developments, including the acquisition of greater cognitive sophistication. There is reason to suspect that early acquired irrational views in the experiential system exist in parallel with more sophisticated views later acquired in the rational system (Epstein, in press-b).

The examination of constructive thinking over the life span is a fruitful area for developmental research, with important practical and theoretical implications. What is the trajectory of the different coping styles measured by the CTI (e.g., Emotional Coping, Behavioral Coping, Categorical Thinking, Esoteric Thinking, Personal Superstitious Thinking, Naive Optimism) over the life span? Preliminary research suggests, surprisingly, that global construct thinking, unlike global intelligence, improves very little, on the average, beyond the age of 10, the earliest age at which the children's CTI has been measured. Of considerable interest, emotional coping was found to decrease in 14-year-old girls and increase in 14-year-old boys. This raises the question of what is being done to adolescent girls and what can be done to correct it. Global constructive thinking was relatively poor among college students who had not had work experience, but it increased when they had experience in the "real" world. Early adolescents (14-year-olds) showed a rise in categorical thinking, which suggested that they may have been attempting to impose a rigid organization on an otherwise too-complicated world. These findings are not only of interest in their own right, but indicate that the children's

CTI is a promising instrument for developmental research on the efficiency of the experiential system.

An important area for further research on constructive thinking is the investigation of the factors that influence it. Correlations between college students and their parents suggest that heredity is not an important variable because parents did not contribute equally to their children's CTI scores. College men and women both exhibited significant correlations of their global constructive thinking with their fathers, whereas only the sons exhibited significant correlations with their mothers. This raises an interesting issue for further research: Why should college women model their constructive thinking after that of their fathers when the constructive thinking of their mothers is just as good?

Another important area for developmental research is the relative influence of the experiential and rational systems on decisional processes as a function of age. It would be interesting, in this regard, to conduct research on heuristic processing as a function of age level. If it is true that the experiential system at its lower reaches is a relatively primitive system, then heuristic processing should differ little in children and adults. However, adults should be more capable of overriding its influence through the use of their rational system. It would be interesting to test this hypothesis as well as to explore procedures for teaching children to override heuristic processing when it is maladaptive. Because heuristic processing is the major way that individuals make decisions in everyday life, and because it biases rational thinking, it is important to improve understanding of this process.

References

Allport, G. W. (1961). *Pattern and growth in personality.* New York: Holt, Rinehart & Winston.

Averill, J. R. (1980). A constructionist view of emotion. In R. Plutchik & H. Kellerman (Eds.), *Emotion, theory, research, and experience: Vol. 1. Theories of emotion* (pp. 305–339). San Diego, CA: Academic Press.

Beck, A. T. (1976). *Cognitive therapy and the emotional disorders.* Madison, CT: International Universities Press.

Block, J. H., & Block, J. (1980). The role of ego-control and ego-resiliency in the organization of behavior. In W. A. Collins (Ed.), *Minnesota Symposia on Child Psychology* (Vol. 13, pp. 39–101). Hillsdale, NJ: Erlbaum.

Cacioppo, J. T., & Petty, R. E. (1982). The need for cognition. *Journal of Personality and Social Psychology, 42,* 116–131.

Catlin, G., & Epstein, S. (1992). Unforgettable experiences: The relation of life-events to basic beliefs about the self and world. *Social Cognition, 10,* 189–209.

Ellis, A. (1973). *Humanistic psychotherapy.* New York: McGraw-Hill.

Emmons, R. A. (1986). Personal strivings: An approach to personality and subjective well-being. *Journal of Personality and Social Psychology, 51,* 1058–1068.

Epstein, A. (1989). *Mind, fantasy, and healing.* New York: Delacorte.

Epstein, S. (1973). The self-concept revisited, or a theory of a theory. *American Psychologist, 28,* 404–416.

Epstein, S. (1976). Anxiety, arousal and the self-concept. In I. G. Sarason & C. D. Spielberger (Eds.), *Stress and anxiety* (pp. 183–224). Washington, DC: Hemisphere.

Epstein, S. (1979a). Natural healing processes of the mind: I. Acute schizophrenic disorganization. *Schizophrenic Bulletin, 5,* 313–321.

Epstein, S. (1979b). The ecological study of emotions in humans. In P. Pliner, K. R. Blankstein, & I. M. Spigel (Eds.), *Advances in the study of communication and affect: Vol. 5. Perception of emotions in self and others* (pp. 47–83). New York: Plenum Press.

Epstein, S. (1980). The self-concept: A review and the proposal of an integrated theory of personality. In E. Staub (Ed.), *Personality: Basic issues and current research* (pp. 82–132). Englewood Cliffs, NJ: Prentice-Hall.

Epstein, S. (1981). The unity principle versus the reality and pleasure principles, or the tale of the scorpion and the frog. In M. D. Lynch, A. A. Norem-Hebeisen, & K. J. Gergen (Eds.), *Self-concept, advances in theory and research* (pp. 27–37). Cambridge, MA: Ballinger.

Epstein, S. (1983a). The unconscious, the preconscious and the self-concept. In J. Suls & A. Greenwald (Eds.), *Psychological perspectives on the self* (Vol. 2, pp. 219–247). Hillsdale, NJ: Erlbaum.

Epstein, S. (1983b). A research paradigm for the study of personality and emotions. In M. M. Page (Ed.), *Personality—Current Theory and Research: 1982 Nebraska Symposium on Motivation* (pp. 91–154). Lincoln: University of Nebraska Press.

Epstein, S. (1984). Controversial issues in emotion theory. *Annual Review of Research in Personality and Social Psychology, 5,* 64–87.

Epstein, S. (1985). The implications of cognitive-experiential self-theory for research in social psychology and personality. *Journal for the Theory of Social Behaviour, 15,* 283–310.

Epstein, S. (1987). Implications of cognitive self-theory for psychopathology and psycho-therapy. In N. Cheshire & H. Thomae (Eds.), *Self, symptoms and psychotherapy* (pp. 43–58). New York: Wiley.

Epstein, S. (1989). Values from the perspective of cognitive-experiential self-theory. In N. Eisenberg, J. Reykowski, & E. Staub (Eds.), *Social and moral values* (pp. 3–22). Hillsdale, NJ: Erlbaum.

Epstein, S. (1990). Cognitive-experiential self-theory. In L. Pervin (Ed.), *Handbook of personality theory and research: Theory and research* (pp. 165–192). New York: Guilford Press.

Epstein, S. (1991a). Cognitive-experiential self-theory: Implications for developmental psychology. In M. Gunnar & L. A. Sroufe (Eds.), *Self-processes and development: Vol. 23. Minnesota Symposia on Child Psychology* (pp. 79–123). Hillsdale, NJ: Erlbaum.

Epstein, S. (1991b). The self-concept, the traumatic neurosis, and the structure of personality. In D. Ozer, J. M. Healy, Jr., & A. J. Stewart (Eds.), *Perspectives in personality* (Vol. 3, Part A, pp. 63–98). London: Kingsley Publishers.

Epstein, S. (1991c). Cognitive-experiential self-theory: An integrative theory of personality. In R. Curtis (Ed.), *The relational self: Convergences in psychoanalysis and social psychology* (pp. 111–137). New York: Guilford Press.

Epstein, S. (1992a). Coping ability, negative self-evaluation, and overgeneralization: Experiment and theory. *Journal of Personality and Social Psychology, 62,* 826–836.

Epstein, S. (1992b). Constructive thinking and mental and physical well-being. In L. Montada, A. H. Filipp, & M. J. Lerner (Eds.), *Life crises & experiences of loss in adulthood* (pp. 385–409). Hillsdale, NJ: Erlbaum.

Epstein, S. (1992c). The cognitive self, the psychoanalytic self, and the forgotten selves: Comment on Drew Westen, the cognitive self, and the psychoanalytic self. Can we put our selves together? *Psychological Inquiry, 3,* 34–37.

Epstein, S. (in press-a). Emotion and self-theory. In M. Lewis & J. Haviland (Eds.), *The handbook of emotions.* New York: Guilford Press.

Epstein, S. (in press-b). Bereavement from the perspective of cognitive-experiential self-theory. In M. S. Stroebe, W. Stroebe, & R. O. Hansson (Eds.), *Sourcebook of bereavement.* New York: Cambridge University Press.

Epstein, S., & Denes-Raj, V. (1992). [The experiential system and errors in conjoint probability judgments]. Unpublished raw data.

Epstein, S., & Erskine, N. (1983). The development of personal theories of reality. In D. Magnusson & V. Allen (Eds.), *Human development: An interactional perspective* (pp. 133–147). San Diego, CA: Academic Press.

Epstein, S., Heier, H., & Denes-Raj, V. (1992). [Individual differences in heuristic responding]. Unpublished raw data.

Epstein, S., & Katz, L. (1992). Coping ability, stress, productive load, and symptoms. *Journal of Personality and Social Psychology, 62,* 813–825.

Epstein, S., Lipson, A., Holstein, C., & Huh, E. (1992). Irrational reactions to negative outcomes: Evidence for two conceptual systems. *Journal of Personality and Social Psychology, 62,* 328–339.

Epstein, S., & Meier, P. (1989). Constructive thinking: A broad coping variable with specific components. *Journal of Personality and Social Psychology, 57,* 332–350.

Erikson, E. H. (1963). *Childhood and society* (2nd ed.). New York: Norton.

Fiske, S. T., & Taylor, S. E. (1991). *Social cognition* (2nd ed.). New York: McGraw-Hill.

Freud, S. (1965). *The interpretation of dreams.* In J. Strachey (Ed. and Trans.), *standard edition.* New York: Basic Books. (Original work published 1900)

Funder, D. C., Block, J. H., & Block, J. (1983). Delay of gratification: Some longitudinal personality correlates. *Journal of Personality and Social Psychology, 37,* 1198–1213.

Horowitz, M. J. (1976). *Stress response syndromes.* Northvale, NJ: Jason Aronson.

Janoff-Bulman, R. (1979). Characterological versus behavioral self-blame: Inquiries into depression and rape. *Journal of Personality and Social Psychology, 37,* 1789–1809.

Janoff-Bulman, R. (1989). Assumptive worlds and the stress of traumatic events: Applications of the schema construct. *Social Cognition, 7,* 113–136.

Kahneman, D., & Tversky, A. (1973). On the psychology of prediction. *Psychological Review, 80,* 237–251.

Katz, L., & Epstein, S. (1991). Constructive thinking and coping with laboratory-induced stress. *Journal of Personality and Social Psychology, 61,* 789–800.

Kirkpatrick, L. A., & Epstein, S. (1992). Cognitive-experiential self-theory and subjective probability: Further evidence for two conceptual systems. *Journal of Personality and Social Psychology, 63,* 534–544.

Kobasa, S. C., Maddi, S. R., & Kahn, S. (1982). Hardiness and health: A prospective study. *Journal of Personality and Social Psychology, 42,* 168–177.

Larsen, R. J., & Diener, E. (1987). Emotional response intensity as an individual difference characteristic. *Journal of Research in Personality, 21,* 1–39.

Lazarus, R. (1991). *Emotion and adaptation.* New York: Oxford University Press.

Markus, H., & Nurius, P. (1986). Possible selves. *American Psychologist, 41,* 954–969.

McCann, I. L., & Pearlman, L. A. (1990). *Psychological trauma and the adult survivor: Theory, therapy and transformation.* New York: Brunner/Mazel.

Miller, D. T., & Gunasegaram, S. (1990). Temporal order and the perceived mutability of events: Implications for blame assignment. *Journal of Personality and Social Psychology, 59,* 1111–1118.

Miller, D. T., Turnbull, W., & McFarland, C. (1989). When a coincidence is suspicious: The role of mental simulation. *Journal of Personality and Social Psychology, 57,* 581–589.

Nisbett, R., & Ross, L. (1980). *Human inference: Strategies and shortcomings of social judgment.* Englewood Cliffs, NJ: Prentice-Hall.

Norem, J. K., & Cantor, N. (1986). Defensive pessimism: "Harnessing" anxiety as motivation. *Journal of Personality and Social Psychology, 51,* 1208–1217.

Rotter, J. B. (1966). Generalized expectancies for internal versus external control of reinforcement. *Psychological Monographs, 80*(1, Whole No. 609).

Sappington, A. A. (1990). The independent manipulation of intellectually and emotionally based beliefs. *Journal of Research in Personality, 24,* 487–509.

Savin-Williams, R. C., & Jaquish, G. A. (1981). The assessment of adolescent self-esteem: A comparison of methods. *Journal of Personality, 49,* 324–333.

Smith, E. R. (1984). Model of social inference processes. *Psychological Review, 91,* 392–413.

Swann, W. B., Jr. (1984). Quest for accuracy in person perception: A matter of pragmatics. *Psychological Review, 91,* 457–477.

Swann, W. B., Jr. (1987). Identity negotiation: Where two roads meet. *Journal of Personality and Social Psychology, 53,* 1038–1051.

Swann, W. B., Jr. (1990). To be known or to be adored: The interplay of self-enhancement and self-verification. In R. M. Sorrentino & E. T. Higgins (Eds.), *Handbook of motivation and cognition: Foundations of social behavior* (Vol. 2, pp. 408–448). New York: Guilford Press.

Taylor, S. E., & Brown, J. D. (1988). Illusion and well-being: A social psychological perspective on mental health. *Psychological Bulletin, 103,* 193–210.

Tversky, A., & Kahneman, D. (1974). Judgment under uncertainty: Heuristics and biases. *Science, 185,* 1124–1131.

Tversky, A., & Kahneman, D. (1982). Judgments of and by representativeness. In D. Kahneman, P. Slovic, & A. Tversky (Eds.), *Judgment under uncertainty: Heuristics and biases* (pp. 84–98). New York: Cambridge University Press.

Westen, D. (1992). The cognitive self and the psychoanalytic self: Can we put our selves together? *Psychological Inquiry, 3,* 1–13.

Index

About the Editors

David C. Funder is professor of psychology at the University of California, Riverside. He received his PhD in psychology from Stanford University. He has been associate editor of the *Journal of Personality and Social Psychology*, and consulting editor to that journal as well as to the *Journal of Personality* and the *Personality and Social Psychology Bulletin*. He is co-editor, with Steve West, of a special issue of the *Journal of Personality* entitled "Consensus, self-other agreement, and accuracy in personality judgment." His research has addressed the cross-situational consistency of behavior, the longitudinal stability of personality, ego-control, attribution theory, and attitude change. His current research focuses on factors that influence the degree to which judgments of personality are accurate.

Ross D. Parke is professor of psychology and director of the Center for Family Studies at the University of California, Riverside. He is past president of Division 7, the Developmental Psychology Division of the American Psychological Association. He has been editor of *Developmental*

Psychology and associate editor of *Child Development.* Professor Parke is author of *Fathers,* co-author of *Child psychology: A contemporary perspective,* editor of *The family: Review of child development research,* Volume 7, and co-editor of *Family–Peer relationships: In search of the linkages,* and *Children in time and place.* His research has focused on early social relationships in infancy and childhood. He is well-known for his early work on the effects of punishment, aggression, and child abuse and for his work on the father's role in infancy and early childhood. His current work focuses on the links between family and peer social systems.

Carol Tomlinson-Keasey is professor of psychology at the University of California, Davis, and Vice Provost for Faculty Relations. She received her PhD in psychology from the University of California, Berkeley. During the last decade, her research on women's development has examined the longitudinal data contained in the Terman Life Cycle Study. From this vantage point, she has contributed to discussions of the contemporary status of women.

Keith Widaman is professor of psychology at the University of California, Riverside. He received his PhD in psychology from Ohio State University. His major research interests involve the growth and development of mental and behavioral abilities and competencies, differential development of these abilities by persons with and without mental retardation, and the identification of factors that moderate development of abilities. He is also interested in multivariate analysis, including factor analysis and structural modeling. He received the R. B. Cattell Award from the Society of Multivariate Experimental Psychology in 1992.